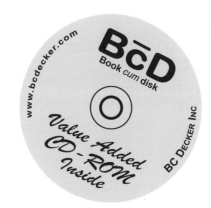

American Cancer Society
Atlas of
Clinical Oncology

Published

Blumgart, Fong, Jarnagin	*Hepatobiliary Cancer (2001)*
Cameron	*Pancreatic Cancer (2001)*
Char	*Tumors of the Eye and Ocular Adnexa (2001)*
Eifel, Levenback	*Cancer of the Female Lower Genital Tract (2001)*
Ginsberg	*Lung Cancer (2002)*
Grossbard	*Malignant Lymphomas (2001)*
Pollock	*Soft Tissue Sarcomas (2001)*
Posner, Vokes, Weichselbaum	*Cancer of the Upper Gastrointestinal Tract (2001)*
Prados	*Brain Cancer (2001)*
Shah	*Cancer of the Head and Neck (2001)*
Silverman	*Oral Cancer (1998)*
Sober, Haluska	*Skin Cancer (2001)*
Wiernik	*Adult Leukemias (2001)*
Willett	*Cancer of the Lower Gastrointestinal Tract (2001)*
Winchester, Winchester	*Breast Cancer (2000)*

Forthcoming

Carroll, Grossfeld	*Prostate Cancer (2002)*
Clark, Duh, Jahan, Perrier	*Endocrine Tumors (2002)*
Droller	*Urothelial Cancer (2002)*
Fuller, Seiden, Young	*Uterine and Endometrial Cancer (2003)*
Ozols	*Ovarian Cancer (2002)*
Raghavan	*Germ Cell Tumors (2002)*
Richie, Steele	*Kidney Tumors (2003)*
Volberding	*Viral and Immunological Malignancies (2003)*
Yasko	*Bone Tumors (2002)*

American Cancer Society
Atlas of
Clinical Oncology

Editors

GLENN D. STEELE JR, MD
Geisinger Health System

THEODORE L. PHILLIPS, MD
University of California

BRUCE A. CHABNER, MD
Harvard Medical School

Managing Editor

TED S. GANSLER, MD, MBA
Director of Health Content, American Cancer Society

American Cancer Society

Atlas of

Clinical Oncology

Lung Cancer

Robert J. Ginsberg, MD

Professor of Surgery and Chairman
Division of Thoracic Surgery
University of Toronto
Chief, Thoracic Surgery
Toronto General Hospital
Toronto, ON

2002
BC Decker Inc
Hamilton • London

BC Decker Inc
P.O. Box 620, LCD 1
Hamilton, Ontario L8N 3K7
Tel: 905-522-7017; 1-800-568-7281
Fax: 905-522-7839; 1-888-311-4987
E-mail: info@bcdecker.com
www.bcdecker.com

ISBN 1–55009–099–2
Printed in Canada

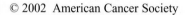

Sales and Distribution

United States
BC Decker Inc
P.O. Box 785
Lewiston, NY 14092-0785
Tel: 905-522-7017; 800-568-7281
Fax: 905-522-7839; 888-311-4987
E-mail: info@bcdecker.com
www.bcdecker.com

Canada
BC Decker Inc
20 Hughson Street South
P.O. Box 620, LCD 1
Hamilton, Ontario L8N 3K7
Tel: 905-522-7017; 800-568-7281
Fax: 905-522-7839; 888-311-4987
E-mail: info@bcdecker.com
www.bcdecker.com

Foreign Rights
John Scott & Company
International Publishers' Agency
P.O. Box 878
Kimberton, PA 19442
Tel: 610-827-1640
Fax: 610-827-1671
E-mail: jsco@voicenet.com

Argentina
CLM (Cuspide Libros Medicos)
Av. Córdoba 2067 – (1120)
Buenos Aires, Argentina
Tel: (5411) 4961-0042/(5411) 4964-0848
Fax: (5411) 4963-7988
E-mail: clm@cuspide.com

Japan
Igaku-Shoin Ltd.
Foreign Publications Department
3-24-17 Hongo
Bunkyo-ku, Tokyo, Japan 113-8719
Tel: 3 3817 5680
Fax: 3 3815 6776
E-mail: fd@igaku-shoin.co.jp

U.K., Europe, Scandinavia,
Middle East
Elsevier Science
Customer Service Department
Foots Cray High Street
Sidcup, Kent
DA14 5HP, UK
Tel: 44 (0) 208 308 5760
Fax: 44 (0) 181 308 5702
E-mail: cservice@harcourt.com

Singapore, Malaysia,Thailand,
Philippines, Indonesia, Vietnam,
Pacific Rim, Korea
Elsevier Science Asia
583 Orchard Road
#09/01, Forum
Singapore 238884
Tel: 65-737-3593
Fax: 65-753-2145

Australia, New Zealand
Elsevier Science Australia
Customer Service Department
STM Division
Locked Bag 16
St. Peters, New South Wales, 2044
Australia
Tel: 61 02 9517-8999
Fax: 61 02 9517-2249
E-mail: stmp@harcourt.com.au
Web site: www.harcourt.com.au

Mexico and Central America
ETM SA de CV
Calle de Tula 59
Colonia Condesa
06140 Mexico DF, Mexico
Tel: 52-5-5553-6657
Fax: 52-5-5211-8468
E-mail: editoresdetextosmex@prodigy.net.mx

Brazil
Tecmedd
Av. Maurílio Biagi, 2850
City Ribeirão Preto – SP – CEP: 14021-000
Tel: 0800 992236
Fax: (16) 3993-9000
E-mail: tecmedd@tecmedd.com.br

Contents

Preface

Prior to my returning home to Canada, my colleagues and I at Memorial Sloan-Kettering Cancer Center (MSKCC), were asked by BC Decker Inc and the American Cancer Society to develop a clinical atlas of lung cancer as part of their *Clinical Atlas of Oncology* series. This is the final product! This monograph, in the form of an atlas, is designed to provide information not only to practicing oncologists, but also to primary care physicians and interested non-physicians on the various aspects of the epidemiology, diagnosis, and current management of this highly malignant disease which is the number one cause of cancer deaths in North America for women and men. Unfortunately, because many believe that this is a "self-inflicted" cancer, lung cancer research and patient advocacy have not enjoyed the emotional and financial support given to other oncologic diseases. Hopefully, in the future, this "lack of interest" by the community will be reversed.

I would like to thank all my former colleagues at MSKCC for their help in developing this atlas. I am also grateful for the assistance provided to me by my secretaries Dorrell Granderson at MSKCC, and Liz Doherty, at the University of Toronto. I would like to thank the American Cancer Society for their support and encouragement and the staff of BC Decker Inc for their encouragement and advice.

Lastly, but certainly not least, I am forever grateful for the continuing love, patience, and unfaltering support provided by my wife, Charlotte, and my children, Karyn, Jordan, and David, during the development of this atlas.

Robert J. Ginsberg, MD
March 2002

Contributors

TIM AKHURST, MBBS
Department of Radiology
Memorial Sloan-Kettering Cancer Center
New York, NY
*Imaging Work-Up of Lung Cancer: Utility and
    Comparison of Computed Tomography and
    FDG Positron Emission Tomography*

CHRISTOPHER G. AZZOLI, MD
Department of Medicine
Memorial Sloan-Kettering Cancer Center
New York, NY
*Advances in the Treatment of Metastatic
    Non-Small Cell Lung Cancer*

PETER B. BACH, MD, MAPP
Department of Medicine
Memorial Sloan-Kettering Cancer Center
New York, NY
Epidemiology of Lung Cancer

ROBERT J. DOWNEY, MD
Department of Surgery
Weill Medical College of Cornell University
Memorial Sloan-Kettering Cancer Center
New York, NY
Follow-up After Lung Cancer Resection

MARK B. FEINSTEIN, MD
Department of Medicine
Weill Medical College of Cornell University
Memorial Sloan-Kettering Cancer Center
New York, NY
Clinical Features of Lung Cancer

ROBERT J. GINSBERG, MD, FRCSC
Division of Thoracic Surgery
Toronto General Hospital
Toronto, ON
*Local and Locoregional Non-Small Cell
    Lung Cancer*
*Palliative and Definitive Local Therapies in
    the Treatment of Recurrent or Metastatic
    Lung Cancer*

ROBERT HEELAN, MD
Department of Radiology
Memorial Sloan-Kettering Cancer Center
New York, NY
*Imaging Work-Up of Lung Cancer: Utility and
    Comparison of Computed Tomography and
    FDG Positron Emission Tomography*

SCOTT A. LAURIE, MD, FRCPC
Department of Medicine
University of Ottawa
Ottawa Regional Cancer Centre
Ottawa, ON
*Local and Locoregional Non-Small Cell
    Lung Cancer*

ROBERT J. KORST, MD
Department of Surgery
Weill Medical College of Cornell University
Memorial Sloan-Kettering Cancer Center
New York, NY
The Future

MARK G. KRIS, MD
Department of Medicine
Weill Medical College of Cornell University
Memorial Sloan-Kettering Cancer Center
New York, NY
The Future

LEE M. KRUG, MD
Department of Medicine
Memorial Sloan-Kettering Cancer Center
New York, NY
Small Cell Lung Cancer

NAEL MARTINI, MD
Department of Surgery
Memorial Sloan-Kettering Cancer Center
New York, NY
In Situ and Occult Lung Cancer

VINCENT A. MILLER, MD
Department of Medicine
Weill Medical College of Cornell University
Memorial Hospital for Cancer and Allied Disease
New York, NY
*Advances in the Treatment of Metastatic
    Non-Small Cell Lung Cancer*

KENNETH K. NG, MD
Department of Medicine
Memorial Sloan Kettering Cancer Center
New York, NY
*Local and Locoregional Non-Small Cell
    Lung Cancer*

JOHN R. PELLETT, MD
Department of Surgery
University of Wisconsin
Madison, WI
In Situ and Occult Lung Cancer

DIANE E. STOVER, MD
Department of Medicine
Weill Medical College of Cornell University
Memorial Sloan-Kettering Cancer Center
Clinical Features of Lung Cancer

KENNETH E. ROSENZWEIG, MD
Department of Radiation Oncology
Memorial Hospital for Cancer and Allied Diseases
Memorial Sloan-Kettering Cancer Center
New York, NY
*Palliative and Definitive Local Therapies in
    the Treatment of Recurrent or Metastatic
    Lung Cancer*

TRACEY WEIGEL, MD
Department of Surgery
University of Wisconsin
Madison, WI
In Situ and Occult Lung Cancer

DOROTHY A. WHITE
Department of Medicine
Weill Medical College of Cornell University
Memorial Sloan Kettering Cancer Center
New York, NY
Prevention and Screening of Lung Cancer

PHILIP W. WONG, MD
Department of Medicine
Albert Einstein Medical College of Yeshiva
    University
Jacobi-North Central Bronx Network
Bronx, NY
Prevention and Screening of Lung Cancer

MAUREEN F. ZAKOWSKI, MD
Department of Pathology
Weill Medical College of Cornell University
Memorial Sloan-Kettering Cancer Center
New York, NY
Pathology

Epidemiology of Lung Cancer

PETER B. BACH, MD, MAPP
ROBERT J. GINSBERG, MD

Epidemiology is the discipline in which the distribution, determinants, and outcomes of disease are observed and evaluated in human populations. The epidemiology of lung cancer is the focus of this chapter, which is divided into six sections: stage at diagnosis, incident lung cancer worldwide, sociodemographic differences in incidence and outcome from lung cancer, environmental risk factors for lung cancer, histologic type and stage of incident lung cancer cases in the United States, and coexisting diseases that predispose individuals to the development of lung cancer.

In the year 2002, an estimated 169,400 people (90,200 males and 79,200 females), in the United States will be diagnosed with lung and bronchus cancer and approximately 154,900 lives (89,200 males and 65,700 females) will be claimed by it.[1]

Lung and bronchus cancer is expected to account for 25 percent of all US female cancer deaths and 31 percent of all male cancer deaths in the year 2002.[4] Lung cancer is the leading form of cancer death in American men since the early 1950s, escalating rapidly until 1991, when the rates began to fall for the first time (Figures 1–1 and 1–2). This decline corresponded with a 30-year lag period between peak tobacco usages by men in 1960s, as well as the release of the first Surgeon General's Report on Smoking and Tobacco Use in 1964. The mortality rates in women continue to increase; however this rate of increase is slower than earlier periods.[5]

STAGE AT DIAGNOSIS OF PRIMARY LUNG CANCER

One of the explanations for the very poor survival of patients with primary lung cancer is that most patients initially present with disease at an advanced stage. In advanced stages, therapy rarely results in cure. For small cell carcinoma, which is staged using a simple scheme—limited or extensive—only 26 percent of newly diagnosed patients have limited-stage disease at the time of diagnosis. The remainder of patients with small cell carcinoma are either incompletely staged (12 percent), or have extensive disease (62 percent). Non-small cell carcinoma is staged using the TNM characteristics and the consensus definitions of the American Joint Committee on Cancer (AJCC) staging system covered elsewhere in this monograph.[6] With the exception of a relatively rare form of adenocarcinoma—bronchioalveolar cell carcinoma (BAC)—most patients who are diagnosed with non-small cell carcinoma also have advanced disease (Table 1–1).

WORLDWIDE INCIDENCE AND MORTALITY OF LUNG CANCER

Lung cancer is the most frequently occurring cancer worldwide, and the incidence of this disease has risen sharply in recent years, likely due to the increased availability of cigarettes. Worldwide, the lung cancer incidence rate is 38 cases per 100,000 men and 11 per 100,000 women. The highest rates among males are observed in Eastern Europe, North America, and Northern Europe. Among women, the highest rates are in North America, Northern Europe, and Micronesia/Polynesia.[2]

Since 1950, lung cancer has increased 10-fold in men and eight-fold in women in Japan. In China, many nonsmoking women exhibit high cancer rates, primarily associated with exposure to hazardous cooking oil vapors and other forms of indoor air pollutants.[3] Recent Canadian statistics on cancer show that one-quarter of new cases (25 percent) and one-third of deaths (31 percent) in males, and almost one-third of new cases (30 percent) and about one-quarter of deaths (23 percent) in females are due to lung cancer alone.[8] The report projects that lung cancer will continue as the leading cause of cancer death among Canadian women in 2001, accounting for approximately 2,000 more deaths compared with breast cancer deaths. This reflects the rapid increase in lung cancer mortality rates among Canadian women over the past 15 years, while age-standardized breast cancer mortality rates declined slightly.

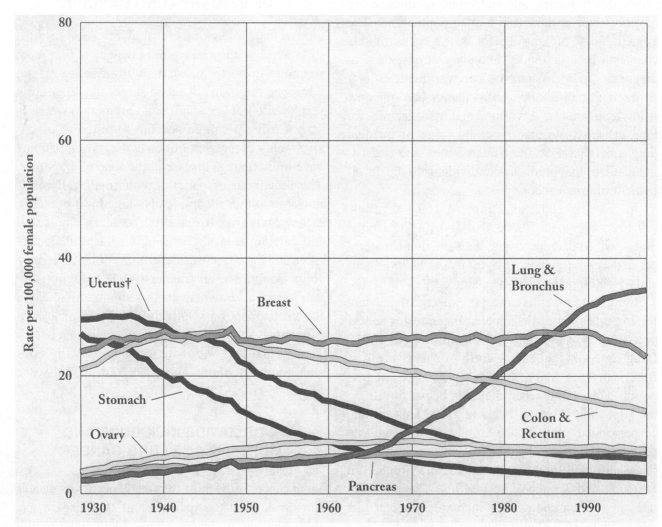

Figure 1–1. Age-adjusted cancer mortality rates for women (1930–1988) in the United States. Source: Vital Statistics of the United States, 1998 – http://www.cancer.org/statistics.

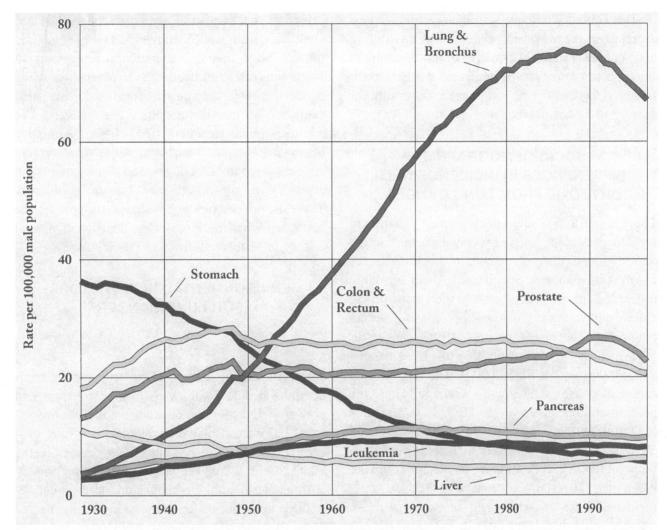

Figure 1–2. Age adjusted cancer mortality rates for men (1930–1988) in the United States. Some authors consider large cell carcinoma to be of neuroendocrine origin, and thus a form of small cell carcinoma. Others argue that most large cell carcinomas are related to adenocarcinoma. Source: Vital Statistics of the United States, 1998 – http://www.cancer.org/statistics.

Table 1–1. STAGE AT DIAGNOSIS FOR THE FIVE MOST COMMON HISTOLOGIES OF NON-SMALL CELL LUNG CANCER					
Cell Type	Stage I (%)	Stage II (%)	Stage III (%)	Stage IV (%)	Incompletely Staged (%)
Squamous cell carcinoma	21	4	27	22	26
Adenocarcinoma	20	4	24	37	16
Bronchioalveolar cell carcinoma (BAC)	48	5	10	12	25
Mixed histology (adenocarcinoma and squamous cell carcinoma)	30	9	25	23	14
Large cell carcinoma*	12	3	26	36	23

Adapted from Surveillance, Epidemiology, and End Results, Division of Cancer Control and Population Sciences, National Center for Health Statistics, Center for Disease Control and Prevention, Stat 3.0, 1992–1997.

*Some authors consider large cell carcinoma to be of neuroendocrine origin, and thus a form of small cell carcinoma. Others argue that most large cell carcinomas are related to adenocarcinoma.

The United Kingdom has achieved the largest decrease in the world in premature deaths due to lung cancer, primarily because of its widespread smoking cessation campaign. Since the 1970s, the United Kingdom's male lung cancer death rate for ages 35 to 54 has halved.[9]

SOCIO-DEMOGRAPHIC DIFFERENCES IN INCIDENCE AND OUTCOME FROM LUNG CANCER

There is substantial socio-demographic variation in incidence rates of lung cancer within the United States—much of which is explained by differences in smoking patterns. Specifically, there are large differences in incidence between men and women, elderly and young persons, and persons of different ethnicities. The incidence rate of lung cancer for U.S. men is nearly twice that of U.S. women (67/100,000 versus 41/100,000). The risk of lung cancer also rises substantially with age, where the peak incidence is in age 75 to 79-year-olds (357/100,000), compared with risk in persons aged 50 to 54 of 58/100,000. Black men are at a substantially higher risk of developing lung cancer than are white men (101/100,000 versus 64/100,000), while incidence rates in white and black women are roughly equal. Incidence rates in American Indians (18/100,000) and persons of Asian or Pacific Island descent (36/100,000) are substantially lower than the national average. The rates are considerably lower among both males and females in other ethnic groups (Table 1–2). Mortality rates are highest in black males and approximately seven- to nine-fold lower rates are seen in Asian/Pacific Island females (see Table 1–2).

The overall probability of survival 5 years after diagnosis of primary cancer of the lung is 16 percent. Survival after diagnosis varies with the socio-demographic factors listed above. Women enjoy substantially better 5-year survival than men (18 percent versus 14 percent). Age at diagnosis is also associated with probability of 5-year survival to a greater extent than can be explained by actuarial patterns alone. For example, persons younger than age 45 at diagnosis experience a 23 percent 5-year survival, while persons over age 65 have only a 14 percent 5-year survival. Racial discrepancies in survival have been well documented in other publications:[10] black patients experience a 12 percent 5-year survival, compared with 16 percent for white patients. This discrepancy in survival is somewhat explained by two factors: there are differences in use of surgical treatment (ie, potentially curative treatment) between black and white patients who are diagnosed in early stages, and black patients, on average, are diagnosed with later-stage disease. There is no compelling evidence supporting the hypothesis that the disease has a different natural history in patients of different ethnicities.[11]

ENVIRONMENTAL RISK FACTORS FOR LUNG CANCER

Tobacco

An overwhelming amount of experimental and epidemiologic data combine to form a coherent and powerful argument that cigarette smoking is the primary risk factor for the development of lung cancer.[12] Only about 15 percent of lung cancer in the United States (27,000 cases per year) are *not* directly attributable to smoking exposure, and the majority of these lung cancers are of the adenocarcinoma cell type. Two specific histologic types (squamous cell carcinoma and small cell carcinoma) essentially do not occur in the absence of this risk factor. In terms of the effect of smoking on risk of lung cancer, the risk increases both with the average number of cigarettes smoked and with the number of years of smoking, with earlier age at initiation, and with unfiltered cigarettes (versus filtered). Risk of lung cancer begins to fall when people stop smoking. Ten years after quitting, the risk of lung cancer is approximately 50 percent of that faced by similar people who continue to smoke. At no time after quitting does the risk of lung cancer return to that of "never-smokers."

Other exposures to tobacco have also been demonstrated to increase the risk of lung cancer substantially. The majority of evidence on environmental tobacco exposure ("second-hand smoke") supports the argument that this exposure increases the risk of lung cancer. In nonsmoking wives of

Table 1–2. INCIDENCE AND MORTALITY RATES* OF LUNG AND BRONCHUS CANCER BY RACE AND ETHNICITY, U.S., 1990–1997					
Gender	White	Black	Asian/Pacific Islander	American Indian	Hispanic
Incidence					
Males	71.9	111.1	51.9	25.1	38.0
Females	43.3	45.8	22.5	13.3	19.4
Total	55.4	73.3	35.5	18.4	27.1
Mortality					
Males	69.5	99.5	34.2	40.9	31.6
Females	34.0	33.0	14.9	19.8	11.0
Total	49.1	60.1	23.4	29.0	19.8

Adapted from Surveillance, Epidemiology, and End Results Program, Division of Cancer Control and Population Sciences, National Center for Health Statistics, Center for Disease Control and Prevention, 2000.
*Rates are per 100,000 and age-adjusted to the 1970 U.S. standard population. Incidence data are from the 11 SEER areas; mortality data are from all states except data for Hispanics exclude deaths from Connecticut, Louisiana, New Hampshire, and Oklahoma.

smoking husbands, the risk of developing lung cancer is 1.3 times that of nonsmoking wives of nonsmokers.[13] Research from the Wolfson Institute of Preventative Medicine provided evidence for a 24 percent greater risk of developing lung cancer in nonsmoker who lives with a smoker compared with a person who does not live with a smoker.[14] Similar high-quality epidemiologic data has demonstrated that the risk of lung cancer is also increased in people who smoke cigars and pipes, with risk increasing with duration and intensity of use. The rising incidence for adenocarcinoma of the lung between 1975 and 1994 and the deteriorating survival may be explained by the changes in tobacco use and the increased use of low-tar filter cigarettes since the 1960s.[15]

Occupational and Environmental Exposures

A number of elements including radon have been linked to the development of lung cancer, and a number of researchers have estimated that up to 15 percent of all lung cancer is associated with environmental or occupational exposures. Common occupational substances have been reviewed by global committees such as the International Agency for Research on Cancer (IARC) and the International Union Against Cancer (UICC) for cancer-causing potential, and many workplace materials have been identified as possible lung carcinogens (Table 1–3). There is also good evidence supporting a relationship between routine exposure to any of nine industrial compounds and an increase in an individual's risk of developing lung cancer: aluminum production byproducts, arsenic (encountered in copper smelting), asbestos, bis(chloromethyl)ether (BCME, encountered in the

Table 1–3. ESTABLISHED OR SUSPECTED LUNG CARCINOGENS	
Established Lung Carcinogens	Suspected Lung Carcinogens
Arsenic (inorganic)	Acrylonitrile
Asbestos	Beryllium
Bis(chloromethyl)ether	Cadmium
Chloromethyl methyl ether	Ceramic fibres
Chromium compounds	Diesel engine exhaust
Gamma radiation	Ferric oxide dust
Ionizing radiation (x-rays)	Insecticides
Mustard gas	Lead
Nickel compounds	
Polycyclic aromatic hydrocarbons	
Radon decay products	
Soots	
Tars	
Tobacco smoke	
Mineral oils	
Vinyl chloride	
Wood dust	

Adapted from International Agency for Research on Cancer. Carcinogen identification and evaluation. http://www.iarc.fr/ (accessed Nov 21, 2001).

textile and painting industries), chromium-derived compounds (encountered in arc welding, and by chromium platers), coke oven emissions (encountered in iron and steel foundries), mustard gas (no longer encountered), impurities associated with nickel (encountered in nickel refineries), vinyl chloride (encountered in vinyl chloride manufacturing).

Asbestos exposure independently increases an individual's risk of developing lung cancer. When combined with smoking exposure, the individual risk far exceeds the sum of the separate effects of smoking and asbestos.

The evidence implicating other exposures is somewhat weaker, largely because of the difficulties involved in controlling for the powerful effects of smoking in observational studies, making subtle correlations difficult to interpret. Despite this limitation, for beryllium, cadmium, crystalline silica, and formaldehyde, there is evidence suggesting that routine exposure to these compounds increases an individual's risk of lung cancer. In addition, air pollution, particularly from exhaust emanating from foundries, diesel-powered machinery and trucks, as well as exposure to electromagnetic fields likely contributes to lung cancer risk.

Exposure to radioactive compounds deserves more in-depth consideration. Uranium and fluorspar miners are exposed at very high levels to the inert gas, radon, that is a byproduct or uranium decay. Exposure to radon at substantially lower levels routinely occurs in residential neighborhoods. Residential exposure is greater in basements and in concrete-containing structures that it is in upper floors of houses or wood-based structures. The epidemiological evidence that the level of exposure for uranium and flurospar miners is sufficient to substantially increase the risk of lung cancer. However, it remains unclear whether exposure to residential radon is also associated with an increased risk of lung cancer. Several case control studies have inconsistent findings, while a recent meta-analysis supports an association.[16]

On-the-job exposure to carcinogens (Table 1–3) is another risk factor for lung cancer with the risk sharply increased when exposure is combined with smoking.

Exposure to ionizing radiation (such as that encountered in nuclear power plants) has not been shown to increase the risk to an individual of developing lung cancer.[17]

Diet

Hypotheses regarding the relationship between consumption of a diet high in fruits, vegetables, and antioxidant nutrients and lowered risk of developing lung cancer has generated much research into dietary factors. The preponderance of case-control studies of vegetable consumption suggested that increased vegetable consumption is associated with decreased risk of lung cancer. Results from case control studies of fruit consumption have been more mixed, with roughly half of the studies suggesting a protective association. Strong evidence from case-control studies may not be reflective of the actual association between dietary factors and risk of developing lung cancer, as in the case of beta-carotene. Multiple case-control and cohort studies consistently identified a protective effect of dietary beta-carotene.[18,19] However, two randomized controlled trials, the Alpha Tocopherol Beta-Carotene (ATBC) Cancer Preventative Study and the Beta-Carotene and Retinol Efficacy Trial (CARET), demonstrated that beta-carotene supplementation among heavy smokers was, in fact, associated with increased risk of lung cancer.[20,21]

HISTOLOGIC TYPES AND STAGE AT PRESENTATION OF INCIDENT LUNG CANCERS

Traditionally, two histologic types describe the majority of primary lung cancers: small cell cancers that represent malignant transformation of neuroendocrine cells, and non-small cell cancers, which are of epithelial origin. Within each of these categories are a number of more specific cell types, including adenocarcinoma and squamous cell carcinoma, which together account for the majority of non-small cell lung cancers. Occasionally, lymphomas, carcinoid tumors, and a multitude of other histologic varieties can originate in the lung parenchyma. In 1996, 40 percent of primary lung cancers in the United States were of the adenocarcinoma type, followed by squamous cell carcinoma (27 percent), and small cell carcinoma (19 percent). The other histologic types each represented less than 10 percent of primary lung cancers (Table 1–4). Age appears to be a contributing risk factor for squamous cell and small cell carcinoma. Compared with other lung cancer subtypes, a smaller number of patients under age 50 years were afflicted with these subtypes of lung cancer.[22] Using a cancer registry, a German study reviewed lung cancer data in young females (14–46 years) for risk factors, stage, histology, therapy, and survival. The most frequently occurring cancer was adenocarcinoma, whereas, squamous cell carcinoma occurred less frequently in this cohort compared with same-age-group males (Table 1–5). A significantly higher proportion of young females were diagnosed with advanced stage IIIB or IV non-small cell lung cancer compared with older females (> 45 years), older males (> 46 years), or same-age-group males.[23] A number of studies have observed a rise in the frequency of occurrence of adenocarcinoma in all patients, and it is the most frequent cell type found in females and younger patients.[22,23] This shift from squamous cell carcinoma to adenocarcinoma may be ascribed to a shift in smoking behavior.

DISEASE ENTITIES ASSOCIATED WITH LUNG CANCER

Three types of disease deserve special mention due to their association with lung cancer risk: cancers of the head and neck, cancers associated with nonmalignant lung tumors, and acquired immunodeficiency syndrome (AIDS). For patients with cancer of the head and neck, a disease also largely attributable to smoking, the risk of developing lung cancer is roughly four times that of age and smoking-matched controls.[24] One study demonstrated that up to 50 percent of lung lesions detected in patients with head and neck cancer were primary cancers of the lung, rather than metastatic spread of the primary tumor.[24] Clinically, it is important to determine whether a new pulmonary mass in a patient with treated head and neck cancer represents metastatic disease, or a potentially resectable and curable primary lung cancer.

A number of lung diseases confer a greater risk of the development of lung cancer—particularly adenocarcinoma. Chronic obstructive pulmonary disease (COPD) is the most common of these diseases, in which patients with predominantly emphysematous lungs face a substantially increased risk of cancer above that due to smoking alone. Patients with healed tuberculosis also face an increased risk at the site of the primary infection (termed "scar carcinoma"), as do patients with silica-induced lung disease. Human immunodeficiency virus (HIV) infection predisposes individuals to the development of a number of malignancies, including Kaposi's sarcoma, lymphoma, and cervical cancer. Whether or not HIV infection increases the likelihood of a patient developing bronchogenic carcinoma remains controversial. A number of studies have demonstrated increased incidence of lung cancer in persons with HIV infection, but most are hampered by substantial bias introduced by differences in surveillance, or differences in sociodemographic characteristics between compared

Table 1–4. HISTOLOGIC FEATURE OF PRIMARY CANCERS OF THE LUNG: CELL TYPES THAT ACCOUNT FOR 1% OR MORE OF ALL LUNG CANCERS	
Histologic Type	**Proportion (%)**
Squamous cell	27
Adenocarcinoma	40
Small cell carcinoma	19
Large cell carcinoma	8
Bronchioalveolar cell carcinoma	4
Mixed adenocarcinoma/squamous cell carcinoma	2
Carcinoid	1

Surveillance, Epidemiology, and End Results (SEER) Program Public-Use Data (1973–1998), National Cancer Institute, DCCPS, Surveillance Research Program, Cancer Statistics Branch, released April 2001, based on the August 2000 submission.

Table 1–5. FREQUENCY OF CELL TYPES BY AGE AT DIAGNOSIS AND GENDER FOR PATIENTS AT LUNGENKLINIK HECKESHORN 1986–1995

Cell Types	Females		Males	
	< 45yrs	> 45yrs	< 45yrs	> 45yrs
Adenocarcinoma	37 (38.5)	386 (28.4)	46 (23.0)	724 (22.0)
Bronchioalveolar carcinoma	6 (6.3)	50 (3.4)	4 (2.0)	51 (1.6)
Squamous cell carcinoma	14 (14. 6)	238 (17.5)	45 (22.5)	1,113 (33.9)
Small cell carcinoma	14 (14. 6)	310 (22.8)	626 (13.0)	16 (18.8)
Large cell carcinoma	15 (15.6)	195 (14.4)	40 (22.0)	482 (14.7)
Carcinoid tumors	9 (9.4)	35 (2.6)	10 (5.0)	22 (0.7)
Others*	1 (1.0)	144 (10.6)	24 (12.5)	278 (8.4)
Total	96 100%	1,358 100%	199 100%	3,286 100%

Data are presented as n (%).

*Mucoepidermoid carcinoma; sarcoma of the lung; lung cancer unknown histology. carcinoma p < 0.01.[6]

groups. A well-managed population-based study conducted in 1998 suggested an increase in risk for patients with HIV infection 6.5 times above the baseline population risk.[25] These findings are similar to a recent investigation comparing cancer rates in AIDS patients with those of the New York State general population. The results exhibit a significantly increased risk of lung cancer with advancing immunodeficiency, in both male and female patients.[26]

REFERENCES

1. Cancer Facts and Figures 2002. American Cancer Society: Atlanta, Georgia, 2002.

2. Parkin Dm, Pisani P, Ferlay J. Global Cancer Statistics. CA Cancer J Clin 1999;49:33–64.

3. Thomson P, Robinson K, Robbe IJ. Lung cancer and indoor air pollution arising from Chinese-style cooking among nonsmoking women living in Shanghai, China. Epidemiology 2000;11(4):481–2.

4. Jemal A, Thomas A, Murray T, Thun M. Cancer Statistics, 2002. CA Cancer J Clin 2002;512:22–52.

5. Ries LAG, Eisner MP, Kosary CL, et al., editors. SEER Cancer Statistics Review, 1973–1998, National Cancer Institute. Bethesda (MD), http://seer.cancer.gov/Publications/CSR1973_1998/, 2001.

6. Mountain CF. Revisions in the international system for staging lung cancer. Chest 1997;111:1710–7.

7. World Health Organization. Cancer in developed countries: assessing the trends. WHO Chron 1985;39:109–11.

8. National Cancer Institute of Canada: Canadian Cancer Statistics 2000. Toronto, Canada, 2000. April 2000, ISSN 0835-2976. Accessed:http://www.cancer.ca and http://www.ncic.ca.

9. Peto R, Darby S, Deo H, et al. Smoking, smoking cessation, and lung cancer in the UK since 1950: combination of national statistics with two case-control studies. BMJ. 2000;321(7257):323–9.

10. King TE, Brunetta P. Racial disparity in rates of surgery for lung cancer. N Engl J Med 1999;341:1231–3.

11. Bach PB, Cramer LD, Warren JL, Begg CB. Racial differences in treatment of early stage lung cancer. N Engl J Med 1999;341:1198–205.

12. The health consequences of smoking: cancer. A report of the Surgeon General; 1982; DHHS Publication number 82-50179 ed., US Department of Health and Human Services.

13. Blot WJ, Fraumeni JF Jr. Passive smoking and lung cancer. J Natl Cancer Inst 1986;77:993–1000.

14. Hackshaw AK, Law MR, Wald NJ. The accumulated evidence on lung cancer and environmental tobacco smoke. BMJ 1997;315:980–8.

15. Maryska LG, Janssen-Heijnen , Jan-Willem W, et al. Is there a common etiology for the rising incidence of decreasing survival with adenocarcinoma of the lung? Epidemiology 2001;12:256–8.

16. Frumkin H, Samet JM. Radon. CA Cancer J Clin. 2001;51:337–44.

17. Ernster VL, Mustacchi P, Osann KE. Epidemiology of lung cancer. In: Murray JF, Nadel JA, editors. Textbook of respiratory medicine. 2nd ed. Philadelphia (PA): W.B. Saunders Company; 1994. p. 504–27.

18. Boffetta P, Agudo A, Ahrens W, et al. Multicenter case-control study of exposure to environmental tobacco smoke and lung cancer in Europe. J Natl Cancer Inst 1998; 90(19):1440–50.

19. Mayne ST, Janerich DT, Greenwald P, et a. Dietary beta-carotene and lung cancer risk in US nonsmokers. J Natl Cancer Inst 1994;86:33–8.

20. Hennekens CH, Buring JE, Manson JE, et al. Lack of effect of long-term supplementation with beta-carotene on the

incidence of malignant neoplasms and cardiovascular disease. N Engl J Med 1996;334:1145–9.

21. Omenn GS, Goodman GE, Thornquist MD, et al. Effects of a combination of beta-carotene and vitamin A on lung cancer and cardiovascular disease. N Engl J Med 1996;334:1150–5

22. Day GL, Blot WJ. Second primary tumors in patients with oral cancer. Cancer 1992;70:14–9.

23. Lienert T, Serke M, Schönfeld N, Loddenkemper R. Lung cancer in young females. Eur Respir J 2000;16:986–90.

24. Malefatto JP, Kasimis BS, Moran EM, Wuerker RB. The clinical significance of radiographically detected pulmonary neoplastic lesions in patients with head and neck cancer. J Clin Oncol 1984;2:625–30.

25. Parker MS, Leveno DM, Campbell TJ, et al. AIDS-related bronchogenic carcinoma: fact or fiction? Chest 1998; 113:154–61.

26. Gallagher B, Wang Z, Schymura MJ, Kahn A, Fordyce EJ. Cancer incidence in New York State acquired immunodeficiency syndrome patients. Am J Epidemiol 2001;154: 544–56.

2

Prevention and Screening of Lung Cancer

PHILIP W. WONG, MD
DOROTHY A. WHITE, MD

Lung cancer is the most common cause of cancer death for both men and women in the United States and is a major problem worldwide.[1] Five-year survival remains low at 16 percent.[2] The poor prognosis in lung cancer treatment is due in large part to the advanced stage of most cancers at the time of diagnosis. Since large numbers of current and former smokers remain at risk for lung cancer, the death toll from this disease can be expected to continue to rise unless there is a new approach. Preventive strategies aimed at cessation of cigarette smoking will need to be employed in a systematic fashion to decrease the number of persons at risk for the disease. Unfortunately, even after cigarette smoking ceases, the risk of developing lung cancer remains high in an individual for many years.[3] Thus, interventions, such as chemoprophylaxis to prevent development of cancer in ex-smokers and screening to provide earlier diagnosis of lung cancers that do develop, are also needed to improve survival. The lack of widespread preventive and screening strategies for lung cancer, as compared to other major cancers, has been due in large part to pessimism regarding the ability to impact this disease. Recent scientific advances and re-assessment of existing data, however, are bringing about a change in these attitudes, offering new promise for improved outcome. This chapter will summarize the current knowledge regarding prevention, screening, and early diagnosis of lung cancer.

PREVENTION

Lung cancer is unique among the common cancers because risk factors for its development can be identified in most cases. This provides an opportunity to intervene either to prevent the cancer if the risk factor can be eliminated or modified, or to identify individuals in whom screening or early diagnostic interventions would be beneficial. The recognized risk factors for development of lung cancer are indicated in Table 2–1 with the strategies available to combat them.

Cigarette Smoking

Cigarette smoking alone accounts for at least 85 to 90 percent of all lung cancer cases.[1] Although the incidence of smoking in the United States has decreased since the 1960s, approximately one-quarter of the adult population smokes, with almost equal numbers of men and women smoking (Figure 2–1).[4] Unfortunately, the decrease in smoking has recently started to plateau. This is due to increasing smoking prevalence among high school students and women and girls. The percentage of smokers remains high in many other countries.

Table 2–1. RISK FACTORS IN LUNG CANCER AND PREVENTIVE STRATEGIES	
Risk Factors	**Preventive Strategies**
Cigarette smoking	Smoking cessation program
	Education
	Advertising restrictions
	Law and taxation
Passive smoking	Education
	Strict smoking regulations
Diet	Fruit and vegetable consumption
	chemoprevention
Occupational exposures	Workplace regulation
	Education
Pre-existing lung diseases	Early detection
Family history of lung cancer	Early detection
	genetic markers

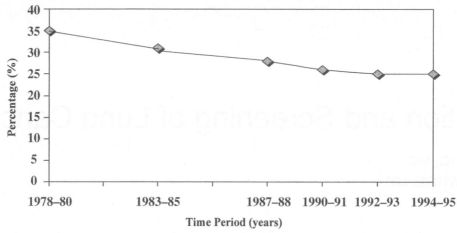

Figure 2–1. Trends in cigarette smoking among North American adults across all races, National Health Interview Surveys, United States, 1978–1995. Prevalence is age-adjusted to the 1990 U.S. standard population. Since the 1960s, there has been a declining percentage of smokers in the United States, but this decline has begun to plateau. (Adapted from Wingo PA, Ries LAG, Giovino GA, et al. Annual report to the nation on the status of cancer 1973–1996, with a special section on lung cancer and tobacco smoking. J Natl Cancer Inst 1999;91:675–90.)

Premalignant exfoliative cytologic changes in the bronchial epithelium can be demonstrated in proportion to the duration and amount of cigarette use.[5] There is a 10-fold increase in the incidence of lung cancer among smokers compared to nonsmokers.[6] Persons who inhale deeply or begin smoking at an earlier age are at increased risk of developing cancer. In those who quit, there is a progressively declining risk of development of lung cancer as the duration of abstinence lengthens, but the cancer risk of ex-smokers remains elevated relative to the risk of a lifetime nonsmoker even in cases of up to 30 years of abstinence (Table 2–2).[7] Lower cancer death risk is observed among those quitting earlier in life.[3] The benefit of decreased smoking in North American adults (a trend which began in the 1960s) resulted in a plateau of the cancer incidence rates in the mid-

1980s, and in the most recent years has resulted in a slight decrease in incidence (Figure 2–2).

Smoking often begins at a young age, and in most cases first use of tobacco occurs before high school graduation. Smoking by family members and friends is strongly associated with smoking initiation in adolescence. Smokers develop tolerance to the adverse effects of nicotine. Several years after starting to use tobacco, consumption typically increases from a few cigarettes per day to up to 50 cigarettes per day. Seventy percent of adolescents who smoke three or more cigarettes a day will become dependent smokers for two or three decades.[8] Measures to prevent initiation of smoking in adolescents are education, changes in societal attitudes, and legislative controls. Educational efforts need to be directed to teenagers and parents, and public health initiatives should try to change societal views of the desirability of smoking. Controlled advertising for tobacco, regulation of distribution of cigarettes, and taxation of tobacco may also reduce consumption.

Smoking Cessation

Once started, cigarette smoking is highly addictive and difficult to stop. However, most patients who stop smoking tend to do so on their own or with self-help materials. For some patients, more intervention

Table 2–2. RELATIVE RISK OF LUNG CANCER IN CURRENT AND FORMER SMOKERS		
Smoking Category		Relative Risk
Never-smokers		1.0
Current smokers		15.8–16.3
Former smokers		
Years of abstinence:	1–9	5.9–19.5
	10–19	2.0–6.1
	≥ 20	1.9–3.7

(Adapted from Samet JM. Health benefits of smoking cessation. Clin Chest Med 1991;12:673.)

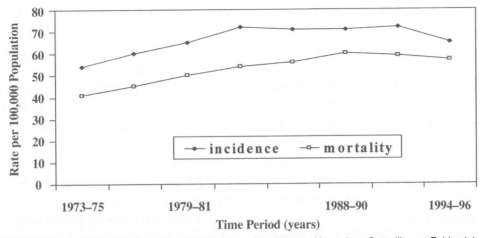

Figure 2–2. Incidence and death rates of cancer of the lung and bronchus: Surveillance, Epidemiology and End Results (SEER), 1973–1996 among North American white and black races. In the mid-1980s (about 20 years after the decline in smoking), the incidence of lung cancers began to plateau and in recent years to decrease. (Adapted from Wingo PA, Ries LAG, Giovino GA, et al. Annual report to the nation on the status of cancer 1973–1996, with a special section on lung cancer and tobacco smoking. J Natl Cancer Inst 1999;91:675–90.)

will be necessary or helpful. Approaches to smoking cessation have included physician advice, individual and group counseling, hypnosis, acupuncture, behavioral therapy and, most recently, pharmacologic interventions. The overall success rate of all types of intervention has been between 20 and 40 percent abstinence at 12 months. Although these success rates are not ideal, they still result in a major impact on the future health of those who have stopped smoking.

The Agency for Health Care Policy and Research (AHCPR) has recently produced a comprehensive guideline on smoking cessation which provides a starting point in dealing with smoking cessation in the office setting.[9] This recommends identifying all smokers, diagnosing nicotine dependence, providing self-help smoking cessation brochures and advice tailored to all smokers, referring recalcitrant smokers to specialized clinics, and using nicotine replacement therapy (NRT) or bupropion in combination with brief counseling and active follow-up. Physicians are encouraged to identify smokers regularly (at every visit) by using smoking status as a vital sign. This maneuver has been shown to trigger the clinician to initiate discussions about quitting. Physicians are also encouraged to establish whether nicotine dependence is present. The Fagerstrom score is a quick approach for the busy clinician.[10] This includes nine questions, with the two key questions being: (1) does the patient

smoke within 5 minutes of awaking? and (2) Does the patient smoke greater than 25 cigarettes per day? Those who answer yes to both questions are highly dependent on nicotine.

The success rate of physician advice has been up to 10 percent with occasional improved success in special situations, such as with cardiac patients, where quit rates may reach 40 percent.[11,12] For behavioral therapy, quit rates average 20 percent. The cessation rates at 1 year for the American Lung Association and American Cancer Society programs were 16 percent and 22 percent, respectively.[13]

Pharmacologic Therapy

The two approaches to drug therapy currently available are nicotine replacement therapy (NRT) and bupropion. These may be given alone or in combination. Nicotine is a highly addictive psychoactive drug that is both a stimulant and a euphoriant. It leads to a release of systemic norepinephrine and elevates brain dopamine levels. Some of its effects are a boost in energy, improved concentration, euphoria, anorexia, and physiologic and psychologic dependence. Smoking delivers nicotine to the alveolar structure of the lung where it is directly absorbed into arterial blood and quickly delivered to the brain. Within a few seconds of inhaling smoke, the blood level of nicotine changes from low to high. Nicotine levels then decrease quickly by redistribution and subsequently more slowly by metabolism. The half-life of nicotine is approximately 2 to 4 hours. The typical smoker delivers 200 to 300 boluses of nicotine to the brain each day. The rapid rise in levels is connected with the euphoria and addiction while withdrawal symptoms are believed related to a decrease in nicotine levels below a certain threshold. Administering nicotine replacement at a level above the withdrawal threshold may prevent the onset of withdrawal symptoms while avoiding the peak levels and reducing the addiction.

Nicotine replacement is available as chewing gum, transdermal patch, nasal spray, and inhaler (Table 2–3). NRT can lead to a doubling of the smoking cessation rate compared to placebo, and should be encouraged for all patients attempting to quit, particularly for smokers heavily dependent on nicotine (Figure 2–3).[14,15] All preparations are essentially equally effective. Nicotine blood levels similar to those maintained in moderate smokers require relatively high doses of the currently available formulations. In clinical practice, most nicotine replacement results in only partial replacement of the nicotine levels achieved by smoking cigarettes. Fixed doses of nicotine replacement, as given by the patch, are the most likely to be effective in the early stages of smoke cessation. Those using only as-needed doses of the gum, nasal spray, or oral inhaler will likely under-dose themselves and have a higher risk of relapse. If cravings or withdrawal symptoms occur with the patch, an increased dose should be considered. If there are only occasional breakthrough symptoms, use of the gum at those times may be helpful. Nicotine nasal spray can also be a useful

adjunct to the patch, particularly with its very rapid uptake of nicotine similar to a cigarette, which relieves withdrawal symptoms and craving quickly. There is less experience with the nicotine inhaler, which delivers nicotine to the buccal mucosa—not the lung. It can also be used as an adjunct to the patch and may provide oral tactile stimulation similar to a cigarette. Sole therapy with gum or the inhalers may be suitable for very light cigarette smokers.

NRT is relatively safe and well tolerated. Nicotine replacement is associated with dose-related side effects including nausea, palpitations, headache, and sweating. Mild transitory skin irritation is seen in a significant number of patients using the patch, and a contact dermatitis occurs in a small percentage of smokers. Nightmares and sleep disturbance are sometimes seen and removal of the patch before bed can be helpful. NRT is not appropriate for use in patients with Buerger's disease, Prinzmetal's angina, or demonstrated sensitivity to nicotine. Two studies have evaluated the safety of the transdermal patch in those with coronary artery disease, and neither study found any evidence of increased toxicity.[16,17] Patients with coronary artery disease should, however, be cautioned that they cannot continue to smoke while using the patch. Another concern for nicotine replacement is the potential for addiction to the therapy. The addiction potential appears very low and some consider this a safer addiction than tobacco.

Bupropion is the first non-nicotine-containing agent to be approved by the FDA for smoking cessation. It is a non-tricyclic antidepressant that has both dopaminergic and adrenergic actions. The Zyban form of bupropion (GlaxoWellcome: Research Triangle Park, NC) was developed for smoking cessation and

Table 2–3. NICOTINE REPLACEMENT THERAPY				
Type	Onset (min.)	Dose	Advantages	Problems
Patch	50	< 15 cig/day—7 to 14 mg/day < 20 cig/day—15 to 21 mg/day < 40 cig/day—21 to 35 mg/day < 40 cig/day—42 mg/day	Constant dose Easy dose	Local skin irritation if used at night Sleep disturbances
Gum	30	Light smokers—2 mg Heavy smokers—4 mg 2 sticks/hour	Quick onset Easy to vary dose	Jaw pain Dental problems Swallowing leads to GI effects
Nasal spray	10	1–2 doses/hour 8–10 doses/day	Quick onset Easy to vary dose	Nasal symptoms Difficult to use with nasal congestion
Inhaler	30	4 mg/cartridge 6–8 cartridges/day	Quick onset	Local irritation Oral stimulation

comes with a smoker support program. The suggested dose is 150 mg/day for 3 days then 300 mg/day, beginning 1 week prior to cessation and continuing for 7 to 12 weeks. Its mechanism of action is not clear, and its efficacy may not be related to its antidepressant effect. Rates of quitting with bupropion were approximately double that seen with placebo.[18,19] There are several contraindications for the use of bupropion, including seizure disorders, history of anorexia or bulimia, and uncontrolled hypertension. The drug was generally well tolerated, with the most common adverse events being insomnia and dry mouth. It is a choice in patients who have failed or do not want to use NRT.

Passive Smoke Exposure

Nonsmokers who are exposed to environmental tobacco smoke, referred to as passive smokers, have an increased risk of lung cancer. A meta-analysis of 37 published epidemiologic studies of lung cancer risk showed an excess risk of lung cancer of 24 percent among nonsmokers who lived with a smoker,[20] and also demonstrated tobacco-specific carcinogens in the blood and urine of nonsmokers exposed to environmental smoke. Specific strategies to prevent lung cancer from passive smoking are education of both smokers and nonsmokers about the risk, and stringent smoking restrictions in the workplace and other public places.

Diet

Epidemiologic studies strongly suggest that consumption of fruits and vegetables rich in beta-carotene are associated with lower lung cancer risk in women and men.[21] It is hypothesized that antioxidant vitamins in fruits and vegetables prevent carcinogenesis by passively interfering with DNA oxidase. Vitamin A was also found to inhibit experimental tracheobronchial squamous cell metaplasia and tumors.[22] These observations led to large trials studying the effect of dietary supplementation. In the Physician Health Study, 22,071 male physicians were randomly assigned to receive aspirin 325 mg, beta-carotene 50 mg, or both, or placebo, with a 12-year follow-up.[23] The incidence of lung cancer was identical in all groups. The Alpha-tocopherol, Beta-

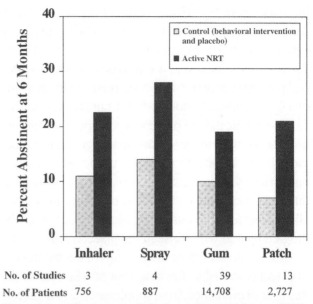

Figure 2–3. Effectiveness of nicotine replacement therapy (NRT). Abstinence rates are based on averages obtained from several studies. Use of nicotine replacement therapy approximately doubles the abstinence success rate compared to placebo. (Data adapted from Rennard SI, Daughton DM. Nicotine replacement therapy: what are the options today? J Respir Dis 1998;19:S20–S25.)[14]

carotene Lung Cancer Prevention Study Group (ATBC study) found no reduction in the incidence of lung cancer among male smokers after 5 to 8 years of dietary supplementation with alpha-tocopherol or beta-carotene.[24] Total mortality was actually increased in those who received beta-carotene than in those who did not. In another trial, the Carotene and Retinol Efficacy Trial (CARET), 4 years of supplementation with beta-carotene and vitamin A had no benefit in male ex-smokers or asbestos workers and may have had an adverse effect on the incidence of lung cancer in those who still continued to smoke.[25]

Other trials have looked at the use of vitamin A in the prevention of second primary cancers and found mixed results. Pastorino and colleagues tested high-dose vitamin A on 307 patients with resected stage I non-small cell lung cancer and showed a greater number of patients with either recurrence or new primary tumors in the treated group.[26] There was, however, no significant difference in the overall survival. Another group prospectively studied 86 smokers for bronchial squamous metaplasia, documented by bronchial biopsies, randomized to isotretinoin or placebo, and observed no effect of intervention. A resultant decline in metaplasia occurred with smoking cessation.[27] Preliminary work by Hong and colleagues at M.D. Anderson suggested that patients with potentially cured head and neck cancer who were treated with 13-*cis*-retinoic acid had a reduced incidence of second primary cancers.[28] However, preliminary analysis of a recent phase III, double-blind, randomized trial of 13-*cis*-retinoic acid to prevent second primary tumors in patients with stage I non-small cell lung cancer indicates no benefit in reduction of incidence of second primary tumors. Subgroup analysis suggested that lung cancer recurrence and mortality may actually be increased in current smokers treated with the drug compared with those in the placebo arm.

Thus at present there are no current chemopreventive agents available for lung cancer. The reason for this lack of protection from supplements in the face of the epidemiologic data on the beneficial effect of fruits and vegetables in the diet is unknown. It may be related to the higher pharmacologic doses in the trials compared to dietary consumption, or to some other constituents of diet that accompany the vitamins in the diet. The use of beta-carotene or vitamin A and E should be discouraged based on their lack of efficacy and the potential increased risk. The use of a diet high in vegetables and fruit, however, should be encouraged and seems prudent for cancer prevention.

Non-Tobacco Carcinogens

Associations of specific environmental or chemical exposure to excess lung cancer risk has been recognized. The International Agency for Research on Cancer provides an extensive list of these chemicals and substances.[29] These include asbestos, radon, arsenic, bis(chloromethyl)ether, chromium, nickel, and polycyclic aromatic compounds, among others. Asbestos is the best-recognized environmental cause of lung cancer. Approximately 1 to 5 percent of lung cancers can be attributed to asbestos exposure alone. Chronic asbestos exposure increases the risk of developing both mesothelioma and lung cancer with risk ratios of about 2:15.[30] Synergy between smoking and asbestos exposure has been shown, and it is estimated that there is a 50-fold increased risk for heavy smokers who are subject to chronic, heavy asbestos exposure without protective measures compared with the non-smoking, non-asbestos-exposed male population.[6]

Lung cancers due to radon exposure were demonstrated in studies of miners who worked in poorly-ventilated uranium and non-uranium mines. A dose-related increased risk with radon exposure was established in both smoking and nonsmoking underground miners. In the past decade, domestic radon exposure has become a public concern. In the United States there are an estimated 5,000 to 36,000 excess lung cancer deaths attributed to indoor radon exposure.[30] Radon has a synergistic interaction with cigarette smoking which increases the risk of lung cancer.

The number of cancers attributed to other carcinogens is not well defined. Preventive strategies to minimize environmental carcinogen exposure are workplace standards and quality control programs, home monitoring for radon in high-risk areas, medical monitoring and follow-up of exposed individuals. Risk reduction of confounding factors like smoking.

Family History

Although smoking is highly linked to the development of lung cancer, only a small percentage of smokers will develop cancer. This has suggested the possibility of a genetic factor. Family studies have shown slightly increased lung cancer risk in relatives of lung cancer patients compared with those with no family history of lung cancer—supporting a concept of genetic susceptibility.[31,32] In one study, there was evidence of codominant inheritance occurring in younger patients with lung cancer.[33] Recognition of inherited predisposition to cancer (although not a major risk factor) is important because of the possibilities for early diagnosis, prevention of high-risk smoking, and also to provide insight into the mechanism of carcinogenesis.

Pre-Existing Lung Disease

A meta-analysis of several population-based studies on the relation of pre-existing lung disease to lung cancer in nonsmokers found an increased risk, even after correction for other factors.[34] An estimated risk of 13 percent for lung cancer among lifetime nonsmokers and 16 percent among former smokers was attributed to the presence of prior lung disease. A four- to five-fold increase in lung cancer diagnosis has been documented when airflow obstruction is present, compared with normal airflow with all other risk factors, such as smoking, occupational exposure, family history, and age being controlled.[35] It has been theorized that pre-existing lung disease can heighten susceptibility to carcinogenic insults by the presence of impaired local immune perveillence, ineffective carcinogen clearance, and possibly chronic inflammatory processes that potentiate carcinogenesis. Early detection of lung cancer may be particularly important in this group where the ability to undergo extensive surgery is limited.

SCREENING FOR LUNG CANCER

Lung cancer is most commonly diagnosed on chest radiographs taken for incidental reasons or because of the presence of symptoms of an advanced lung cancer. This has resulted in only five to 20 percent of cancers being discovered at an early stage. There is a consensus that the earlier a cancer is discovered, the greater the chances of survival. Patients with a stage I lung cancer have a 40 to 80 percent survival at 5 years whether the tumor is discovered by accident or by screening.[36,37] Currently in the United States, systematic screening for lung cancer is not recommended by any major medical association, even though a large part of the population is at risk (greater than 100 million smokers and ex-smokers) and lung cancer is a major cause of cancer deaths. This is also the case in most countries of the world— with the exception of Japan, where screening is in widespread practice. This lack of screening has been based on a general acceptance that screening is not worthwhile because it has yet to demonstrate a reduction in mortality in a randomized trial.

Four randomized screening trials in the 1970s and 1980s were performed. Johns Hopkins University, the Mayo Clinic, and Memorial Sloan-Kettering Cancer Center (MSKCC) performed National Cancer Institute (NCI) sponsored studies, and there was also a fourth study from Czechoslovakia.[38–42] These studies included over 35,000 participants. All demonstrated that periodic screening resulted in a significant shift toward earlier diagnosis and markedly increased rates of resectability. There was also lengthened survival from the time of diagnosis

and lower case fatality. However, no disease-specific mortality benefit from screening smokers for lung cancer could be documented. There has been controversy regarding the interpretation of these studies. Some have raised concerns that mortality did not improve because the increased detection of cancer was only of incidental "benign" cancers that would not have led to death. Others maintain that these studies have limitations and do not clearly settle the issue of the effectiveness of screening.

In the MSKCC and Johns Hopkins studies, no benefit was observed from adding sputum cytology to annual chest radiographs.[39,40] In both the screened and unscreened groups, however, 5-year survival rates of cancer were higher than anticipated (35% versus 12%) and this has been ascribed to be due to the effect of screening radiographs in both groups. In the Mayo clinic study, all participants underwent prevalence screening with chest radiography and sputum cytology.[41] There were 91 prevalence cases of cancer (0.83%) and the 5-year cancer-free rate of these cases was nearly 40 percent. Subjects were then randomized to radiographs and sputum cytology every 4 months versus annually. More lung cancers were found in the screened group and there was a shift toward lower stages and better resectability in the screened group. The 5-year survival of lung cancer in the screened group was higher than in controls (33% versus 15%). Because there were more lung cancers and therefore deaths from lung cancer in the screened group, there was no mortality advantage found. The reason for more lung cancers in the screened group remains unclear. The Czechoslovakian study, like the Mayo Clinic study, began with a prevalence screen and then randomization to a screened or control group.[42] The control group was not told to obtain yearly chest radiography or sputum cytology. The study period was only for 3 years, with follow-up for an additional 3 years, during which time both groups had annual chest radiographs. This study was also complicated by the occurrence of a larger number of lung cancer cases in the screened group than in the control group.

A large NCI randomized trial known as the Prostate, Lung, Colon, Ovary Trial in which 148,000 men and women aged 60 to 74 years are enrolled is ongoing. Participants will undergo an initial chest radiograph followed by yearly radiographs for 3 years. The control group will not undergo chest radiographs. The groups, unfortunately, are not balanced for smoking histories, and low-risk patients are being randomized, so it is possible that a definitive answer will not be obtained. At this point, the effectiveness of screening annual chest radiographs is unclear. Many clinicians do perform yearly chest radiographs in high-risk patients based on the data showing that earlier stage cancers may be found.

Several advances recently have been explored to improve screening:

Spiral CT of the Chest

Current technology has advanced to the stage that rapid, relatively low-cost, low-dose spiral CT of the chest can be performed that can detect nodules in the 2- to 3-mm range. The amount of radiation is similar to that of mammography. Several recent studies in Japan, Germany, and the United States have documented the ability of low-dose spiral CT scans to detect lung cancers that cannot be seen on a chest radiograph, and almost all of these cancers are detected in an early stage (Figure 2–4). Keneko and colleagues screened 1,369 Japanese subjects who had at least 20-pack-year smoking histories using

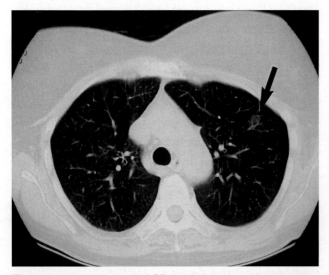

Figure 2–4. Low-dose spiral CT can detect very early cancers, as shown above. This lesion, which was resected and confirmed as malignant, was not detected on a chest radiograph. Preliminary studies indicate that many of the lesions identified by chest CT are stage I cancers with a favorable prognosis.

spiral CT.[43] Fifteen cancers were discovered, including eleven not seen with chest radiography. Fourteen were classified in stage I.[44] Another group of Japanese investigators found similar results, with greater than 80 percent of cancers found to be stage I lesions. Henschke and colleagues reported on low-dose spiral CT as part of the early lung cancer action project (ELCAP).[45] They screened 1,000 symptom-free volunteers, aged 60 years or older with at least 10 pack years of cigarette smoking. Non-calcified nodules were detected in 23 percent at baseline, compared with 7 percent by chest radiograph. Nodules below 5 mm in size were observed with serial CT and evaluated for growth. Those 6 to 10 mm in size were assessed on an individual basis, and those greater than 11 mm went for biopsy. Cancer was found in 2.7 percent (27 cases) and 23 were stage I. Biopsies were performed on 31 patients, of which four were benign.

A study is also under way at the Mayo Clinic, which includes smokers 50 years of age or older, current or former smokers of 20 pack years, with life expectancy of at least 5 years, and no prior cancer within the last 5 years. A total of 15,000 participants have been enrolled. Low-dose fast-spiral CT is performed at the time of enrollment and yearly for 3 years. Sputum cytology is performed on a yearly basis. Preliminary data show indeterminate nodules were found in 51 percent of the cases. Eleven cancers have been detected—10 by CT and one by sputum cytology.[46]

Spiral CT appears to be a promising new screening tool with the potential to find small cancers that can be resected. A major challenge of this approach is to avoid unnecessary procedures for benign nodules. Ongoing studies may be very beneficial in determining exactly who should be screened, how often the scans should be done, and the characteristics of benign versus malignant nodules. Preliminary data indicate that the problem of benign nodules might be less significant on the subsequent scans where a baseline is available. Preliminary data from the second yearly CT of patients from the ELCAP study indicated that of the patients with new nodules, 27 percent were malignant.[47] Additionally, advances in other imaging techniques, such as positron emission tomography (PET), may help to distinguish benign and malignant lesions.

Sputum Cytology

In the NCI screening studies cited above, sputum cytology diagnosed 25 percent of cancers and was the only means of detection in 15 percent of lung cancer cases.[39,41] In cases where the sputum was normal but the radiograph abnormal, the survival at 5 years was 85 to 90 percent. The histology was usually squamous cell lung cancer (Figure 2–5). Other groups have also demonstrated that patients with normal sputum cytology but abnormal radiographs had a very high survival rate.[48,49] Tockman and colleagues have suggested that use of sputum for screening might be extended by adding a specialized procedure such as the employment of monoclonal antibodies (Mo Ab) directed at antigens that are associated with lung cancer.[50] Using archived sputum specimens from subjects who developed lung cancer after documented moderate dysplasia during the Johns Hopkins study, Tockman used a Mo Ab to analyze sputum specimens.[50] He demonstrated positive staining on smears as early as 48 months prior to the diagnosis of cancer using standard cytology criteria. Studies are under way to prospectively validate this technique. In a preliminary report in those with resected stage I lung cancer, this Mo Ab sputum test demonstrated a sensitivity of 77 percent and specificity of 82 percent for detection of a second lung primary tumor.[51]

Investigators are also examining sputum and other respiratory specimens for biomarkers indicative of premalignant changes in an effort to identify individuals at very high risk for developing lung cancer. Elucidating molecular biologic events may be the key to improving the sensitivity of sputum evaluation and may lead to effective chemoprevention strategies.

Fluorescence Bronchoscopy

Standard bronchoscopy has been shown to be useful in localizing radiographically occult lesions. However, carcinoma in situ (CIS) and microinvasive tumors can be difficult to identify. Lam and others have shown that the autofluorescence spectra of areas of dysplasia and CIS differ from normal bronchial tissue.[52] The laser-induced flourescence endoscope (LIFE) bronchoscopy system has been developed and approved by the FDA for use in identifying abnormal bronchial tissue. This bronchoscope uses a helium-cadmium laser using blue light at 442 nm for illumination (instead of white light), and allows enhanced visualization of areas of dyplasia and CIS

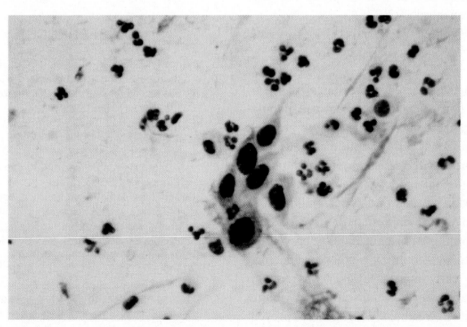

Figure 2–5. Cytologic analysis of sputum from a smoker shows a cluster of hyperchromic, irregularly-shaped cells with a high nuclear-to-cytoplasmic ratio in a background of inflammation. This is a characteristic squamous cell carcinoma—the type of cancer that usually can be detected with screening using sputum cytology. (Papanicolaou; × 1000 original magnification)

(Figure 2–6). The autofluorescence bronchoscope may have a role in screening trials when the sputum cytology shows moderate or severe dysplasia, or in those when sputum demonstrates malignant cells but no lesions are visible on chest radiographs.

A multicenter study evaluating the sensitivity of the fluorescent bronchoscope in localizing premalignant and malignant endobronchial lesions showed a 271 percent increased sensitivity in detecting lesions when compared to white-light examination.[52] The sensitivity for intraepithelial neoplasia (moderate to severe dysplasia or CIS) is about 6 times greater than with conventional bronchoscopy. Limitations of this procedure are that it is time-consuming, there is increased cost due to the need for many biopsies to eliminate false-positives, and it requires specialized skill and training. This technique is likely to be applicable only if the incidence of cancer in the screened population is high. One such population is smokers with severe chronic obstructive pulmonary disorders. In one study, moderate dysplasia or worse was found in 27.5 percent of such patients, including CIS in 1.7 percent.[35] The risk of developing a second lung primary for a patient with Non-small cell lung cancer (NSCLC) who has undergone a potentially curative resection is almost 5 percent per year, and these patients may also be a target group for auto-fluorescence bronchoscopy.[53]

CONCLUSION

There is much evidence of a preclinical phase of lung cancer. Clones of endobronchial cell populations develop genetic mutations, leading to progressively more malignant cells and ultimately to invasive disease. Structurally, cells move through phases of hyperplasia to mild, moderate, and severe dysplasia to carcinoma in situ and invasive carcinoma. This progression provides an opportunity to try to disrupt the cycle and promote normalization by prevention of smoking and by minimizing other risk factors. The finding of early signs of dysplasia by sputum cytology may allow interventions aimed at finding carcinoma in situ or treatment with agents to prevent progression of malignancy. The screening CT scan, sputum cytology, and the autofluorescent broncho-scope remain promising tools for early detection of

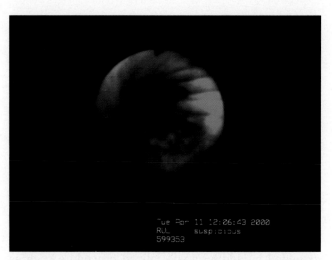

Figure 2–6. Fluorescence bronchoscopy can detect intraepithelial neoplasia with a much higher sensitivity than conventional bronchoscopy. An area where the fluorescence is abnormal and suspicious for cancer can be seen at 5 o'clock.

cancer in select populations. Progress is needed to identify the right target groups for these approaches. Ultimately, our understanding of the genetic damage that occurs may allow development of better and more sensitive markers to detect populations at high risk, those in whom chemoprevention is needed and for whom aggressive screening is beneficial. All these avenues need to be vigorously pursued to reduce the mortality from lung cancer.

REFERENCES

1. Wingo PA, Ries LAG, Giovino GA, et al. Annual report to the nation on the status of cancer 1973–1996, with a special section on lung cancer and tobacco smoking. J Natl Cancer Inst 1999;91:675–90.
2. Landis SH, Murray T, Bolden S, Wingo PA. Cancer statistics, 1999. CA Cancer J Clin 1999;49:8–31.
3. Halpern MT, Gillespie BW, Warner KE. Patterns of absolute risk of lung cancer mortality in former smokers. J Natl Cancer Inst 1993;85:457–64.
4. Centers for Disease Control and Prevention. State-specific prevalence of cigarette smoking among adults, and children's and adolescents' exposure to environmental tobacco smoke—United States, 1996. MMWR Morb Mortal Wkly Rep 1997;46:1038–43.
5. Auerbach O, Hammond EC, Garfinkel L. Changes in the bronchial epithelium in relation to cigarette smoking, 1955–1960 vs. 1970–1977. N Engl J Med 1979;300:381–6.
6. Hammond EC, Selikoff IJ, Seidman H. Asbestos exposure, cigarette smoking and death rates. Ann NY Acad Sci 1979;330:473–90.
7. Samet JM. Health benefits of smoking cessation. Clin Chest Med 1991;12:669–79.

8. Parran TV. The physician's role in smoking cessation. J Respir Dis 1998;19:S6–S12

9. Fiore MC, Bailey WC, Cohen SJ, et al. Smoking cessation. Clinical Practice Guideline No. 18. Rockville (MD): US Dept. of Health and Human Services, Public Health Service, Agency for Health Care Policy and Research; April 1996. Publication No. AHCPR96–0692.

10. Fagerstrom KO. Measuring degree of physical dependence to tobacco smoking with reference to individualization of treatment. Addict Behav 1978;3:235–41.

11. Cummings SR, Coates TJ, Richard RJ, et al. Training physicians in counseling about smoking cessation: a randomized trial of the "Quit for Life" program. Ann Intern Med 1989;110:640–7.

12. Schwartz JL. Methods of smoking cessation. Clin Chest Med 1991;12:737–53.

13. Lando HA, McGovern PG, Barios FX, et al. Comparative evaluation of American Cancer Society and American Lung Association smoking cessation clinics. Am J Public Health 1990;80:554–9.

14. Rennard SI, Daughton DM. Nicotine replacement therapy: what are the options today? J Respir Dis 1998;19(84): S20–S25.

15. Fiore MC, Smith SS, Jorenby DE, et al. The effectiveness of nicotine patch for smoking cessation: a meta-analysis. JAMA 1994;27:1940–7.

16. Joseph AM, Norman SM, Ferry LH, et al. A randomized trial of transdermal nicotine for smoking cessation in cardiac patients. N Engl J Med 1996;335:1792–8.

17. Working Group for the Study of Transdermal Nicotine in Patients with Coronary Artery Disease. Nicotine replacement therapy for patients with coronary artery disease. Arch Intern Med 1994;154:989–95.

18. Hurd RD, Sachs DPL, Glover ED, et al. A comparison of sustained release bupropion and placebo for smoking cessation. N Engl J Med 1997;337:1195–202.

19. Jorenby DE, Leischow SJ, Nides MA, et al. A controlled trial of sustained-release bupropion, a nicotine patch, or both, for smoking cessation. N Engl J Med 1999;340:685–91.

20. Hackshaw AK, Law MR, Wald NJ. The accumulated evidence on lung cancer and environmental tobacco smoke. BMJ 1997;315:980–8.

21. Ziegler RG, Mayne ST, Swanson CA. Nutrition and lung cancer. Cancer Causes Control 1996;7:157–77.

22. Saffiotti U, Montesano R, Sellakumar AR, Borg SA. Experimental cancer of the lung. Inhibition by vitamin A of the induction of tracheobronchial squamous metaplasia and squamous cell tumors. Cancer 1967;20:857–64.

23. Hennekens CH, Eberlein K. A randomized trial of aspirin and β-carotene among US physicians. Prev Med 1985;14: 165–8.

24. The Alpha-Tocopherol, Beta-Carotene Cancer Prevention Study Group. The effect of vitamin E and beta-carotene on the incidence of lung cancer and other cancers in male smokers. N Engl J Med 1994;330:1029–35.

25. Omenn GS, Goodman GE, Thornquist MD, et al. Effects of a combination of beta-carotene and vitamin A on lung cancer and cardiovascular disease. N Engl J Med 1996;334: 1150–5.

26. Pastorino U, Infante M, Maioli M, et al. Adjuvant treatment of stage I lung cancer with high-dose vitamin A. J Clin Oncol 1993;11:1216–22.

27. Lee JS, Lippman SM, Benner SE, et al. Randomized placebo-controlled trial of isotretinoin in chemoprevention of bronchial squamous metaplasia. J Clin Oncol 1994;12:937–45.

28. Hong WK, Benner SE, Lippman SM. Evolution of aerodigestive tract 13-cis-retinoid acid chemoprevention: the M.D. Anderson experience [review]. Leukemia 1994;8:S33–S37.

29. International Agency for Research on Cancer. Overall evaluations of carcinogenicity: an updating of IARC monographs from Volumes 1 to 42, Supplement 7. Lyon, France: IARC; 1987.

30. National Research Council. Comparative dosimetry of radon in mines and homes. Washington (DC): National Academy Press; 1991.

31. Ooi WL, Elston RC, Chen VW, et al. Increased familial risk for lung cancer. J Natl Cancer Inst 1986;76:217–22.

32. Sellers TA, Ooi WL, Elston RC, et al. Increased familial risk for non-lung cancer among relatives of lung cancer patients. Am J Epidemiol 1987;126:237–46.

33. Sellers TA, Bailey-Wilson JE, Elston RC, et al. Evidence for mendelian inheritance in the pathogenesis of lung cancer. J Natl Cancer Inst 1990;82:1272–9.

34. Brownson RC, Alavanja MCR, Caporaso N, et al. Epidemiology and prevention of lung cancer in nonsmokers. Epidemiol Rev 1998;20:218–36.

35. Kennedy T, Proudfoot S, Franklin W, et al. Cytopathological analysis of sputum in patients with airflow obstruction and significant smoking histories. Cancer Res 1996;56:4673–8.

36. Naruke T, Tsuchiya R, Kondo H, et al. Implications of staging in lung cancer. Chest 1997;112(Suppl)4:242–8.

37. Mountain CF, Dresler CM. Regional lymph node classification for lung cancer staging. Chest 1997;111:1718–23.

38. Berlin NI, Buncher CR, Fontana RS, et al. The National Cancer Institute Cooperative Early Lung Cancer Detection Program. Results of the initial screen (prevalence). Early lung cancer detection: introduction. Am Rev Respir Dis 1984;130:545–9.

39. Melamed MR, Flehinger BJ, Zaman MB, et al. Screening for early lung cancer. Results of the Memorial Sloan-Kettering study in New York. Chest 1984;86:44–53.

40. Frost JK, Ball WC Jr, Levin ML, et al. Early lung cancer detection: results of the initial (prevalence) radiologic and cytologic screening in the Johns Hopkins study. Am Rev Respir Dis 1984;130:549–54.

41. Fontana RS, Sanderson DR, Woolner LB, et al. Screening for lung cancer. A critique of the Mayo Lung Project. Cancer 1991;67:1155–64.

42. Kubik A, Polak J. Lung cancer detection. Results of a randomized prospective study in Czechoslovakia. Cancer 1986;57:2427–37.

43. Keneko M, Eguchi K, Ohmatsu H, et al. Peripheral lung cancer screening and detection with low dose spiral CT versus radiography. Radiology 1996;201:798–802.

44. Sone S, Takashima S, Li F, et al. Mass screening for lung cancer with mobile spiral computed tomography scanner. Lancet 1998;351:1242–5.

45. Henschke CI, McCauley DI, Yankelevitz DF, et al. Early Lung Cancer Action Project: overall design and findings from baseline screening. Lancet 1999;354:99–105.

46. Jett JR, Swensen SJ, Midthun DE, et al. Screening for Lung Cancer: Mayo Clinic study with low-dose spiral CT scan (SCT) and sputum cytology (prevalence screen). Am J Respir Crit Care Med 2000;161:A13.

47. McGuiness G, Najidich D, Miettinen O, et al. Early Lung Cancer Action Project: findings from repeat annual screening. Am J Respir Crit Care Med 2000;161:A13.

48. Bechtel JJ, Kelley WR, Petty TL, et al. Outcome of 51 patients with roentgenographically occult lung cancer detected by sputum cytology testing. Arch Intern Med 1994;154:975–80.

49. Saito Y, Nagamota N, Shin-Ichiron O, et al. Results of surgical treatment from roentgenographically occult bronchogenic squamous cell carcinoma. J Thorac Cardiovasc Surg 1992;104:401–7.

50. Tockman MS, Gupta PK, Myers JD, et al. Sensitive and specific monoclonal antibody recognition of human lung cancer antigen on preserved sputum cells: a new approach to early lung cancer detection. J Clin Oncol 1988;6: 1685–93.

51. Tockman MS, Mulshine JL, Piantadosi S, et al. Prospective detection of preclinical lung cancer: results from two studies of heterogeneous nuclear ribonucleoprotein A2/B1 overexpression. Clin Cancer Res 1997;3:2237–46.

52. Lam S, MacAulay C, Hung J, et al. Detection and localization of early lung cancer by imaging techniques. J Thorac Cardiovasc Surg 1991;105:1035–40.

53. Pairolero PC, Williams DE, Bergstralk EJ, et al. Postsurgical stage I bronchogenic carcinoma: morbid implications of recurrent disease. Ann Thorac Surg 1984;38:331–8.

3

Pathology

MAUREEN F. ZAKOWSKI, MD

The recognition and description of pulmonary cancer dates back to 1810, and by 1872 Bennett had fully described the clinical aspects based on an analysis of 39 cases. Karl Rokitansky (1804–1878) recognized several gross types of lung lesions, but the earliest microscopic studies were those of Langerhans, Machiafava, and Malassez in the 1870s.

A monograph reviewing 374 cases of carcinoma was written by Adler in 1912, and a review by Sweller in 1929 referred to the rising incidence of lung cancer. By 1940, the incidence of lung cancer was noted to have increased markedly in the previous two decades, and irritating inhalations, tobacco use, coal tar products, and dusts were thought to be implicated.[1]

The common types of cancer included under the heading of bronchogenic carcinoma include: squamous cell carcinoma, adenocarcinoma, with the distinctive subtype of bronchioalveolar carcinoma, small cell carcinoma, and large cell carcinoma. Current data suggest that adenocarcinoma is the most frequently encountered type[2] of primary lung cancer, and it is the most common type found in women. This increase in adenocarcinoma is accompanied by a relative decrease in squamous cell carcinoma and small cell carcinoma. These changes in frequency rates may reflect changes in smoking patterns as well as changes in the histologic criteria used to diagnose lung cancer.[2]

While the incidence of lung cancer is declining significantly in men, the decline in women has been much slower. The death rate for this disease is falling sharply for men since the 1990s; however, deaths in women in the same time period are increasing.

Synchronous lung carcinomas and multiple primary tumors are well described[3] with squamous cell carcinoma being the most common subtype associated with multiple primaries.

The diagnosis of lung cancer is made by examining histologic or cytologic specimens from the lung itself or from suspected metastases. Seventy-five percent of lung cancers are diagnosed by cytologic methods,[4] including fine-needle aspiration, bronchial brushes and washes, and examination of sputum. Problems in making an accurate pathologic diagnosis include poor laboratory technique, overinterpretation of reactive processes, and misidentification of tumors metastatic to the lung as primary lung cancers.

As discussed by Colby and colleagues, the histology of lung tumors is not homogeneous, and most tumors show cellular heterogeneity at the light microscopic, histochemical or electron microscopic level.[5] Nonetheless, the WHO classification is based on the light microscopic findings (Table 3–1). Since the distinction between small cell carcinoma and non-small cell carcinoma is usually straightforward histologically, tumor heterogeneity is not often a clinical issue.

ADENOCARCINOMA

Adenocarcinoma, the lung tumor least closely associated with smoking, accounts for almost 40 percent of primary tumors. Often peripherally located, it may involve the pleura and be associated with scarring (Figure 3–1) and pleural effusion. The theory that peripheral adenocarcinomas can arise in areas of

Table 3–1. WHO LUNG CANCER HISTOLOGIC CLASSIFICATION

PREINVASIVE LESIONS
Squamous dysplasia
Carcinoma in situ
Atypical adenomatous hyperplasia
Diffuse idiopathic pulmonary neuroendocrine cell hyperplasia

MALIGNANT LESIONS
Squamous cell carcinoma
  Variants
    Papillary
    Clear cell
    Small cell
    Basaloid

Small cell carcinoma
  Variants
    Combined small cell carcinoma

Adenocarcinoma
  Acinar
  Papillary
  Bronchioloalveolar carcinoma
    Non-mucinous
    Mucinous
    Mixed mucinous and non-mucinous or indeterminate cell type
  Solid adenocarcinoma with mucin
  Adenocarcinoma with mixed subtypes
  Variants
    Well-differentiated fetal adenocarcinoma
    Mucinous ("colloid") adenocarcinoma
    Mucinous cystadenocarcinoma
    Signet-ring adenocarcinoma
    Clear cell adenocarcinoma

Large cell carcinoma
  Variants
    Large cell neuroendocrine carcinoma
    Combined large cell neuroendocrine carcinoma
    Basaloid carcinoma
    Lymphoepithelioma-like carcinoma
    Clear cell carcinoma
    Large cell carcinoma with rhabdoid phenotype

Adenosquamous carcinoma

Carcinomas with pleomophic, sarcomatoid or sarcomatous elements
    Carcinomas with spindle and/or giant cells
    Pleomorphic carcinoma
    Giant cell carcinoma
    Carcinosarcoma
    Pulmonary blastoma
    Others

Adapted from Travis WD, Colby TV, Corrin B, et al. Histological typing of lung and pleural tumours. 3rd ed. (World Health Organization International Histological Classification of Tumours.) Berlin: Springer-Verlag Berlin, 1999.

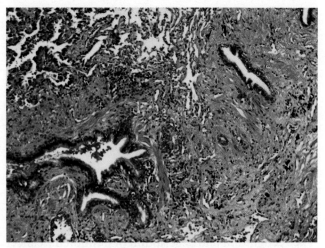

Figure 3–1. Abnormal glandular structures of adenocarcinoma in background of dense fibrous tissue (scar carcinoma). Uninvolved lung is seen in upper left corner. (H & E stain; ×20 original magnification)

Adenocarcinoma is a glandular epithelial malignancy with acinar, papillary, bronchioalveolar, or solid growth patterns. It is often associated with mucin production, although special stains may be needed to detect mucin, particularly in poorly-differentiated tumors. Mucin detection can sometimes distinguish solid adenocarcinoma from otherwise identical-appearing large cell carcinoma.

Gross Findings

Adenocarcinomas are usually peripherally located, well-circumscribed masses. They may be found in association with fibrosis and pleural puckering (Figure 3–2). The penetration of the pleura, which may require elastic stains to document, is important

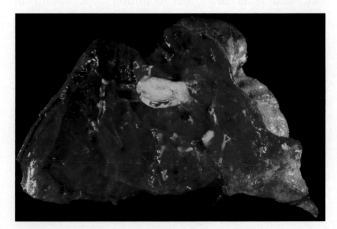

Figure 3–2. Well-circumscribed adenocarcinoma in periphery of lung. This tumor is associated with pleural puckering.

scarring such as seen with tuberculosis or infarctions or other injuries is a very old one. The concept of scar carcinoma suggests that preneoplastic epithelial changes in the area of scarring lead to the development of carcinoma.[6] Some investigators suggest that the scar development is secondary to the carcinoma.[7]

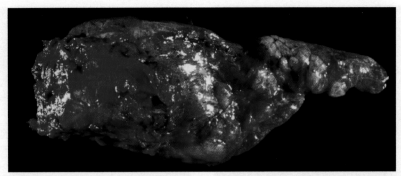

Figure 3–3. Adenocarcinoma of left upper lobe of lung, extending through pleura and involving chest wall.

information in tumor staging. Tumors may grow through the pleurae to the chest wall (Figures 3–3 and 3–4). The tumors are grayish white in color, with areas of hemorrhage and necrosis (Figures 3–4 and 3–5). They may have a glistening or mucoid cut surface when sufficient mucin production is present (Figure 3–6). These peripherally located tumors are not often found in association with a bronchus, but can be associated with malignant pleural effusions (Figures 3–7 and 3–8); for this reason sputum samples are less often positive for adenocarcinoma than for squamous cell carcinoma.

Microscopic Findings

The usual bronchial adenocarcinoma is gland forming, and areas of well-differentiated tumor can merge into and coexist with poorly-differentiated foci. Special stains such as mucicarmine or PAS may be needed to demonstrate intracellular mucin (Figure 3–9). Papillary or tubular formations may be evident (Figures 3–10 to 3–13). Adenocarcinoma can have unusual patterns: clear-cell, signet ring-cell, and spindle-cell features can all be found. Adenocarcinoma must be distinguished pathologically from mesotheliomas. This can be very challenging on cytologic specimens and frequently requires additional studies be performed for accurate classification.

The cells of adenocarcinoma are more uniform than those of squamous cell carcinoma or large cell carcinoma. Cells are usually large, with large nuclei, a high nucleus-to-cytoplasmic ratio, and prominent eosinophilic nucleoli (Figure 3–14). The cytoplasm may appear vacuolated, reflecting the mucin production. Unlike squamous cell carcinoma, the cytoplasmic borders are often poorly defined or indistinct. Histologically, tumors are graded as well, moderately or poorly differentiated, with the majority showing moderate differentiation. It is usually not necessary to use immunohistochemical stains to identify adenocarcinoma, but they may prove useful in separating primary from metastatic tumors or in identifying mesothelioma.[8]

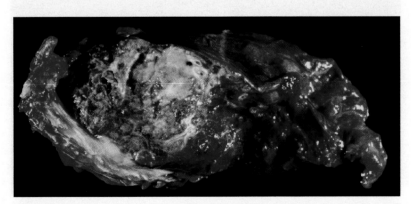

Figure 3–4. Cut surface of tumor in Figure 3–4 showing chest-wall musculature and rib involvement. Note necrotic appearance of the tumor.

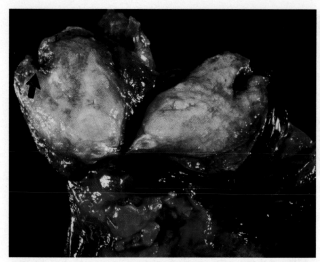

Figure 3–5.   Peripheral adenocarcinoma involving pleura. The cut surface of the tumor is smooth and glistening. Note previous biopsy site (*arrow*).

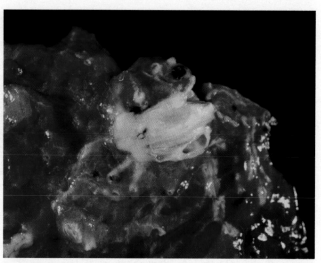

Figure 3–6.   Peripheral adenocarcinoma surrounding, and adherent to, pulmonary artery. Note cut surface showing anthracotic lymph nodes.

BRONCHIOLOALVEOLAR CARCINOMA

Bronchioloalveolar carcinoma (BAC) is a distinctive subtype of peripheral adenocarcinoma which spreads along pre-existing alveolar septae and does not invade lung parenchyma, thus preserving the underlying pulmonary architecture. Two main cell types are found in BAC—mucinous and non-mucinous; the majority of tumors are non-mucinous. Bronchorrhea, considered a classic sign of BAC, is actually rarely seen.[9]

Gross Findings

BAC is usually present in the lung as grayish areas of consolidation, sometimes with central scarring.

Unlike with other bronchogenic carcinomas, hemorrhage and necrosis are not generally seen, and pleural invasion is uncommon (Figures 3–15 and 3–16). The pneumonic form of BAC is usually seen with the mucinous type, and an entire lobe of lung may become consolidated.

Microscopic Findings

Adenocarcinoma of the lung can contain areas that resemble BAC and areas of atypical type II alveolar cell hyperplasia can appear difficult to distinguish from BAC. The term BAC should be reserved for those tumors that grow along the pre-existing frame-

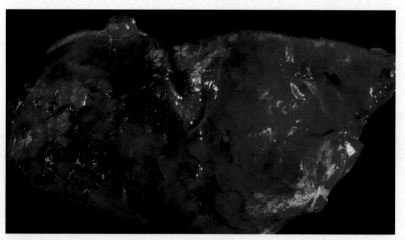

Figure 3–7.   Adenocarcinoma associated with a pleural defect. Again, anthracotic pigment deposition is seen.

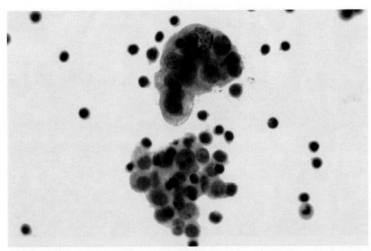

Figure 3–8.   Cluster of cells of adenocarcinoma in pleural fluid. The cytoplasm contains vacuoles. (Pap stain; ×150 original magnification)

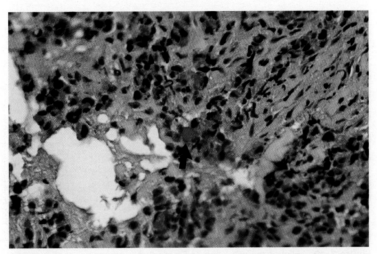

Figure 3–9.   Mucin stain on histologic section of adenocarcinoma. Note intracellular mucin (*arrow*). (Mucicarmine stain; ×40 original magnification)

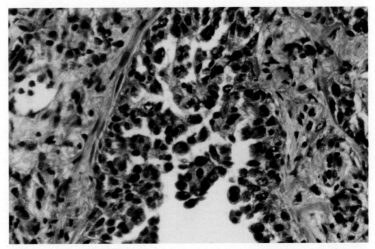

Figure 3–10.   Medium-power photomicrograph of pulmonary adenocarcinoma. Papillary projections are noted in a gland-like lumen. (H & E stain; ×40 original magnification)

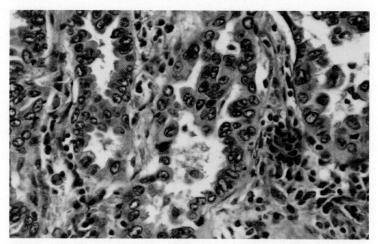

Figure 3–11.   Abnormal glandular structures of adenocarcinoma. Note large, irregularly shaped cells with large nuclei and prominent nucleoli. (H & E stain; ×40 original magnification)

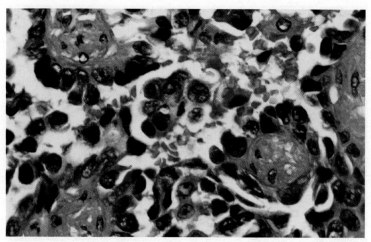

Figure 3–12.   Higher magnification of Figure 3–11, emphasizing abnormally shaped clusters of cells of adenocarcinoma similar to that seen in fluid in Figure 3–8. (H & E stain; ×60 original magnification)

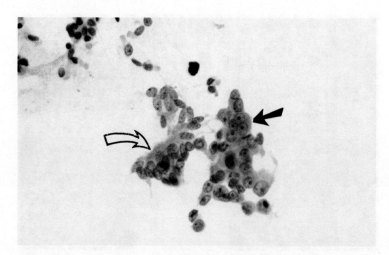

Figure 3–13.   Bronchial brush specimen of adenocarcinoma. Note the malignant cells with large nuclei and prominent nucleoli (*arrow*) adjacent to benign bronchial cells with cilia (*open arrow*). (Pap stain; ×150 original magnification)

work and do not demonstrate areas of invasion (Figures 3–17 to 3–19).

Mucinous BACs are usually very well differentiated and are made up of goblet cells which are mucin producing. The non-mucinous type is composed of type II cells or Clara cells (Figure 3–20). The tumor may appear as papillary clusters, acinar formations or single cells. The cells may project into the alveolar lumen and may have a protruding nucleus. The nucleus may show longitudinal grooves or inclusions (Figure 3–21) and psammoma bodies may be present. Mitotic figures and bizarre cell shapes are uncommon. The non-mucinous type of BAC may have large nuclei, and more atypical forms may have prominent nucleoli with the nucleus protruding in a hobnail pattern.[10] There is an overall uniformity to the cells of BAC. There may be interstitial thickening and fibrosis and an inflammatory component present in these tumors. Mucinous BAC is characterized by tall columnar cells with uniform nuclei. Mucin is seen in the cytoplasm and the inflammatory component is less pronounced than in the non-mucinous type (Figure 3–22). Because BAC are well-differentiated adenocarcinomas with nuclear uniformity, the cytologic diagnosis may be difficult. The cytologic picture may include large three-dimensional groups with papillae, and the nuclei may show inclusions and grooves as seen in other papillary tumors.

SQUAMOUS CELL CARCINOMA

Squamous cell carcinoma of the lung is defined as a malignant epithelial tumor with features of squamous differentiation such as keratin formation and intercellular bridges. These features are most notable in well-differentiated tumors. In contrast to adenocarcinoma, the majority of these tumors arise centrally from major bronchi and ulcerate through the mucosa. Most central squamous cell carcinomas are between 3 and 5 cm in size when detected.[11] Because of their central location, diagnosis by cytologic examination of sputum, bronchial brushes and washes, or endoscopic biopsies can be performed with generally satisfactory results.

Gross Findings

Tumor masses are usually grayish white to yellow and can show central cavitation, necrosis and hemorrhage (Figures 3–23 to 3–26). The texture can be firm or gritty and may be surrounded by areas of obstructive consolidation. Involvement of a bronchus can often be demonstrated (Figure 3–27).

Microscopic Findings

The microscopic appearance of the tumor depends on the degree of differentiation, and there may be

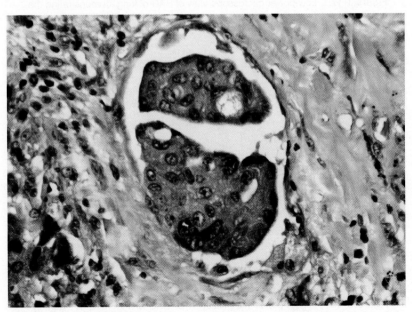

Figure 3–14. Cluster of large cells of pulmonary adenocarcinoma in vascular space in lung. Note the prominent nucleoli. (H & E stain; ×60 original magnification)

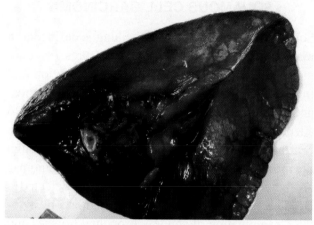

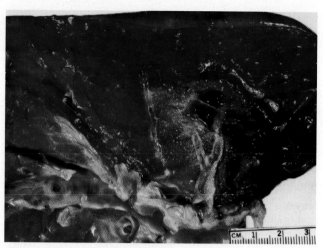

Figure 3–15.   Gross resection specimen of right lung. BAC is present in the superior segment of the lower lobe. The lung appears inflated due to the involvement by tumor.

Figure 3–16.   Cut surface of Figure 3–15 showing the consolidated pneumonic appearance of the BAC.

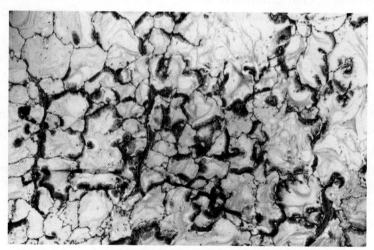

Figure 3–17.   Low-power microscope view of BAC of lung, demonstrating the preservation of the alveolar architecture. (H & E stain; ×20 original magnification)

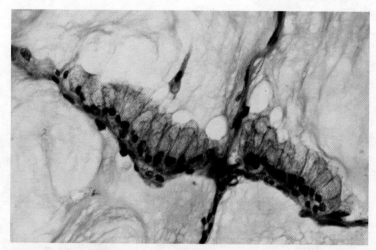

Figure 3–18.   Higher-power magnification of BAC of Figure 3–17, demonstrating tall, columnar, mucin-filled cells arranged along alveolar septae. (H & E stain; ×20 original magnification)

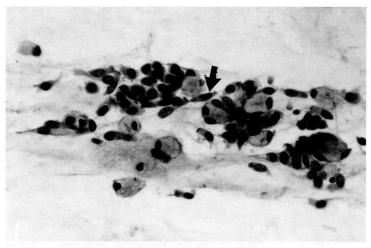

Figure 3–19. FNA of BAC demonstrating well-differentiated, mucin-filled tumor cells. Note the interspersed normal bronchial cells (*arrow*). (Pap stain; ×150 original magnification)

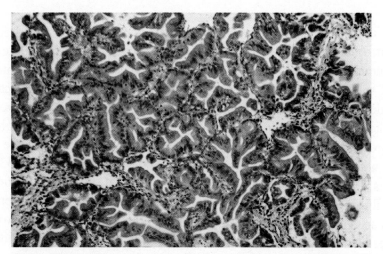

Figure 3–20. Medium-power magnification of non-mucinous BAC. (H & E stain; ×40 original magnification)

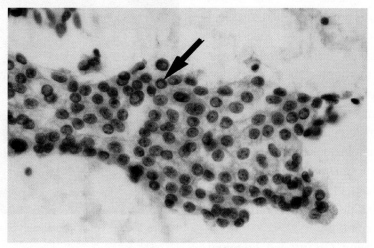

Figure 3–21. FNA of BAC showing nuclear grooves and inclusions (*arrow*) in a non-mucinous tumor. (Pap stain; ×150 original magnification)

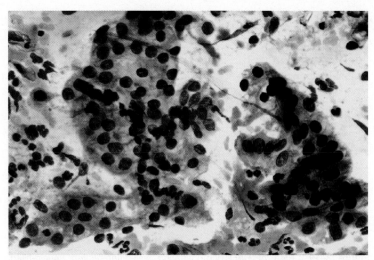

Figure 3–22. FNA of mucinous type of BAC where enlarged mucin-containing cells are present along with benign bronchial epithelial cells. Note relatively clean background. (Pap stain; ×150 original magnification)

variation from area to area. It is not uncommon to find areas of glandular differentiation—making the diagnosis adenosquamous carcinoma. The tumor usually grows as large solid nests of cells that have generous amounts of dense eosinophilic cytoplasm, and which may be quite sizeable with large, hyperchromatic nuclei (Figure 3–28). The nuclei are irregular in shape and may not show prominent nucleoli. Unlike adenocarcinoma, the nuclear-to-cytoplasmic ratio may be low with this tumor. Gaps may be seen between adjacent cells accounting for the intercellular bridges. The intercellular bridges correspond to desmosomal attachments demonstrated with electron microscopy. Keratin may be seen as pinkish orange homogeneous blobs (Figures 3–29 and 3–30). Inflammation and necrosis are often found in association with squamous cell carcinoma. Fine-needle aspiration specimens taken from central necrotic zones may show only this tumor necrosis. Bizarre cell shapes and "tadpole"-shaped cells may be found (Figure 3–31). The diagnosis of squamous cell carcinoma is usually made histologically or cytologically without the use of immunohistochemistry.

There are variants of squamous cell carcinoma including small cell variant, clear cell type, papillary and verrucous types, basaloid type (Figure 3–32), and pleomorphic/giant cell type.[12]

Squamous cell carcinoma is graded histologically as well, moderately and poorly differentiated.

Assessment of histologic grade is not consistently reproducible among pathologists; in an attempt at M.D. Anderson Cancer Center to correlate grade with survival, no statistical significance was found.[13] Other studies observed different results.[14]

The cytologic and histologic appearances of squamous cell carcinoma are similar regardless of the site of origin (Figure 3–33). Unlike adenocarcinoma, which often has a distinct appearance in different organs, there is no difference in appearance of squamous cell carcinoma from, for example, the cervix or lung. Unlike carcinoma in situ, changes

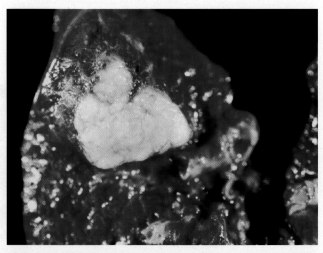

Figure 3–23. Gross photograph of squamous cell carcinoma of right upper lobe of lung. The tumor is located somewhat centrally and there is no pleural involvement. Cut surface of the tumor is smooth, firm, and dense. Necrosis and hemorrhage are not obvious.

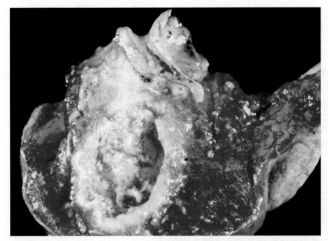

Figure 3–24. Large necrotic cavitating squamous cell carcinoma. This large tumor mass is located in the right upper lobe of the lung and is in continuity with a bronchus.

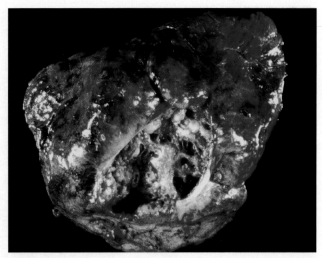

Figure 3–25. Large necrotic cavitating lesion of squamous cell carcinoma.

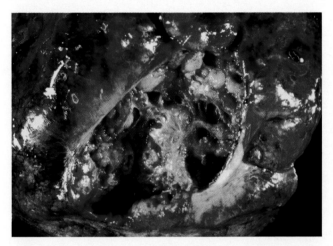

Figure 3–26. Closer view of Figure 3–25 showing cavitation and necrosis. This squamous tumor reached the pleura and was associated with puckering.

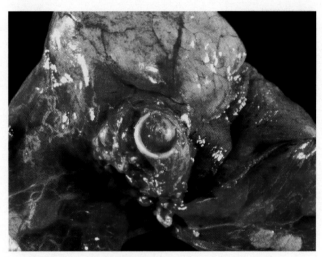

Figure 3–27. Right main stem bronchus showing subtotal obliteration by squamous cell carcinoma.

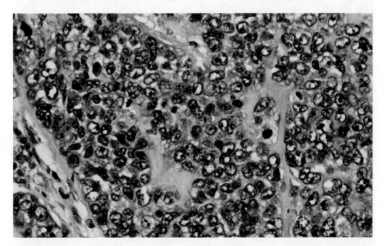

Figure 3–28. Medium-power microscopic view of squamous cell carcinoma. Histologically, the cells grow in large nests. The cells are large with hyperchromatic nuclei. (H & E stain; ×40 original magnification)

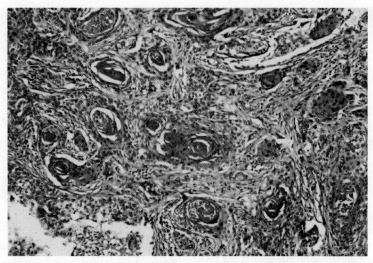

Figure 3–29.   Nests of keratin "pearls" in a well- to moderately-differentiated squamous cell carcinoma. (H & E stain; ×20 original magnification)

can be identified in tissue samples; it may be difficult to determine histologically if a squamous cell carcinoma of the lung is primary or metastatic.

LARGE CELL CARCINOMA

Undifferentiated large cell carcinoma is a non-small cell carcinoma that displays no evidence of squamous or glandular maturation with light microscopy.[15] The definition is one of exclusion and necessitates extensive sampling.[16] These tumors may be central or peripheral and exist in several subtypes.

Gross Findings

Large necrotic masses with pleural involvement may be seen. There is no characteristic gross appearance.

Microscopic Findings

There is a wide spectrum of appearance histologically. The tumor usually grows in sheets and nests and may be associated with desmoplastic stroma[16] (Figure 3–34). The most commonly identified form is a uniform type with sheets of closely packed cells with a

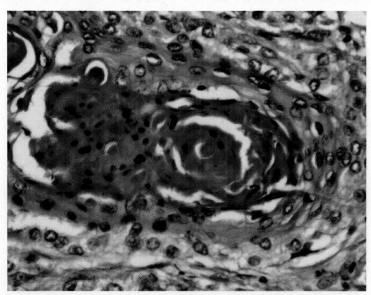

Figure 3–30.   Higher-power view of Figure 3–29 showing the well-formed swirls of keratin. (H & E stain; ×60 original magnification)

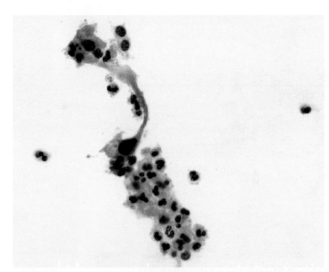

Figure 3–31. Keratinized "tadpole" cell of squamous carcinoma. (Pap stain; ×150 original magnification)

high nuclear-to-cytoplasmic ratio[17] and areas of necrosis (Figure 3–35). According to Mackay, a mucin stain must always be applied to tumors with this appearance because it will be positive in approximately one-half of patients suspected of having undifferentiated large cell carcinoma, thus placing the patient in the adenocarcinoma category.[17] Other forms include pleomorphic giant cell type, spindle cell, clear cell, and lymphoepithelioma-like carcinoma.[16]

Pathologists also identify a specific large cell neuroendocrine tumor that is differentiated from other large cell tumors and other neuroendocrine tumors (small cell tumors). This specific entity appears to have a very poor prognosis. It differs from small cell neuroendocrine tumors in histologic appearance (larger cells with abundant cytoplasm) and response to chemotherapy (poorer). There is another variant of large cell tumors that has neuroendocrine features without being classified as large cell neuroendocrine tumor.

SMALL CELL CARCINOMA

Small cell carcinoma is a malignant epithelial tumor with the cytologic features of scant cytoplasm, finely granular chromatin, absent or inconspicuous nucleoli, and frequent mitosis.[18] The pathologic diagnosis of small cell carcinoma should be made on light microscopic findings, although immunohistochemical stains and electron microscopy are helpful additional studies. This is an aggressive neoplasm and that is reflected in the high-grade morphology.

Gross Findings

Since most patients with small cell carcinoma are not treated surgically, the gross findings of this tumor are most often seen at autopsy. Usually arising centrally around the hilum, the cut surface is grayish white with areas of necrosis. Frequent lymph node involvement is present. Bronchial mucosa involvement is uncommon. Endobronchial lesions are uncommon but reported.[19,20]

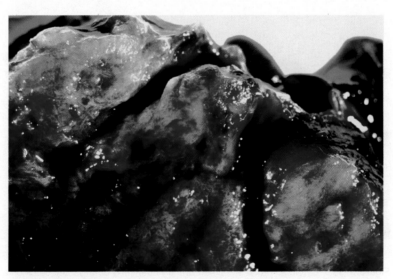

Figure 3–32. Gross photograph of basaloid type of squamous carcinoma showing a lobulated, glistening, cut surface.

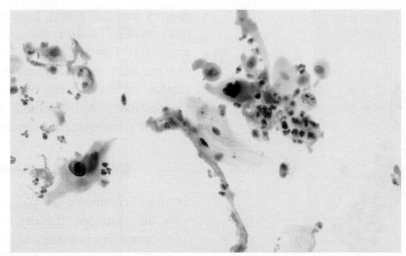

Figure 3–33. Single cells of squamous carcinoma exfoliated in sputum. Note dark nuclei, orangeophilic cytoplasm, and inflammatory background. (Pap stain; ×150 original magnification)

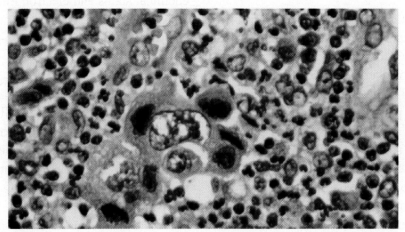

Figure 3–34. Large pleomorphic tumor cells of large cell carcinoma in a histologic section of lung. Note leukocytes surrounding tumor cells. (H & E stain; ×60 original magnification)

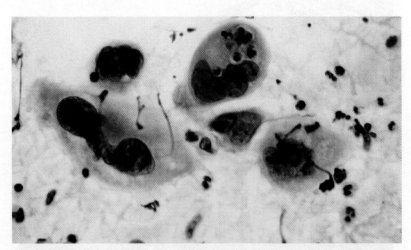

Figure 3–35. Cytologic brush specimen of individual cells of large cell carcinoma. Note high nuclear-to-cytoplasmic ratio and bizarre nuclear shapes. (Pap stain; ×150 original magnification)

Microscopic Findings

The specimens submitted for pathologic study from patients with small cell carcinoma are usually small biopsies, often obtained via bronchoscopic biopsy or by fine-needle aspiration. These specimens are often artifactually distorted, showing crushing, fragmentation and, in the case of cytology, air-drying. This can make definitive diagnosis difficult and may lead to the under-recognition of small cell carcinoma in larger and better-preserved specimens. Non-small cell carcinoma can be mistaken for small cell carcinoma in a limited biopsy sample that shows crush and distortion. Additional samplings may be necessary in diagnosing this cancer.

Small cell carcinoma usually appears at low magnification as monotonous sheets of hyperchromatic cells with foci of necrosis (Figure 3–36). The individual tumor cells are small, but still 2 to 2.5 times the size of lymphocytes. At higher magnification, the atypia of each cell can be appreciated. These round-to-oval cells have a high nucleus-to-cytoplasm ratio with scant amounts of cytoplasm barely visible (Figure 3–37). Rosettes may be present (Figure 3–38). The mitotic count is very high and individual cell necrosis or karyorrhexis is common (Figure 3–39). DNA from broken-down cells may accumulate in blood vessel walls, giving a streaking blue appearance (Figure 3–40). Small cell carcinoma can coexist with large cell carcinoma and is commonly found combined with better-differentiated non-small cell tumors such as squamous cell carcinoma (Figures 3–41 and 3–42). Fine-needle aspiration specimens from small cell carcinoma have a similar appearance to tissue but may be somewhat better preserved (Figures 3–43 and 3–44). In 1981, the WHO modified the classification of small cell carcinoma to three subtypes: oat cell, intermediate, and combined types. Oat cell type is considered by some to be an artifact due to necrosis or histological processing.[21] In 1988, the International Association for the Study of Lung Cancer (IASLC) proposed that small cell carcinoma be divided into three categories: small cell carcinoma, mixed small cell/large cell carcinoma, and combined small cell carcinoma which has components of squamous cell and/or adenocarcinoma. It has been shown that pathologists are more likely to agree on a diagnosis of pure small cell carcinoma than on combined or mixed subtypes.[18] Cytoplasmic dense core granules are seen with electron microscopy, but can be absent in up to 20 percent of cases (Figure 3–45). The assumption that small cell carcinoma is a neuroendocrine tumor is the basis for the classification schemes that put it on the undifferentiated end of a spectrum of tumors that include carcinoid and atypical carcinoid.[17]

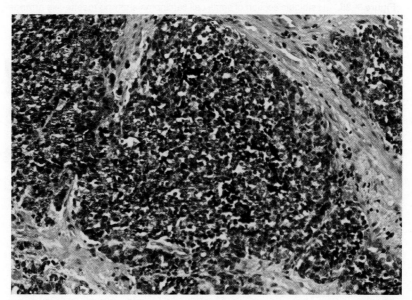

Figure 3–36. Medium-power photomicrograph of monotonous, small, hyperchromatic cells of small cell carcinoma arranged in a nesting pattern. (H & E stain; ×40 original magnification)

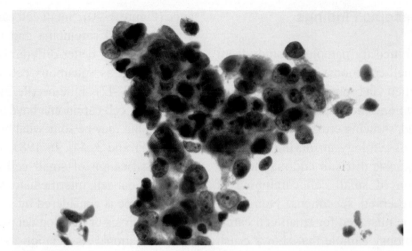

Figure 3–37.   Cytologic preparation of small cell carcinoma, showing scant, barely-visible cytoplasm and tight clustering and molding of tumor cells. (Pap stain; ×150 magnification)

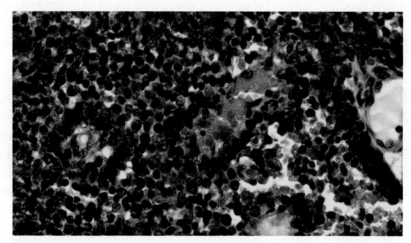

Figure 3–38.   Histologic section of small cell carcinoma showing rosette-like arrangement of cells. (H & E stain; ×20 original magnification)

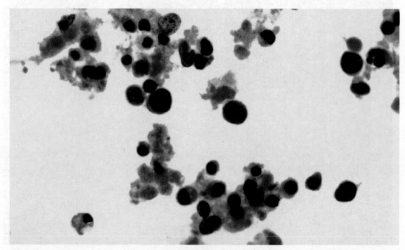

Figure 3–39.   Cytologic specimen of small cell carcinoma showing individual cell degeneration and necrosis; nuclear detail is no longer visible. (Pap stain; ×150 original magnification)

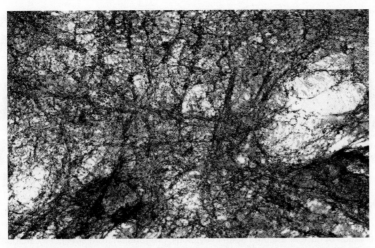

Figure 3–40. Streaks of nuclear material imparting a characteristic appearance to a cytologic specimen of small cell carcinoma. (H & E stain; ×40 original magnification)

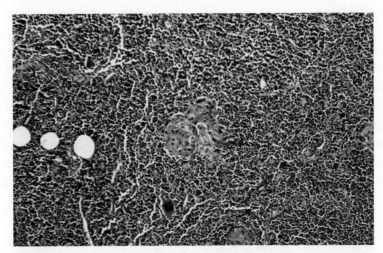

Figure 3–41. Medium-power photomicrograph of histologic section of small cell carcinoma with area of squamous differentiation. (H & E stain; ×20 original magnification)

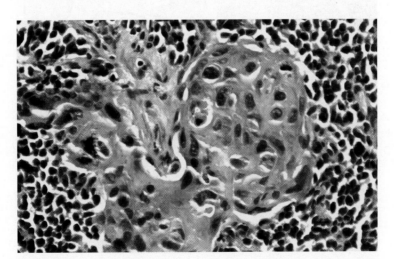

Figure 3–42. Higher-power view of squamous pearl from Figure 3–41. Note similarity to Figure 3–30. (H & E stain; ×60 original magnification)

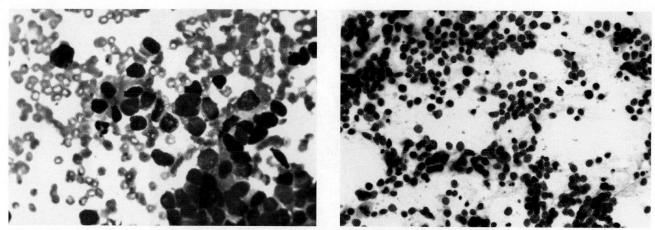

Figure 3–43/44.   Better preservation of nuclear features seen in cytologic preparation from small cell carcinoma. (H & E stain; ×150 original magnification; H & E stain; ×60 original magnification)

LARGE CELL NEUROENDOCRINE CARCINOMA

Also on the spectrum of neuroendocrine tumors is large cell neuroendocrine carcinoma. Large cell neuroendocrine carcinoma is a poorly-differentiated high-grade carcinoma that shows evidence of neuroendocrine differentiation by light microscopy. It is an aggressive tumor with a poor prognosis. Immunohistochemistry or electron microscopy is used to confirm the endocrine features of this tumor. These tumors have been classified in the past as intermediate cell neuroendocrine carcinoma, atypical carcinoid, and intermediate small cell carcinoma, among other designations. According to Colby and colleagues,[18] large cell neuroendocrine carcinoma has taken longer to be recognized as a distinct entity than other tumors because: it requires special confirmatory studies, reliable endocrine markers are only more recently available, the tumor itself is uncommon, it is harder to diagnose than other entities, and many of these tumors were diag-

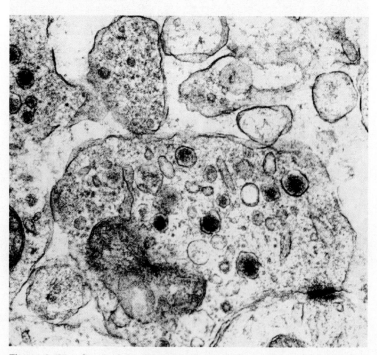

Figure 3–45.   Small, dark, dense neurosecretory granules seen in electron micrograph of small cell carcinoma.

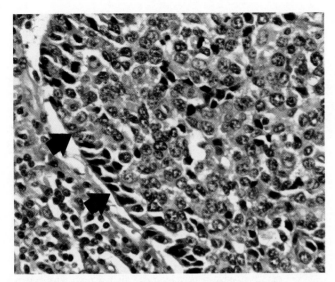

Figure 3–46. Histologic section of large cell neuroendocrine carcinoma (LCNEC) demonstrating high nuclear grade and peripheral palisading (*arrows*) of cells. (H & E stain; ×40 original magnification)

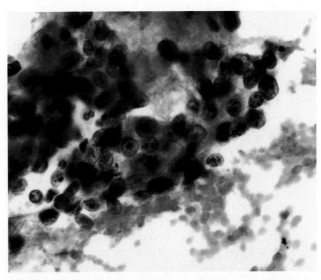

Figure 3–47. Cytologic preparation of large cell neuroendocrine carcinoma (LCNEC). Note prominent nucleoli and generous amounts of cytoplasm. (Pap stain; ×150 original magnification)

nosed as other types (atypical carcinoid intermediate variant of small cell carcinoma, etc) in the past.

Gross Findings

These tumors can be central or peripheral and can be quite large, with areas of necrosis and hemorrhage; the cut surface is tan to white. Lymph node metastases are common at time of presentation.

Microscopic Findings

Large cell neuroendocrine carcinomas are defined by histologic criteria. There are no cytologic criteria yet proposed for these tumors. In general, they have the light-microscopic features of all neuroendocrine tumors: organoid, palisading, or rosette appearance (Figure 3–46) at low power, and in addition, large tumor cells with a low nuclear-to-cytoplasmic ratio with coarse or open chromatin and prominent nucleoli (Figure 3–47). Mitosis and necrosis are frequent. These tumors stain immunohistochemically for chromogranin, synaptophysin, Neuron specific enclase (NSE), bombesin, keratin and CEA (Figure 3–48). Electron microscopy shows dense core granules. The differential diagnosis includes non-small cell carcinomas and intermediate small cell carcinoma and atypical carcinoid.

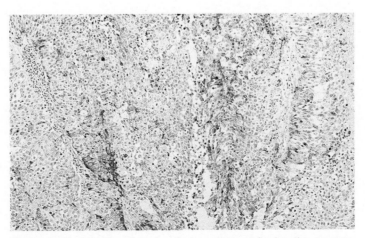

Figure 3–48. Positive stain for chromogranin confirming the neuroendocrine nature of LCNEC. (Chromogranin; ×20 original magnification)

CONCLUSION

The diagnosis of lung cancer can be made on cytology preparations as well as surgically biopsied material. Close cooperation among pathologists, radiologists, and clinicians is essential.

REFERENCES

1. Glaxo Wellcome, American Cancer Society—Cancer Facts & Figures 1999.
2. Gazdar AF, Linnoila RI. The pathology of lung cancer—changing concepts and newer diagnostic techniques. Semin Oncol 1988;15:214–25.
3. Carey FA, Donnelley SC, Walker WS, et al. Synchronous primary lung cancers: prevalence in surgical material and clinical implications. Thorax 1993;48:344–6.
4. Colby TV, Koss MN, Travis WD. Atlas of tumor pathology: Morphologic diagnosis and heterogeneity of carcinoma of the lung. Washington (DC): Armed Forces Institute of Pathology; 1995. p. 135.
5. Colby TV, Koss MN, Travis WD. Atlas of tumor pathology: Morphologic diagnosis and heterogeneity of carcinoma of the lung. Washington (DC): Armed Forces Institute of Pathology. 1995. p. 137.
6. Colby TV, Koss MN, Travis WD. Atlas of tumor pathology: Carcinoma of the lung: Overview, incidence, etiology, and screening. Washington (DC): Armed Forces Institute of Pathology; 1995. p. 95.
7. Shimosato Y, Suzuki A, Hashimoto T, et al. Prognostic implications of fibrotic focus (scar) in small peripheral lung cancers. Am J Surg Pathol 1980;4:365–73.
8. Colby TV, Koss MN, Travis WD. Atlas of tumor pathology: Adenocarcinoma of the lung (excluding bronchioloalveolar carcinoma.) Washington (DC): Armed Forces Institute of Pathology; 1995. p. 194.
9. Daly RC, Trastek VF, Pairolero PC. Bronchoalveolar carcinoma: factors affecting survival. Ann Thorac Surg 1991; 51:368–77.
10. Colby TV, Koss MN, Travis WD. Atlas of tumor pathology: Bronchioloalveolar carcinoma. Washington (DC): Armed Forces Institute of Pathology; 1995. p. 206.
11. Mackay B, Lukeman J, Ordonez N. Tumors of the lung: major problems in pathology. Philadelphia (PA): WB Saunders Company; 1991. p. 166.
12. Colby TV, Koss MN, Travis WD. Atlas of tumor pathology: Squamous cell carcinoma and variants. Washington (DC): Armed Forces Institute of Pathology; 1995. p. 167–72.
13. Mackay B, Lukeman J, Ordonez N. Tumors of the lung: Major problems in pathology. Philadelphia (PA): WB Saunders Company; 1991. p. 176.
14. Carter D. Squamous cell carcinoma of the lung: an update. Semin Diagn Pathol 1985;2:226.
15. Mackay B, Lukeman J, Ordonez N. Tumors of the lung: Major problems in pathology. Philadelphia (PA): WB Saunders Company; 1991. p. 190.
16. Colby TV, Koss MN, Travis WD. Atlas of Tumor Pathology: Large cell carcinoma. Washington (DC): Armed Forces Institute of Pathology; 1995. p. 259.
17. Mackay B, Lukeman J, Ordonez N. Tumors of the lung: Major problems in pathology. Philadelphia (PA): WB Saunders Company; 1991. p. 191.
18. Colby TV, Koss MN, Travis WD. Atlas of tumor pathology: Small cell carcinoma and large cell neuroendocrine carcinoma. Washington (DC): Armed Forces Institute of Pathology; 1995. p. 235.
19. Watkin SW, Soorae AJ, Green JA. Bronchoscopic "resection" of small cell carcinoma. Endoscopy 1989;21:186.
20. Blackman F, Chung HR, McDonald RJ, et al. Oat cell carcinoma with multiple tracheobronchial papillomatous tumors. Chest 1983;83:817.

4

Clinical Features of Lung Cancer

MARC B. FEINSTEIN, MD
DIANE STOVER, MD

Lung cancer is the leading cause of cancer-related mortality in the United States, accounting for over 21 percent of all cancer deaths.[1] Yet despite recent strides in understanding the etiology and treatment of this disease, the survival rate has not changed appreciably over the past 30 years. Since there are no effective screening procedures, most patients are diagnosed at a late stage when surgical cures are no longer possible. Although certain signs and symptoms are characteristic of lung cancer, most of these are nonspecific and are easily overlooked until evidence of more advanced disease is apparent. Furthermore, approximately 15 percent of lung cancer patients present to physicians without any symptoms at all.[2] This chapter will review the clinical manifestations of lung cancer, emphasizing the symptoms and signs attributable to the primary malignancy. Those that are related to antineoplastic therapy are beyond the scope of this discussion.

The symptoms and signs of lung cancer can be divided into four general groups:

1. Symptoms and signs due to the primary tumor, such as coughing, hemoptysis, and wheezing
2. Symptoms and signs attributed to the intrathoracic, extrapulmonary extension of the primary tumor, such as pain, dysphagia, and superior vena cava syndrome
3. Symptoms and signs due to extrathoracic metastases, such as bone pain and weight loss
4. Symptoms and signs not attributable to direct or metastatic spread, such as malignant cachexia and neuromuscular weakness

SYMPTOMS AND SIGNS DUE TO THE PRIMARY TUMOR

Cough and Sputum

Cough has repeatedly been found to be the most common symptom at presentation among patients with lung cancer. Although 70 to 90 percent of patients will experience coughing at some point during their clinical illness, only 20 percent are affected at the time of diagnosis.[3] Symptoms are found more commonly in the setting of centrally located tumors rather than peripheral ones. Coughing is usually chronic and may vary in intensity from day to day. The mechanism by which coughing occurs varies; it may result from a "foreign-body" irritative effect of the tumor, poor drainage due to an obstructing tumor, or a secondary infection.

Hemoptysis

The expectoration of any blood whatsoever, regardless of the amount, denotes hemoptysis. It is most common in the setting of centrally located tumors.[3] In an Israeli study which retrospectively looked at 208 patients with hemoptysis, small cell lung cancer was the most common lung cancer involved, followed in decreasing frequency by squamous cell carcinoma and adenocarcinoma. Metastatic tumors associated with hemoptysis include breast cancer, malignant melanoma, and lymphoma.[4]

Bleeding, usually minimal in severity, is due to ulceration of tumor into the bronchial mucosa. Massive hemoptysis of greater than 200 cc of blood per 24 hours, as a result of direct invasion of blood vessels, is rare. Patients with hemoptysis often experience heaviness, gurgling, or vague chest discomfort that may help localize the source of bleeding. The differential diagnosis includes bronchiectasis, bronchitis, tuberculosis, and foreign bodies, all of which should be excluded by a prompt diagnostic work-up. Bronchoscopy alone reveals a diagnosis in 42 percent of patients with hemoptysis; diagnostic yield is greater among patients with mild hemoptysis or in patients who have abnormal chest radiographs. When both computed tomography (CT) of the chest and bronchoscopy are employed, the diagnostic yield increases to 93 percent.[4]

Dyspnea

Dyspnea is common in lung cancer and is likely multifactorial in etiology. Airway obstruction, atelectasis, post-obstructive pneumonitis, or lymphatic carcinomatosis can produce physiologically significant hypoxemia that often results in shortness of breath. The presence of a pleural effusion should be considered in patients without hypoxemia. Dyspnea, from whatever cause, is usually more severe in the presence of clinically significant emphysema or congestive heart failure.

SYMPTOMS AND SIGNS DUE TO EXTRAPULMONARY TUMOR EXTENSION

Chest Pain

Approximately one-half of lung cancer patients report experiencing chest pain at some point during the course of their illness.[5] Although the lung itself possesses no pain receptors, peribronchial autonomic nerves can transmit vague sensations of discomfort via the vagus nerve. Most commonly, pain is described as a dull, intermittent ache on the side of the tumor, lasting for several minutes to hours at a time. In contrast to the lung, pain receptors do exist in the pleura, mediastinum, and large blood vessels. Therefore, severe chest pain requiring narcotics is almost always the result of pleural metastases, and, if constant or penetrating in character,

may indicate direct invasion of the mediastinum, or bony structures surrounding the pleural space. Superior sulcus tumors are often associated with pain in the shoulder or arm secondary to invasion of the brachial plexus. Brachial plexus invasion may also result in upper extremity weakness, atrophy, or paresthesia. Pleuritic chest pain usually ceases with the onset of a pleural effusion (discussed below).

Pleural Effusion

Large unilateral pleural effusions, particularly those that accommodate more than half the hemithorax, should raise suspicion for malignancy. Effusions secondary to the extension of a peripheral tumor or metastases to the pleura are usually exudative, and often bloody. Chylothorax, resulting from lymphatic obstruction, occurs rarely in lung cancer. However, malignancy is a relatively frequent cause of chylothorax. In a series of studies examining the factors responsible for chylothorax, about 50 percent of these factors were attributable to tumors. Lung cancer comprised less than 25 percent of these malignancies.[6]

Occasionally, cancer patients develop effusions due to congestive heart failure, pulmonary infarction, or pulmonary infection. These are usually smaller in size and resolve with correction of the underlying medical condition.

Superior Vena Cava Syndrome

The superior vena cava is a thin-walled structure with low intraluminal pressures, and is thereby particularly vulnerable to extrinsic compression by tumor. The symptoms of superior vena cava (SVC) syndrome occur when blood flow through this vessel is interrupted, resulting in increased vascular pressure. These include edema of the face, neck, upper torso and breasts; headache; visual distortion; conjunctival edema and erythema; and dilation of collateral veins (Figure 4–1). Patients may complain of tightening of their shirt collar, or that the skin over affected regions has taken on a cyanotic hue. Symptoms generally worsen with bending forward or lying supine.

Prior to 1949, malignancies caused only one-third of all cases of SVC syndrome. The remainder

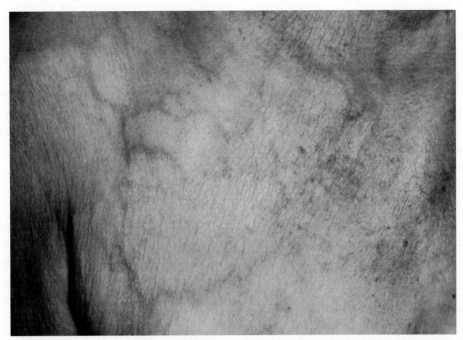

Figure 4–1. Superior vena cava syndrome in an elderly man with non-small cell lung cancer. Note the dilation of collateral veins.

were due to conditions such as aortic aneurysms (usually from syphilis), tuberculosis, and fibrotic mediastinitis. Currently, however, malignancy is associated with 87 to 97 percent of cases.[7] Right-sided tumors cause obstruction more commonly than left-sided ones. Tumors in the superior sulcus, because of their proximity to the superior vena cava, also commonly cause SVC syndrome.

Lymphadenopathy

The initial spread of lung cancer is most typically to the regional hilar and mediastinal lymph nodes; however, the extension of tumor to axillary, supraclavicular, and scalene lymph nodes is also common. Palpable lymphadenopathy, if present, is particularly useful to establish the diagnosis of lung cancer. If malignant cells are found on a successful percutaneous biopsy, the need for invasive and potentially risky procedures, such as bronchoscopy, mediastinoscopy, or an open lung procedure, can be avoided. In a California study, the sensitivity and specificity of fine-needle aspiration for detecting malignancy in palpable supraclavicular lymph nodes was 97 percent and 98 percent, respectively.[8]

Hoarseness

Hoarseness of the voice occurs as a presenting symptom in less than 10 percent of lung cancer patients. The most common cause is compression of the left recurrent laryngeal nerve by tumor and/or mediastinal adenopathy. If lung cancer is suspected, direct laryngoscopy should be performed to rule out vocal cord paralysis.

Dysphagia

Another rare complication of lung cancer is dysphagia. In one series involving 615 consecutive hospital admissions for bronchogenic carcinoma, dysphagia was present in 2.2 percent of patients.[9] Compression of the esophagus by tumor indicates tumor invasion of the posterior mediastinal compartment—usually by massive lymph node involvement. This usually implies that the tumor is unresectable.

Pericardial Effusion/Tamponade

A new-onset arrhythmia or electrocardiographic abnormality in lung cancer should raise suspicion for pericardial disease. Although direct invasion by tumor is the usual cause, pericardial effusion or tamponade can also result from irradiation, drugs, or infection. In the case of radiation, pericardial thickening and/or an effusion can occur as late as 20 years after the completion of treatment. Possible symptoms include palpitations, dyspnea, cough, light-headedness, chest pain, and diaphoresis. Physical examination can show jugular venous distension, diminished heart sounds, and/or a pericardial rub. In the case of chronic pericarditis with pericardial thickening, a pericardial knock may be heard.

SYMPTOMS DUE TO EXTRATHORACIC METASTASES

Central Nervous System Involvement

In autopsy series, central nervous system metastases are found in approximately 20 percent of lung cancer patients at death.[10] Patients usually present with seizures or other focal neurologic abnormalities, such as headache, hemiplegia, personality changes, cerebellar disturbances, or difficulty speaking. Rarely, a metastasis may cause a cranial mononeuropathy or phrenic nerve palsy with hemidiaphragmatic paralysis. Although lung cancer, particularly small cell carcinoma, is among the most common cause of brain metastases, it is important to also rule out other malignancies that commonly spread to the central nervous system. Examples would include thyroid, breast, and colon cancer.

Spinal Cord Compression

Lung cancer is the most common cause of spinal cord compression. Impingement on the spinal cord occurs either through direct extension of a vertebral metastasis or by invasion of a para-spinal mass through the intervertebral foramen. The thoracic spine is most often affected, followed by the lumbosacral spine and cervical spine. The most common symptom is localized back pain that can persist for weeks before the diagnosis of cord compression is made. Rarely, radicular pain may be present in a dermatomal distribution. If spinal cord compression is suspected, physical exam should be a guide to determine the level of spinal cord involvement. In general, neurologic findings are present two vertebrae below the site of compression. Loss of sensation to pinprick or temperature often occurs before changes in motor function. Affected regions may manifest increased spasticity or motor weakness. Deep tendon reflexes may be increased. Loss of the anal wink reflex, as well as sphincter tone, are usually late findings.

Spinal cord compression can result in the irreversible loss of nerve function and, as such, is considered an oncologic emergency. In patients in whom this is suspected, magnetic resonance imaging (MRI) of the spine should be performed as soon as possible to confirm the diagnosis and to guide treatment. Treatment of spinal cord compression includes corticosteroids (most often dexamethasone), radiotherapy—usually to an area extending several vertebrae above and below the site of compression, or surgical decompression by laminectomy.

SYMPTOMS AND SIGNS NOT ATTRIBUTABLE TO DIRECT OR METASTATIC SPREAD

Also called paraneoplastic syndromes, these conditions do not result from any physical effects of the primary tumor or its metastases. In some cases, the underlying mechanisms are well understood, resulting either from peptide release by malignant cells, or by immunologic cross-reactivity between tumor cells and normal tissue. Often, however, the pathophysiology is not understood. Most paraneoplastic conditions resolve with treatment of the underlying malignancy. Below are reviewed the most common paraneoplastic phenomena and their relevant clinical findings. A summary of these is presented in Table 4–1.

Clubbing and Hypertrophic Osteoarthropathy

First described by Hippocrates, clubbing is present in a wide array of disorders, but is most commonly seen in lung cancer (Table 4–2). Although clubbing continues to arouse the curiosity of experienced clinicians and investigators alike, its etiology remains entirely unknown. Under normal conditions, the soft tissue that separates the base of the fingernail bed from the distal phalanx is less than 2 mm thick. With early clubbing, changes in blood volume and interstitial fluid can increase the thickness of connective tissue in the nail bed to 3 to 4 mm.[11] These changes can extend laterally around the fingertips and distally to the tip of the nail bed.

One of the most useful early findings in clubbing is an increase in the sponginess of the soft tissue at the base of the nail. Skin surrounding the cuticle often appears smooth, flushed, or glossy. Clubbing can also be detected by placing together the dorsal surfaces of the distal digits of similar fingers. A diamond-shaped aperture, typically present at the base of the fingernails, is obliterated in clubbing. Furthermore, the proximal edge of a clubbed fingernail is often palpable. With severe clubbing, the overall shape of the fingernail is altered to produce typical "parrot's beak," "watchglass," or "drumstick" types of deformities (Figure 4–2).

Clubbing is sometimes associated with hypertrophic osteoarthropathy (HOA), although either condition can occur in the absence of the other (see

Table 4–1. PARANEOPLASTIC NEUROLOGIC SYNDROMES AND THEIR ASSOCIATED TUMOR TYPES		
	Tumor Type	
Syndrome	Lung Cancer	Other Malignancies
Constitutional symptom		
Clubbing and HOA	Non-small cell	Hepatoma Mesothelioma
Fatigue and cachexia	All types	All types
Neuromuscular syndromes		
Central nervous system syndromes		
Subacute cortical cerebellar degeneration	Small cell Adenocarcinoma	Ovary Breast Hodgkin's disease
Visual paraneoplastic syndromes	Small cell	Ovary
Peripheral nervous system syndromes		
Eaton-Lambert syndrome	Small cell Adenocarcinoma Undifferentiated	Breast
Sensory neuropathy/encephalomyelitis	Small cell	Breast
Endocrine syndromes		
Hypercalcemia	Squamous cell	Breast Kidney Ovary Multiple myeloma Lymphoma
Syndrome of inappropriate ADH	Small cell	Pancreatic carcinoma Lymphoma Thymoma
Cushing's syndrome	Small cell	Thymus Pancreas Pheochromocytoma Medullary thyroid
Cutaneous syndromes		
Dermatomyositis-polymyositis	All types	Ovary Breast Stomach Colon
Acanthosis nigrans	All types	Stomach Colon
Sign of Leser-Trélat	Squamous cell Adenocarcinoma	Hodgkin's disease T-cell lymphoma Sarcomas Breast Cervical

Table 4–2. CONDITIONS COMMONLY ASSOCIATED WITH DIGITAL CLUBBING
Intrathoracic
Bronchogenic carcinoma*
Metastatic lung cancer*
Hodgkin's disease
Mesothelioma*
Bronchiectasis*
Lung abscess
Empyema
Cystic fibrosis
Interstitial fibrosis
Pneumoconiosis
Arteriovenous malformations
Cardiovascular
Congenital cyanotic heart disease
Subacute bacterial endocarditis
Infected aortic bypass graft*
Hepatic and gastrointestinal
Hepatic cirrhosis*
Inflammatory bowel disease
Carcinoma of esophagus or colon
Miscellaneous
Hereditary clubbing

* Hypertrophic osteoarthropathy accompanies clubbing in these conditions (see text for details).

Table 4–2).[11] Any or all of the following changes in the distal extremities characterizes HOA:

1. Periosteal new-bone formation, especially in the long bones
2. Symmetric arthritic changes in the joints and periarticular tissues
3. Thickening of the soft tissues in the face or distal one-third of the arms and legs
4. Neurovascular changes, such as chronic erythema, paresthesia, and increased sweating

As with clubbing, the pathogenesis of hypertrophic osteoarthropathy is unknown. Occasionally, HOA is discovered radiographically by the incidental finding of subperiosteal bone formation. More commonly, patients with HOA complain of the insidious onset of achiness and stiffness of the extremities or distal joints that is relieved by elevation. The distal extremities often appear enlarged and edematous. Skin over the affected region may feel warm and appear thickened (Figure 4–3). Bony tenderness is commonly present over the distal long bones, such as the radius and ulna. Clubbing, if present concurrently, is often subtle and mild in severity, but may help distinguish HOA from other causes of swollen, painful extremities.

Fatigue and Cachexia

Fatigue and malaise are, in many cases, the most common symptom of cancer patients.[12] Moreover, fatigue may be the initial and only presenting symptom of lung cancer patients. Its etiology is multifactorial, and can be complicated by anemia, treatment with chemotherapy and/or radiation, humoral mediators, and depression. Fatigue is usually present in the absence of confounding neuromuscular syndromes (discussed below).

Weight loss is a presenting feature in at least one-third of patients with lung cancer, and, in some studies, is an independent indicator of poor prognosis. Patients can demonstrate profound weight loss—often without anorexia, disappearance of subcutaneous fat, and loss of skin turgor. Although the mechanism by which cachexia develops may vary with the type of underlying tumor, the presence of circulating humoral factors and an increase in the basal metabolic rate are thought to play a role. Inflammatory cytokines, which are elevated in animal models, have been implicated in lung cancer and include tumor necrosis factor-α, interleukin-1β, and interleukin-6. Treatment is symptomatic and may include parenteral nutrition and appetite stimulants. In several controlled trials, significant improvements in appetite, food intake, and weight were shown among patients taking megestrol acetate as opposed to those taking placebo.[13,14]

Neuromuscular Syndromes

As many as one-third of lung cancer patients develop clinically evident neuromuscular abnormalities, but

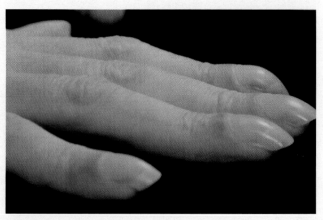

Figure 4–2.   Clubbing of the fingers.

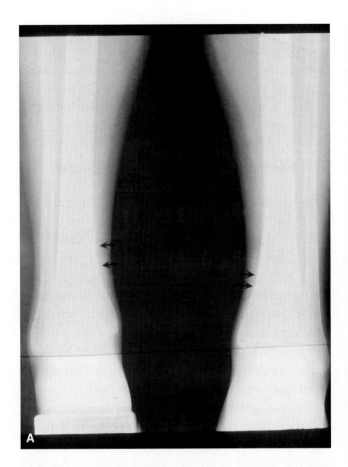

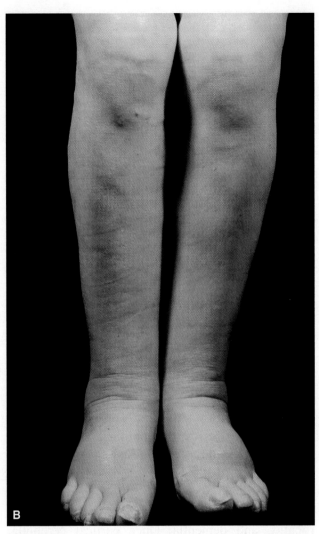

Figure 4–3. Hypertrophic osteoarthropathy in a patient with non-small cell lung cancer. *A*, Radiography of the tibia demonstrates periosteal new bone formation at arrows. *B*, Increased thickness of the subcutaneous soft tissues of the lower extremities. This effect is more pronounced distally than proximally.

the prevalence of subclinical neuromuscular disease may be much higher. In a study involving 100 patients with lung cancer, 99 percent had abnormal muscle histology.[15] Symptoms can develop in any part of the nervous system, and any pathologic process may be involved (Table 4–3). These disorders are further complicated by the fact that they can occur in the absence of any malignancy or can precede the diagnosis of malignancy by months to years. Several features are similar among all neurologic paraneoplastic syndromes. First, the onset of neuromuscular symptoms usually precede the diagnosis of cancer, often by more than a year; second, the neuromuscular symptoms are often more disabling than those directly attributable to the tumor; and third, discovery and treatment of the underlying cancer often leads to improvement of the neuromuscular symptoms.

Although some overlap occurs, cancer-associated neuromuscular diseases can be categorized into central nervous system and peripheral nervous system syndromes:

Central Nervous System Syndromes

Paraneoplastic Cerebellar Degeneration. Paraneoplastic cerebellar degeneration is most closely associated with adenocarcinoma and small cell lung cancer, as well as ovarian cancer, breast cancer, and Hodgkin's disease.[16,17] Despite increasing knowledge of its pathogenesis, it remains a very rare complication of malignancy; only about 300 cases have been reported. However, morphometric studies performed at autopsy indicate that patients who die of cancer generally have fewer Purkinje's cells in their

Table 4–3. PARANEOPLASTIC NEUROLOGIC SYNDROMES

Central nervous system
    Subacute cortical cerebellar degeneration
    Visual paraneoplastic syndrome
    Limbic encephalitis
    Necrotizing myelopathy
    Central pontine myelinosis
Peripheral nervous system
    Myasthenia syndrome
    Sensory neuropathy
    Motor neuropathy
    Sensorimotor neuropathy
    Neuromyotonia

cerebellum than those who die of other diseases.[18] In approximately 50 percent of cases, this syndrome is associated with any of four different antibodies targeting cerebellar Purkinje's cell proteins.[19] The best described of these is anti-Yo.

Symptoms of paraneoplastic cerebellar degeneration usually precede the diagnosis of cancer by several months to a year; in some cases, the cancer may elude detection for 3 to 4 years. Typically, patients develop difficulty walking that worsens over several weeks and progresses to incoordination of the arms and legs, dysarthria, and nystagmus. Neurologic findings are usually bilateral and symmetrical. In many cases, non-cerebellar deficits may develop, including sensorineural hearing loss, peripheral neuropathy, and dementia. Once cortical cerebellar degeneration has reached its peak, symptoms usually stabilize and remain unchanged despite treatment, or even cure, of the underlying malignancy. Diagnosis is most commonly made on clinical grounds alone, although CT and MRI scans may show diffuse cerebellar atrophy. As the presence of autoantibodies is found in only 50 percent lung cancer of patients with paraneoplastic cerebellar degeneration, they are of little use as a screening tool.[20,21] Treatment with immunosuppressive medications or plasmapheresis is not helpful.[17]

Visual Paraneoplastic Syndromes. Cancer-associated retinopathy, manifested as rapidly progressive binocular vision loss, is a very rare complication of lung cancer, occurring predominantly in small cell lung cancer and ovarian cancer. Jacobson and colleagues suggest the characteristic triad of photosensitivity, ring-scotomatous visual field loss, and attenuated retinal arteriole caliber is most char-

acteristic of this syndrome.[22] Studies involving the sera of patients with cancer-associated retinopathy have identified antibodies against a protein whose amino acid sequence is similar to the cone-specific protein, visinin. These activate lymphocytes that consequently invade and infiltrate retinal tissues.[23]

Peripheral Nervous System Syndromes

Eaton-Lambert Syndrome. The association between Eaton-Lambert syndrome and cancer is well established: approximately 70 percent of males and 25 percent of females with this condition harbor an underlying malignancy.[24] The risk of malignancy is low among patients with Eaton-Lambert syndrome under age 40, but risk increases steadily with age. Small cell lung cancer occurs 80 percent of the time a malignancy is present. Adenocarcinomas of the lung and breast cancer are also associated with this syndrome, albeit much less frequently.

Eaton-Lambert syndrome results from the action of IgG antibodies against voltage-sensitive calcium ion channels common to small cell lung cancer cells and the normal neuromuscular junction.[25] As with myasthenia gravis, patients complain of fatigability and weakness that may be out of proportion to objective physical findings. They may possess clinical features suggestive of an underlying lung cancer, such as a history of smoking, an unexplained rise in the erythrocyte sedimentation rate, or other paraneoplastic phenomena. On examination, there is weakness of the proximal extremities; legs are usually affected more than arms. Deep tendon reflexes are decreased to absent. However, unlike myasthenia, muscle strength increases with repeated muscle movement. The diagnosis of Eaton-Lambert syndrome is usually confirmed by electromyography. Among patients found to have Eaton-Lambert syndrome in the absence of a known malignancy, there is currently no general consensus regarding cancer screening.

Sensory Neuropathy and Encephalomyelitis. First described in 1948, paraneoplastic sensory neuropathy is one of the oldest and best characterized of the paraneoplastic neuromuscular syndromes, yet it is extremely rare. In a 15-year period at the Mayo Clinic, only 26 patients were diagnosed with this syndrome. Of these, 19 had small cell lung cancer, four had breast cancer, and three had other neoplasms.[26] Over 75 percent of patients were female, a noteworthy statistic since only 16 percent of patients with small cell lung cancer in general are women. The natural history of sensory neuropathy is often unrelated to that of the primary tumor. Inflammation in the dorsal root ganglia results in neuronal loss, as well as degeneration and fibrosis of the dorsal columns. Symptoms, which can be rapidly progressive, include pain, paresthesia, and unsteadiness of gait. There is loss of sensation to temperature, vibration, and pressure. Autonomic instability can result in hypotension, impotence, and constipation.

Sensory neuropathy is now believed to be the most common component of a group of neuromuscular syndromes that are united by the presence of an antibody, anti-Hu, which binds the nuclei of cerebral cortical neurons. Anti-Hu is extremely specific and has not been found in patients with lung cancer not associated with neurologic symptoms. Of 71 patients studied at the Memorial Sloan-Kettering Cancer Center with anti-Hu-associated neuromuscular symptoms, 74 percent had sensory neuropathy, but in only 62 percent did it dominate the course of the disease. Motor neuron dysfunction was present in 20 percent of patients, although never without other neurologic findings. Limbic encephalopathy was a prominent feature in 20 percent, cerebellar disease in 15 percent, brain stem and/or cranial nerve involvement in 14 percent, and autonomic dysfunction in 10 percent.[27] Symptoms may also include loss of memory that often develops into a severe dementia syndrome, as well as confusion, personality changes, hallucinations, depression, and partial complex seizures. Clinically, the anti-Hu-associated neuromuscular disorders are usually progressive. Roughly one-third of patients develop respiratory failure that requires mechanical ventilation. Severe autonomic instability, including cardiac arrhythmias, may develop. Diagnosis rests on recognition of the clinical picture as well as relevant diagnostic tests. Electromyography may demonstrate nonspecific abnormalities of voluntary motor unit activation. Cerebrospinal fluid abnormalities vary, but may include pleocytosis and protein elevation. The presence of anti-Hu is helpful in confirming a diagnosis. However, as this is an insensitive test, it should not be used as a screening technique.

Endocrine Syndromes

Lung cancer cells, especially those of small cell lung cancer, are able to produce a broad array of peptides that possess functional similarities to biologically active hormones. However, since cancer cells often lack certain key steps in the pathway that leads to the production of hormones, these peptides are usually distinct and less active than their normal counterparts. Listed below are the most common paraneoplastic endocrine syndromes associated with lung cancer, and their respective clinical signs and symptoms:

Hypercalcemia

Hypercalcemia of malignancy occurs in approximately 10 to 15 percent of lung cancer patients. It is most prevalent in squamous cell carcinoma and is relatively rare in small cell carcinoma. In the vast majority of cases, hypercalcemia results from the release of parathyroid hormone-related peptide (PTHrP) by malignant cells. Eight of 13 amino acids on the amino terminus are identical with those of parathyroid hormone (PTH), thereby allowing PTHrP to bind the PTH receptor unhindered.[28] The net effect is increased bone reabsorption, decreased bone formation, and increased tubular reabsorption of calcium by the kidney. Bone metastases are usually absent.

Diagnosis is typically not difficult, as most patients already have been diagnosed with lung cancer by the time hypercalcemia develops. High serum calcium levels can precipitate weakness, lethargy, nausea, vomiting, constipation, and abdominal pain; patients may complain of polyuria. At high calcium levels (> 13 mg/dl), renal insufficiency develops, and patients may develop calcification of the skin, vessels, lungs, heart, and stomach. The presence of hypercalcemia is a poor prognostic finding in lung cancer; the interval between the detection of hypercalcemia and death usually does not exceed 6 months.[29] Therefore, it is rare to find any complications of chronic hypercalcemia, such as kidney stones.

Syndrome of Inappropriate Antidiuretic Hormone (SIADH)

Abnormalities of serum sodium levels are common among patients with small cell lung cancer, and are most typically recognized as syndrome of inappropriate antidiuretic hormone (SIADH). Classically, the presence of SIADH has been associated with elevated serum levels of arginine vasopressin (AVP). Its secretion is considered "inappropriate" when it occurs in the context of normal or decreased plasma osmolality. AVP, also known as antidiuretic hormone, is elevated in up to 60 percent of patients with small cell lung cancer. However, only about 14 percent of such patients manifest clinically significant hyponatremia.[30–32] SIADH can also occur in the setting of other malignancies, such as: tumors of the pancreas, lymphoma, and thymoma, and has been described in a wide number of nonmalignant pulmonary and central nervous system disorders, as well as numerous medications (Table 4–4).

In general, the rate at which sodium concentration falls in SIADH is more relevant to developing neurologic symptoms than the absolute magnitude of the fall. When hyponatremia is mild or develops over the course of several weeks, symptoms may include anorexia, nausea, or vomiting. However, when hyponatremia develops acutely, patients may develop cerebral edema and severe neurologic sequelae, including irritability, confusion, lethargy, and seizures.

The diagnosis is dependent on excluding other potential causes of hyponatremia, such as hypovolemia, diuretic use, hyperlipidemia, hypothyroidism, and adrenocortical insufficiency. Classically, serum osmolality is reduced while urine osmolality is inappropriately elevated. The presence of SIADH is further supported by a positive water-load test. Patients are asked to consume a water load (20 ml/kg of body weight, up to 1,500 ml) in 10 to 20 minutes. Normally, at least 80 percent of this water load should be excreted within 5 hours, and the urine osmolality should decrease to below 100 mmol/L. Failure to do so is diagnostic of SIADH. The water-load test should not be performed, however, unless the serum sodium concentration is at a safe level (above 125 mmol/L).

Cushing's Syndrome

Cushing's syndrome, resulting from ectopic ACTH release, is traditionally associated with small cell lung cancer, occurring in approximately 5 percent of cases. As with hypercalcemia, the rapid natural history of small cell lung cancer prevents many features of chronic Cushing's syndrome (Figure 4–4). Classic symptoms, such as central obesity, striae, and moon facies, do occur, albeit rarely. More commonly, the presence of elevated cortisol levels is first suspected by the presence of characteristic metabolic abnormalities, including hyperglycemia, hypokalemia, and metabolic alkalosis.

Cutaneous Syndromes

Dermatomyositis-Polymyositis

An inflammatory condition of unknown origin involving the muscles and skin, dermatomyositis is associated with malignancy in approximately 25 percent of cases.[33] Both conditions are usually diagnosed within a year of each other. In most case reports, the types of malignancies associated with these conditions parallel those observed in the general population, with tumors of the lung and breast being the most common. Conversely, in the Orient, nasopharyngeal carcinoma is seen most commonly in both the general and dermatomyositis population.

Table 4–4. CONDITIONS ASSOCIATED WITH SIADH
Malignant neoplasms
Small cell lung cancer
Pancreatic carcinoma
Lymphoma
Thymoma
Nonmalignant pulmonary disorders
Pneumonia
Tuberculosis
Lung abscess
Empyema
Chronic obstructive pulmonary disease (COPD)
Central nervous system disorders
Head trauma
Subdural hematoma
Subarachnoid hemorrhage
Meningitis
Systemic lupus erythematosus
Drugs
Chlorpropamide
Cyclophosphamide
Carbamazepine
Vinblastine
Vincristine
Narcotics
Tricyclic antidepressants

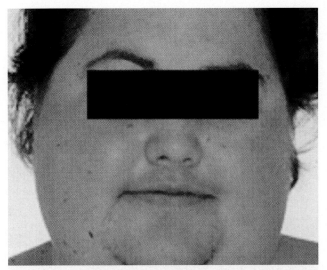

Figure 4–4. Moon facies in a patient with Cushing's syndrome. Note the round, plethoric face, hirsutism, and increased supraclavicular fat pads.

Dermatomyositis typically occurs between ages 40 and 60, and is more common in women than in men. Overall, malignancy-associated dermatomyositis comprises 8 percent of all cases of myositis. Patients complain of pain and weakness in the proximal musculature of the arms and legs. They may have difficulty standing up, lifting heavy objects, and—if the pharyngeal muscles are affected—dysphagia. The skin rash is classically a heliotrope-colored erythema involving the face, neck, arms, and hands. Telangiectasia may be seen surrounding the eyes or fingernails (Gottron's sign) (Figure 4–5). The diagnosis is suggested by the presence of elevated serum creatine kinase, lactate dehydrogenase, and serum glutamic-oxaloacetic transaminase (SGOT). However, a muscle biopsy is usually required for confirmation. Treatment of the underlying malignancy is not always effective in resolving the skin and muscle findings.

Acanthosis Nigricans

Acanthosis nigricans is a velvety hyperpigmentation found most commonly in the neck, groin, and flexor surfaces (Figure 4–6). Although associated with malignancy, particularly lung cancer and gastrointestinal tumors, the presence of acanthosis nigricans is a nonspecific finding. It has also been linked to a number of endocrinopathies not related to malig-

nancy, including insulin-resistant diabetes, acromegaly, and Stein-Leventhal syndrome.

Sign of Leser-Trélat

The sign of Leser-Trélat, also called acquired ichthyosis, is characterized by the sudden appearance of seborrheic keratosis on the shoulder or trunk (Figure 4–7). This skin manifestation is named after the physicians Ulysse Trélat of France and Edmund Leser of Germany, whose names are associated with the belief that the sudden appearance of seborrheic keratosis reflects internal malignancy. Although the incidence and underlying pathophysiology of acquired ichthyosis is unknown, various case reports have noted an association with adenocarcinoma,

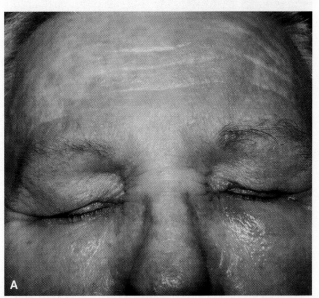

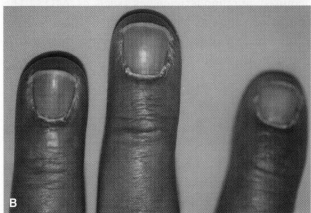

Figure 4–5. Dermatomyositis in a patient with non-small cell lung cancer. *A,* Heliotrope-colored erythema involving the face. *B,* Telangiectasia surrounding the fingernails (Gottron's sign).

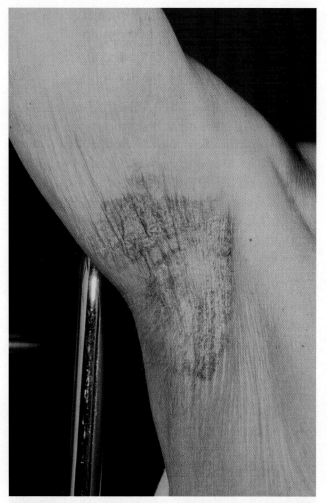

Figure 4–6.   Acanthosis nigricans in the axilla of a patient with non-small cell lung cancer.

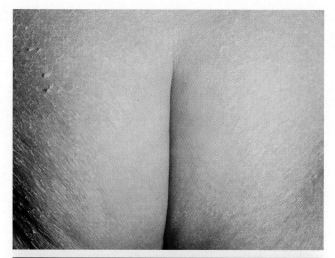

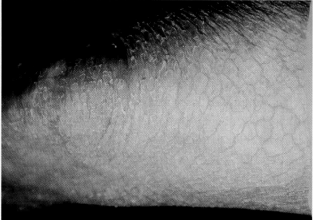

Figure 4–7.   Acquired ichthyosis (sign of Leser-Trélat). Sudden appearance of seborrheic keratosis in a patient with non-small cell lung cancer.

particularly of gastrointestinal origin, squamous cell lung cancer, Hodgkin's disease, T-cell lymphoma, and sarcomas. It is also seen in the setting of acquired immunodeficiencies, such as AIDS. The course of acquired ichthyosis usually parallels the natural history of the underlying tumor, thus resolving with successful treatment.

SUMMARY

Lung cancer is the leading cause of cancer mortality in the United States. It is hoped that this review will allow the reader to organize the diverse, nonspecific, and often subtle manifestations of lung cancer into a clinically useful framework.

REFERENCES

1. Harras A, Edwards BK, Blot WJ, et al (eds). Cancer rates and risks. Bethesda (MD): Cancer Statistics Branch, The National Cancer Institute.
2. Filderman AE, Shaw C, Matthay RA. Lung cancer part I: etiology, pathology, natural history, manifestations, and diagnostic techniques. Invest Radiol 1986;21:80–90.
3. Hyde L, Hyde CI. Clinical manifestations of lung cancer. Chest 1974;65:299–306.
4. Hirshberg B, Biran I, Glazer M, Kramer M. Hemoptysis: etiology, evaluations, and outcome in a tertiary referral hospital. Chest 1997;112:440–4.
5. Farber SM, Mandel W, Spain DM. Diagnosis and treatment of tumors of the chest. New York (NY): Grune & Stratton; 1960.
6. Light RW. Pleural Diseases (2nd Ed.) Philadelphia (PA): Lea & Febiger; 1990.

7. Fincher RE. Superior vena cava syndrome: Experience in a teaching hospital. South Med J 1987;80:1243–5.

8. Ellison E, LaPuerta P, Martin SE. Supraclavicular masses: results of a series of 309 cases biopsied by fine needle aspiration. Head & Neck 1999;21:239–46.

9. Stankey RM, Roshe J, Sogocio RM. Carcinoma of the lung and dysphagia. Dis Chest 1969;55:13–7.

10. Fried BM. Tumors of the lungs and mediastinum. Philadelphia (PA): Lea & Febiger; 1958.

11. Hansen-Flaschen J, Nordberg J. Clubbing and hypertrophic osteoarthropathy. Clin Chest Med 1987;8:287–9.

12. Okuyama T, Tanaka K, Akechi T, et al. Fatigue in ambulatory patients with advanced lung cancer: prevalence, correlated factors, and screening. J Pain Symptom Manage 2001;22:554–64.

13. Tchekmedyian NS, Hickman M, Siau J, et al. Treatment of cancer anorexia with megestrol acetate: impact on quality of life. Oncology 1990;4:185–92.

14. Loprinzi CL, Ellison NM, Schaid DJ, et al. Controlled trial of megestrol acetate for the treatment of cancer anorexia and cachexia. J Natl Cancer Inst 1990;82:1127–32.

15. Gomm SA, Thatcher N, Barber PV, Cumming WJ. A clinicopathological study of the paraneoplastic neuromuscular syndromes associated with lung cancer AJM 1990;75: 577–95.

16. Cao Y, Abbas J, Wu X, et al. Anti-Yo positive paraneoplastic cerebellar degeneration associated with ovarian carcinoma: case report and review of the literature. Gynecol Oncol 1999;75:178–83.

17. Graus F, Dalmau J, Valldeoriola F, et al. Immunological characterization of a neuronal antibody (anti-Tr) associated with paraneoplastic cerebellar degeneration and Hodgkin's disease J Neuroimmunol 1997;74:55–61.

18. Verschuuren J, Chuang L, Rosenblum F, et al. Inflammatory infiltrates and complete absence of Purkinje cells in anti-Yo associated paraneoplastic cerebellar degeneration. Acta Neuropathol 1996;91:519–25.

19. Anderson NE, Rosenblum MK, Posner JB. Paraneoplastic cerebellar degeneration: clinical-immunological correlations. Ann Neurol 1988;24;559–67.

20. Peterson K, Rosenblum MK, Kotanides H, et al. Paraneoplastic cerebellar degeneration: I. A clinical analysis of 55 anti-Yo antibody positive patients. Neurology 1992;42: 1931–7.

21. Hammack JE, Kimmel DW, O'Neill BP, et al. Paraneoplastic cerebellar degeneration: a clinical comparison of patients with and without Purkinje cell cytoplastmic antibodies. Mayo Clin Proc 1990;65:1423–31.

22. Jacobson DM, Thirkill CE, Tipping SJ. A clinical triad to diagnose paraneoplastic retinopathy. Ann Neurol 1990; 28:162–7.

23. Yamagata K, Goto K, Kuo CH, et al. Visinin: a novel calcium binding protein expressed in retinal core cells. Neuron 1990;2:269–76.

24. O' Neill JH, Murray NMF, Newson-Davis, J. The Lambert-Eaton myasthenic syndrome: a review of 50 cases. Brain 1988;111:577–96.

25. Sher E, Pandiella A, Clementi F. Voltage-operated calcium channels in small cell lung carcinoma cell lines: pharmacological, functional, and immunological properties. Cancer Res 1990;50:3892–6.

26. Chalk CH, Windebank AJ, Kimmel DW, McManis PG. The distinctive clinical features of paraneoplastic sensory neuronopathy. Can J Neurol Sci 1992;19:346–51.

27. Dalmau J, Graus F, Rosenblum MK, Posner JB. Anti-Hu—associate paraneoplastic encephalomyelitis/sensory neuronopathy. A clinical study of 71 patients. Medicine 1992; 71:59–72.

28. Tsuchihashi T, Yamaguchi K, Miyake Y, et al. Parathyroid hormone-related protein in tumor tissues obtained from patients with humoral hypercalcemia of malignancy. J Natl Cancer Inst 1990;82:40–4.

29. Campbell JH, Ralston S, Boyle IT, et al. Symptomatic hypercalcaemia in lung cancer. Respir Med 1991;85:223–7.

30. Bondy P, Gilby E. Endocrine function in small cell undifferentiated carcinoma of the lung. Cancer 1982;50:2147–53.

31. Hainsworth J, Workman R, Greco F. Management of the syndrome of inappropriate antidiuretic hormone secretion in small cell lung cancer. Cancer 1983;51:161–5.

32. List A, Hainsworth J, Davis B, et al. The syndrome of inappropriate antidiuretic hormone secretion of (SIADH) in small cell lung cancer. J Clin Oncol 1986;4:1191–8.

33. Callen JP. Dermatomyositis and malignancy. Clin Dermatol 1993;11:61–5.

5

Diagnosis and Staging

ROBERT J. KORST, MD

Once history, physical examination, and radiologic findings suggest the diagnosis of non-small cell lung cancer (NSCLC), important information must be ascertained prior to initiation of therapy. First, the diagnosis needs to be confirmed histopathologically, and second, the tumor must be clinically staged. Clinical staging is a process that encompasses all staging maneuvers/procedures that are performed prior to attempted treatment. Accurate clinical staging is mandatory because the treatment of NSCLC is stage-dependent. Diagnosis and staging usually occur concurrently, and many of the same modalities are used for both. Several important principles should be followed during the clinical staging process:

1. Although history, physical examination, and radiologic studies may indicate a particular clinical stage, tissue should be obtained for confirmation whenever possible in most situations. This principle is especially relevant when staging the mediastinal lymph nodes, given that enlarged lymph nodes demonstrated on computed tomography (CT) may represent inflammatory changes. Notable exceptions, however, include brain, adrenal, and some bony metastases, where specific radiologic studies may be diagnostic.

2. The clinical stage should be accurately determined using the minimum number of examinations and procedures. This goal is best accomplished by adopting a strategy in which evaluations for more advanced disease are performed first. If distant metastases are suspected, these should be definitively diagnosed prior to an attempt to stage locoregional disease, because if

distant metastases are detected, no further staging procedures are indicated.

3. When a patient's clinical stage is unclear despite appropriate staging maneuvers, the patient should be given "the benefit of the doubt" and assigned the lowest possible clinical stage. Although this policy may subject some patients with more advanced disease to surgical resection, more importantly, patients with earlier stage disease will be less likely to be denied resection because of equivocal clinical staging.

DIAGNOSIS

If physical examination or imaging studies suggest distant metastatic disease (M1), in many instances the suspected metastatic lesion should be removed for biopsy instead of the primary lesion. This approach will both diagnose as well as stage the patient with one procedure. An exception is the patient with relatively inaccessible M1 disease, such as brain metastases, where the pulmonary lesion should be approached for diagnosis.

When M1 disease is not suspected, histologic confirmation of NSCLC may be obtained using a variety of techniques, ranging from noninvasive (sputum cytology) to highly invasive (thoracotomy). Although uncommon, exploratory thoracotomy may still be needed to establish the diagnosis when clinical data suggest NSCLC, but other less invasive attempts at biopsy have proved inconclusive. At thoracotomy, attempts should be made to diagnose the tumor by removing as little normal lung as possible (Tru-cut or excisional biopsy), but occasionally lobectomy may be needed to confidently rule out the presence of tumor. This latter circumstance may occur when a large mass is encountered in a patient at risk for malignancy, and less invasive biopsy attempts show only inflammation and/or atypical cells. In the vast majority of cases, however, the histologic diagnosis of NSCLC can be made using less invasive techniques.

Diagnostic Procedures

Sputum Cytology

Although used routinely in past decades, the examination of expectorated cells in the sputum is rarely performed today given the widespread availability of fiberoptic bronchoscopy and percutaneous fine-needle aspiration. Many patients with NSCLC, especially those with earlier stages of disease, will require bronchoscopy as part of the staging process, essentially eliminating the need for cytologic evaluation of expectorated sputum. Occasionally, a positive diagnosis obtained by sputum cytology may spare the patient any further procedures. An example is the patient who presents with a lung mass and multiple brain metastases suspected on imaging studies. Confirmation of malignant cells in the spu-

tum would eliminate the need for further diagnostic and staging procedures.

The diagnostic yield of sputum cytology is dependent on several factors, including tumor location, size and histology, the experience of the cytopathologist, and the quality of the sputum specimen.[1] Larger, centrally located tumors are most likely to be diagnosed using sputum cytology, as are squamous and small-cell types (Figure 5–1). The number of specimens needed to optimize the diagnostic yield is three, which are best produced in the early morning on 3 consecutive days.[2] False-positive results occur rarely, but are most common in patients with acute pulmonary inflammatory conditions.[3]

In recent years, research has focused on attempts to improve the diagnostic yield of sputum cytology. Such efforts have evaluated the role of sputum immunostaining using antibodies against lung cancer-specific epitopes,[4] as well as the use of the polymerase chain reaction (PCR) to detect oncogene and tumor suppressor gene mutations in expectorated cells.[5] Malignancy-associated changes (MACs) are cellular changes present in nonmalignant cells which may indicate that a malignancy is also present.[6] In addition, other investigators have focused on techniques to improve the sputum induction

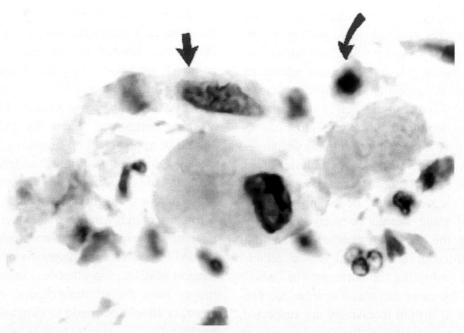

Figure 5–1. Microscopic examination of expectorated sputum from a 79-year-old male with an endobronchial lesion in the bronchus intermedius. The curved arrow indicates a normal bronchial epithelial cell, while the straight arrow confirms the diagnosis of squamous cell carcinoma in this patient.

process itself, in an attempt to improve the adequacy of sputum specimens. One example is the use of inhaled agents to facilitate sputum mobilization.[7]

Bronchoscopy

Flexible, fiberoptic bronchoscopy has become an essential tool in the diagnosis and staging of the patient with NSCLC, and has essentially replaced rigid bronchoscopy which is now mainly reserved for selected therapeutic purposes. The flexible bronchoscope is an effective means for visualization of the entire tracheobronchial tree out to the proximal sub-segmental bronchi. In addition to establishing the diagnosis of lung cancer, bronchoscopy rules out additional endobronchial lesions, which may affect the treatment plan.

Several techniques are available to the bronchoscopist for establishing a lung cancer diagnosis. If an endobronchial lesion is visible, it should be directly brushed for cytology and a biopsy specimen taken (Figure 5–2). If no endobronchial tumor is seen, but external airway compression is noted, transbronchial needle aspiration for cytology may be useful. External compression typically results from hilar or mediastinal nodal disease, and a positive aspiration not only secures the diagnosis, but also aids in proper staging. If the bronchoscopic examination is entirely normal, bronchial washings should be obtained by wedging the tip of the bronchoscope into the segmental bronchus where the tumor is thought to reside, followed by vigorous washing with saline. The washings are then centrifuged, stained, and evaluated by an experienced cytopathologist. Transbronchial biopsy is a technique which may be utilized to obtain tissue from a pulmonary lesion too peripheral to be visualized directly with the bronchoscope. Biopsy forceps are passed into the lesion using fluoroscopy in the anterior-posterior plane as a guide. The fluoroscope is then rotated up to ninety degrees to use parallax to confirm intra-tumoral placement of the forceps. A biopsy specimen is taken and the lesion is then brushed or needle aspirated. If significant bleeding ensues, the tip of the bronchoscope can be wedged into the bronchus until hemostasis is obtained.

Using more than one of the above techniques will improve diagnostic yield.[8] Even if an endobronchial

lesion is visualized and a biopsy specimen taken, it should also be brushed and washed. If performed last, often the washings may collect cells disrupted by the brushing and biopsy. If a transbronchial needle aspiration is to be performed, care must be taken to pass the needle through the bronchial wall at a site remote from any endobronchial tumor. Otherwise, a false-positive result may be obtained.

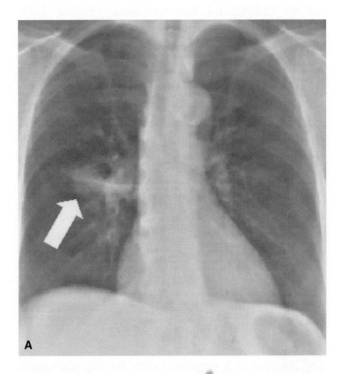

A

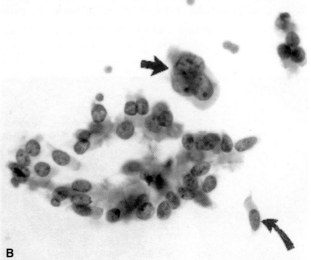

B

Figure 5–2. *A,* A 58-year-old, actively smoking woman underwent bronchoscopy for an abnormal chest radiograph. *B,* Although no endobronchial tumor was apparent, brushings performed in the superior segment of the right lower lobe reveal adenocarcinoma (*straight arrow*). The curved arrow indicates normal bronchial epithelial cells, with visible cilia.

Transthoracic Needle Aspiration for Cytology

When the suspected lung cancer is very peripheral, it is not uncommon that all bronchoscopic maneuvers will fail to provide a definitive diagnosis. In such cases, the lesion may be approached by the interventional radiologist using image-guided transthoracic needle aspiration for cytology (FNA), or core biopsy. Either fluoroscopy or CT guidance can be utilized for this technique (Figure 5–3). While the incidence of pneumothorax may be as high as 50 percent, the majority of cases are minor, require no therapy, and resolve on their own.[9]

The results of transthoracic FNA must be interpreted with caution. Although a normal result is very specific for malignancy, a positive aspiration must be associated with a specific benign diagnosis, such as hamartoma or granulomatous inflammation. If malignant cells are not seen but a specific benign diagnosis is not made, the result must be interpreted as indeterminate.[10] This is especially true when acute or chronic, non-granulomatous inflammation is detected, since many lung cancers may be associated with these findings if an element of bronchial obstruction is present.

STAGING SYSTEM

The purpose of a staging system for any malignant disease is threefold. First, it must provide an estimate of tumor burden and extent of spread; second,

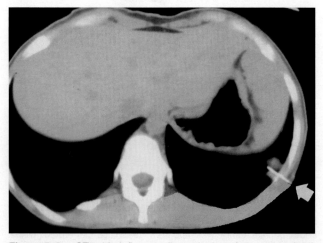

Figure 5–3. CT-guided, fine-needle aspiration of a peripheral, left lower-lobe nodule in a patient who underwent a CT scan for an unrelated purpose. Note the needle (*arrow*) protruding from the lesion.

it must provide prognostic information that can be applied to individual patients; and third, an effective staging system must be able to direct therapy. Patients are first staged based on clinical information, which includes invasive procedures short of resection (eg, mediastinoscopy, thoracoscopy, thoracotomy without resection), and it is on this staging that therapy is based. If surgical resection is performed, patients are then pathologically staged; it is this staging on which the prognosis is based. Most malignancies, NSCLC included, are currently staged according to the T (tumor), N (nodal disease), and M (metastasis) scheme (Table 5–1). The nodal descriptor (N) is based on the lymph node staging map which was adopted by The American College of Surgeons (Figure 5–4) and specifically defines N1, N2, and N3 disease. The AJCC stage groupings for NSCLC were recently refined in 1997 (see Table 5–2) to further reflect prognosis.[11]

Clinical staging of the T descriptor directly affects the treatment plan, since T1, T2, and T3 lesions are usually considered surgically resectable, whereas T4 tumors are not. While assignment of T1 and T2 status is generally fairly accurate based on radiographic findings, discrimination of T3 from T4 may be difficult short of thoracotomy and exploration. For example, T4 involvement of the mediastinal structures may be suggested by clinical or radiographic findings, but in many cases a surgically resectable T3 or even T2 lesion is found at exploration (Figure 5–5).

The N descriptor is difficult to accurately stage without biopsy since lymph nodes may be enlarged due to inflammation and not tumor. Inflamed lymph nodes are usually the result of tumor-associated pneumonitis with or without bronchial obstruction, but not infrequently granulomatous disease is present concurrent with NSCLC. The distinction between N2 and N3 disease is of vital importance since the presence of metastatic N3 lymph nodes (see Table 5–2; Figure 5–6) usually precludes an attempt at surgical resection. Similarly, the distinction of N0-N1 from N2 disease is significant, since many patients with positive N2 mediastinal lymph nodes are treated with induction chemoradiotherapy followed by surgical resection, as opposed to resection alone (if N2 nodes are negative). Although the distinction between N0 and N1 is far less critical, the presence of positive hilar N1 lymph nodes will necessitate the performance of a pneumonectomy in many cases. The status of the N1 nodes usually remains uncertain until thoracotomy is performed since, with the exception of tracheobronchial nodes, (level 10; see Figure 5–4) biopsy of N1 nodes can be difficult.

Table 5–1. TNM STAGING CLASSIFICATION FOR LUNG CANCER

Primary Tumor (T)

TX: Primary tumor cannot be assessed, or tumor proven by the presence of malignant cells in sputum or bronchial washings but visualized by imaging or bronchoscopy

T0: No evidence of primary tumor

Tis: Carcinoma in situ

T1: Tumor 3 cm or less in greatest dimension, surrounded by lung or visceral pleura, without bronchoscopic evidence of invasion more proximal than the lobar bronchus

T2: Tumor with any of the following features of size or extent:
- More than 3 cm in greatest dimension
- Involves main bronchus, 2 cm or more distal to the main carina
- Invades the visceral pleura
- Associated with atelectasis or obstructive pneumonitis that extends to the hilar region but does not involve the entire lung

T3: Tumor of any size that directly invades any of the following: chest wall (including superior sulcus tumors), diaphragm, mediastinal pleura, parietal pericardium; or tumor in the main bronchus within 2 cm, but not involving the main carina; or associated atelectasis or obstructive pneumonitis of the entire lung

T4: Tumor of any size that invades any of the following: heart, great vessels, trachea, esophagus, vertebral body, carina; or separate tumor nodules in the same lobe; or tumor with a malignant pleural effusion

Nodal Involvement (N)

NX: Regional lymph nodes cannot be assessed

N0: No regional lymph node involvement

N1: Metastasis to ipsilateral peribronchial and/or ipsilateral hilar lymph nodes, and intrapulmonary nodes including involvement by direct extension of the primary tumor

N2: Metastasis to ipsilateral mediastinal and/or sub-carinal lymph nodes

N3: Metastases to contralateral mediastinal, contralateral hilar, ipsilateral or contralateral scalene, or supraclavicular lymph nodes

Distant Metastases (M)

MX: Distant metastases cannot be assessed

M0: No distant metastases

M1: Distant metastases present (may include tumor nodules in separate lobes of lung)

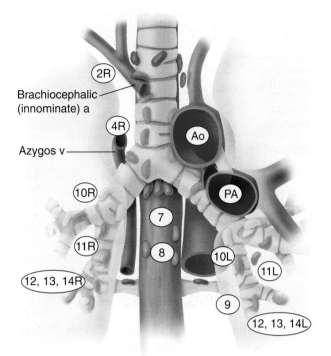

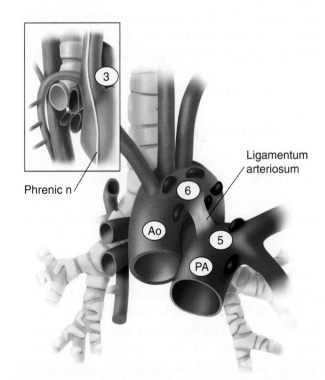

Figure 5–4. Lymph node staging map adopted by The American College of Surgeons. N1: double digit, ipsilateral; N2: single digit, ipsilateral; N3: single or double digit, contralateral. Level 1: highest mediastinal; level 2: upper paratracheal; level 3: pre-vascular and retro-tracheal; level 4: lower paratracheal (including azygos nodes); level 5: subaortic (A-P window); level 6: para-aortic (ascending aorta or phrenic); level 7: sub-carinal; level 8: para-esophageal (below carina); level 9: pulmonary ligament; level 10: hilar; level 11: interlobar; level 12: lobar; level 13: segmental; level 14: sub-segmental. Mountain/Dresler modifications from Naruke/ATS-LCSG map. Adapted with permission from Bristol-Myers Squibb Oncology.

Table 5–2. STAGE GROUPINGS FOR NON-SMALL CELL LUNG CANCER			
Occult carcinoma	TX	N0	M0
Stage 0	Tis	N0	M0
Stage 1A	T1	N0	M0
Stage 1B	T2	N0	M0
Stage 2A	T1	N1	M0
Stage 2B	T2	N1	M0
	T3	N0	M0
Stage 3A	T1	N2	M0
	T2	N2	M0
	T3	N2	M0
	T3	N1	M0
Stage 3B	Any T	N3	M0
	T4	Any N	M0
Stage 4	Any T	Any N	M1

SPECIFIC CLINICAL STAGING PROCEDURES

Prior to initiating therapy, patients with NSCLC must be accurately staged. The best approach to staging is one in which the stage is correctly determined using the minimum number of examinations and procedures. Some of the invasive procedures may be performed at the time of the initial office visit (thoracentesis, scalene node aspiration), while more invasive procedures require anesthesia.

Evaluation for Distant Disease

NSCLC can be an aggressive disease which metastasizes readily. Distant organs most commonly involved include the brain, bones, liver, adrenal glands, and remote regions of the lungs. Systemic symptoms, including significant weight loss, fatigue, and tumor fever usually indicate disseminated disease, as do focal neurologic symptoms and unrelenting bony pain. A complete metastatic work-up should be performed in these individuals and should consist of a brain MRI as well as a bone scan. Most chest CT scans performed for lung cancer extend down through the liver and adrenal glands, making these organs relatively easy to evaluate. In the absence of symptoms or an elevated serum alkaline phosphatase level, routine brain and bone scans are generally not indicated in suspected early-stage disease, given their low yield.[12] However, in cases of more locally advanced but still surgically resectable disease, a thorough metastatic work-up should be completed prior to initiating a complex attempt at resection.[13]

Staging of Locoregional Disease

Cervical Mediastinoscopy

Introduced by Carlens in 1951 (see Figure 5–5), cervical mediastinoscopy is used frequently to stage the mediastinum in patients with NSCLC.[14] Through a small, transverse incision in the suprasternal notch, the mediastinoscope is introduced into the superior mediastinum in the pretracheal plane (Figure 5–7). The anatomy is then delineated, and lymph nodes from level 2 on the right, level 4 and 10 bilaterally, and level 7 are easily removed for biopsy. The extent of mediastinal node dissection to be performed at the time of medi-

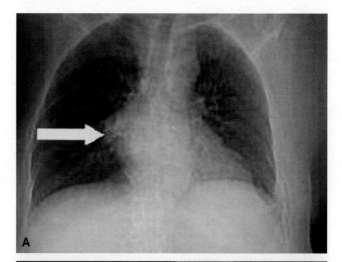

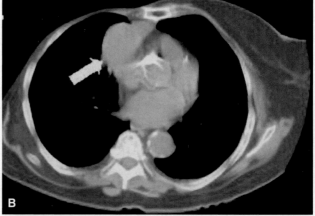

Figure 5–5. Tumors abutting the mediastinum frequently require operative exploration to accurately stage the T descriptor. *A,* A 72-year-old female presented with an asymptomatic right lung mass abutting the heart on routine chest radiography. *B,* CT scan suggests compression of the right atrium with loss of planes between the tumor and pericardium. At thoracotomy, the tumor was classified as T2, since not even the visceral pleura was invaded. Arrows indicate the tumor in both images.

astinoscopy is controversial. However, in order to accurately stage the mediastinum, lymph nodes from the sub-carinal space (level 7), as well as both the ipsilateral paratracheal (N2) and contralateral paratracheal (N3) regions should be removed and examined. It is not acceptable to only perform a biopsy on ispsilateral nodes, since the distinction between N2 and N3 is a crucial one. A positive transbronchial needle aspiration of an ipsilateral node does not rule out contralateral disease and eliminate the need for cervical mediastinoscopy. During the procedure, if the CT scan suggests N3 disease, these should be approached first, because a positive biopsy will eliminate the need for further dissection. Complications are rare, but when they do occur they are mainly related to bleeding or left recurrent laryngeal nerve palsy.[15]

In addition to nodal disease in the mediastinum, cervical mediastinoscopy is also useful in determining the resectability of the primary tumor in selected situations. Tumors which appear as though they may invade the mediastinal structures, such as the trachea on the right side, are especially amenable to mediastinoscopic exploration. Similarly, mediastinal exploration may help discern whether mediastinal disease represents extension of the primary disease into the mediastinum, or nodal metastases.

Indications for mediastinoscopy are controversial and surgeon-specific. Given the high false-positive rate of CT in staging the mediastinum, most surgeons agree that radiographically enlarged lymph nodes (> 1 cm) represent a clear indication for mediastinoscopy. Relative indications include the presence of a large or centrally located primary tumor, and the need for an extended, complex resection, especially in a poor-risk patient.[16] Mediastinoscopy may also be indicated to assess the proximity of the primary tumor to such vital structures as the trachea and superior vena cava. Limitations of the procedure include the inability to excise for biopsy lymph nodes from levels 5 and 6, as well as anterior sub-carinal nodes.

Extended Cervical Mediastinoscopy

Mediastinal lymph nodes not accessible using standard cervical mediastinoscopy include aortopul-

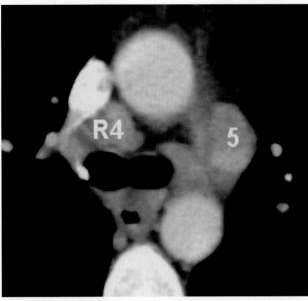

Figure 5–6. N3 mediastinal lymph nodes. A 48-year-old male presented with a left upper-lobe lung mass, with no tissue diagnosis. CT scan demonstrated not only enlarged N2 nodes in the sub-aortic position (level 5), but also contralateral lower paratracheal nodes (R4). Cervical mediastinoscopy was performed as both a diagnostic as well as a staging maneuver to confirm tumor in the right level-4 lymph nodes. The level 5 lymph nodes were not sampled because the treatment plan would not be affected by the result of this procedure.

monary window (level 5) and preaortic (level 6). Usually associated with left upper-lobe tumors, these regions may be accessed using extended cervical mediastinoscopy. Once the standard procedure is completed, the mediastinoscope is redirected between the innominate and left common carotid arterial trunks, over the aortic arch to the aortopulmonary window. Caution needs to be exercised with this approach since manipulation of the great vessels does occur, making this procedure more risky. Nevertheless, in experienced hands extended cervical mediastinoscopy can be performed with minimal morbidity and mortality, eliminating the need for a separate incision.[17]

Anterior Mediastinotomy (Chamberlain Procedure)

More popular than extended cervical mediastinoscopy to provide access to levels 5 and 6 is the left anterior mediastinotomy through the left second interspace. The internal mammary vessels may be divided, but more frequently they are left intact.

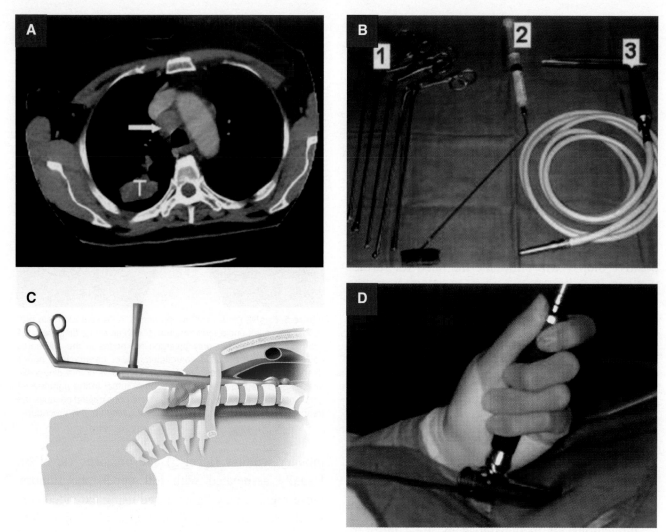

Figure 5–7. Cervical mediastinoscopy. *A,* CT scan of the chest from a 74-year-old female with a biopsy-proven right upper-lobe adenocarcinoma (T) and an enlarged right lower paratracheal lymph node (level 4; *arrow*). *B,* Operative instruments for cervical mediastinoscopy. 1) Biopsy forceps; 2) Fine needle for aspiration; 3) Cervical mediastinoscope with light cord. *C,* Schematic depicting the correct mediastinal plane of dissection used during cervical mediastinoscopy. *D,* Operative photograph depicting the mediastinoscope being inserted through a 1-cm cervical incision.

Similarly, the second costal cartilage can be resected for improved exposure. Typically the pleural space is not entered, but if this occurs the pleural air can be evacuated at the time of closure using a catheter, eliminating the need for a chest tube.

Indications for biopsy of levels 5 and 6 include bulky adenopathy where neoadjuvant therapy would be considered. These levels are usually not routinely removed in the absence of gross adenopathy since a significant cure rate is obtainable even in the presence of limited nodal disease at these stations.[18] In addition to lymph node biopsy, the Chamberlain procedure is useful for assessing the primary tumor in those instances where resectability is questioned

due to proximity to the aorta or main pulmonary artery (Figure 5–8). An anterior mediastinotomy may also be used to rule out pericardial/cardiac invasion when imaging studies are equivocal. Drawbacks of anterior mediastinotomy include significant postoperative pain as well as slight chest wall deformity if the costal cartilage is resected.

Thoracoscopy

Since the advent of video-assisted surgical techniques, thoracoscopy represents another alternative to anterior mediastinotomy and extended cervical mediastinoscopy for biopsy of lymph nodes at levels 5 and 6. Thoracoscopy also provides one of the most thorough examinations of the entire hemithorax (Figure 5–9), including the visceral and parietal pleurae, and allows for the assessment of the primary tumor as well. Typically three or four trocars are placed and single-lung ventilation is performed to allow visualization of the entire pleural space. In addition, a finger may be inserted in place of a trocar to palpate and localize small nodules (Figure 5–10). If pleural metastases are detected, a sclerotic agent may then be placed into the hemithorax to prevent development of pleural effusion (Figure 5–11).

The advantage of thoracoscopy is clearly its versatility, but the procedure does depend on the achievement of one-lung ventilation and the placement of a chest tube in most circumstances. In addition, thoracoscopy does not eliminate the need for cervical mediastinoscopy to assess the superior mediastinal nodes. Despite these drawbacks, video thoracoscopy has replaced anterior mediastinotomy in many surgeons' practices.[19]

Scalene Node Biopsy

Palpable scalene lymph nodes are best sampled using fine-needle aspiration, which can be performed at the initial office consultation. The routine biopsy of non-palpable nodes is no longer advocated, although some

data suggest that the yield of scalene node biopsy is increased in the presence of N2 disease.[20] Scalene nodes are easily sampled at the time of standard cervical mediastinoscopy by simply directing the scope and the dissection toward the ipsilateral scalene fat pad, with the goal of avoiding a second incision.[20]

SPECIAL DIAGNOSTIC AND STAGING SITUATIONS

The previous discussion serves as an adequate guideline for staging the vast majority of patients with NSCLC. However, several distinct clinical situations deserve further mention in more detail because, either they do not adhere to the previously stated principles, or they represent somewhat ambiguous or controversial staging situations.

Tissue Diagnosis of Distant Metastatic Disease

Although tissue confirmation of clinical and radiographic findings should be obtained whenever possible, several situations exist where this may not be necessary, and even contraindicated. The patient that presents with a biopsy-proven NSCLC and has had an MRI of the brain showing a mass lesion does not need tissue from the brain lesion prior to definitive treatment for both. Similarly, a patient with NSCLC who has a positive bone scan with a correlative radiologic study (MRI or plain films) showing a lesion characteristic of metastasis does not necessarily need a bone biopsy unless the radiologic findings

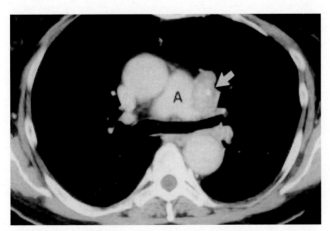

Figure 5–8. Indication for the Chamberlain procedure. CT scan image at the level of the carina from a patient with a primary tumor (*arrow*) abutting the main pulmonary artery (see *A*). Resectability is questioned based on this image, but exploration through a left anterior mediastinotomy (Chamberlain procedure) revealed a plane between the tumor and the pulmonary artery, and a complete resection was performed via a posterolateral thoracotomy.

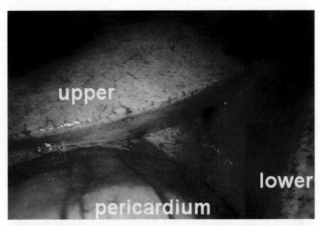

Figure 5–9. Video-assisted thoracic surgery (VATS). Following insertion of the video camera through the eighth intercostal space, the entire hemithorax is visualized.

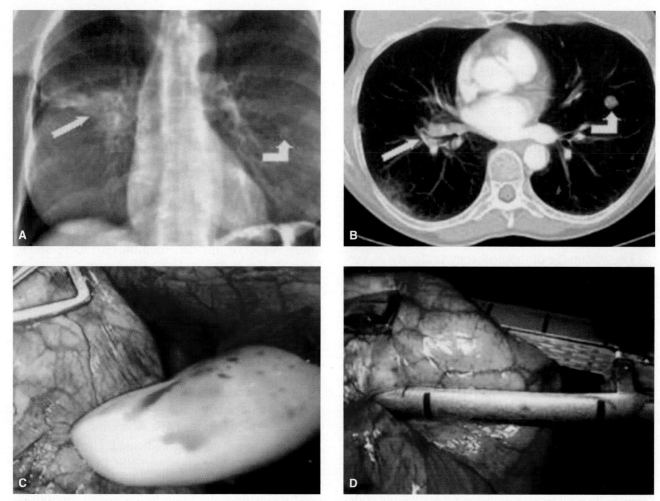

Figure 5–10.   Video-assisted thoracic surgery (VATS) used as a technique to excise a contralateral lung nodule. *A,* A 54-year-old female presented with a chest radiograph revealing a right hilar lung cancer (*straight arrow*) and a contralateral nodule, suspicious for metastasis (*angled arrow*). *B,* CT scan of the chest confirming these lesions. *C,* The operator's finger is inserted through a trocar site to palpate the abnormality for localization purposes. *D,* The automatic stapling device is then used to amputate the lung tissue containing the suspicious nodule.

are equivocal and the lesion is accessible. One commonly encountered situation in the staging of patients with NSCLC is the presence of rib lesions on bone scan. The ribs are not well visualized on MRI, and plain films may not demonstrate an abnormality. If a lesion is appreciated on plain films, a needle biopsy may be attempted using fluoroscopic guidance. In cases where no lesion is demonstrated on plain films, the skin overlying the abnormal rib can be marked in the nuclear medicine department using the bone scan, and the rib can then be sampled using an open technique.

The evaluation of an adrenal nodule in the patient with NSCLC has evolved in recent years to a completely noninvasive approach. Since the incidence of adrenal metastases has been reported to be as high as

nearly 8 percent in patients thought to have disease localized to the chest,[21] and benign adrenal adenomas are not uncommon in the general population, the distinction between a metastatic lesion and an adenoma is not an uncommon dilemma. Traditionally, adrenal lesions necessitated a biopsy for definitive diagnosis. Recent studies, however, have shown that this distinction can accurately be made using MRI, and even thin-cut, non-contrast CT scan, obviating the need for an invasive procedure.[22,23]

Metastatic Disease versus Multiple Primary Lung Tumors

The patient with multiple lung lesions on CT scan presents a complex, though not uncommon, dilemma

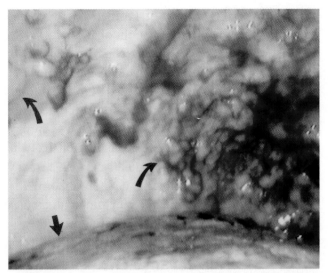

Figure 5–11.   VATS used for the detection of pleural metastases. A 79-year-old male with an extensive smoking history presented with a right upper-lobe lung mass and a small pleural effusion. Cytologic examination of the fluid obtained by thoracentesis was negative for malignant cells, but thoracoscopic examination of the parietal pleurae revealed metastatic tumor (*curved arrows*). The straight arrow indicates the collapsed lung.

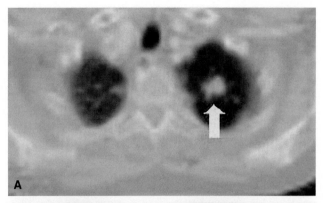

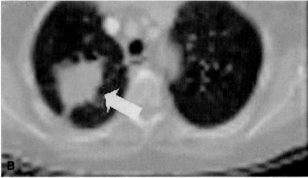

Figure 5–12.   Synchronous primary lung cancers. CT scan from a 76-year-old female shows two separate primary non-small cell lung cancers—one in the right upper lobe and the other at the left apex. Cervical mediastinoscopy was abnormal and the patient underwent sequential lobectomies with mediastinal lymph node dissection. Pathologic staging revealed a T2N0M0 lesion on the right and a T1N0M0 lesion on the left.

for the clinician. In the setting of a dominant, stellate lung mass bearing the radiographic appearance of a primary tumor with multiple smaller lesions in the lung fields, the most efficient strategy for diagnosis and staging is to perform a biopsy of one of the smaller lesions to confirm not only histology, but the presence of metastatic disease. If this biopsy demonstrates a benign lesion, the larger lesion may then need to be sampled.

When two malignant lung tumors of similar histologies have been documented, either ipsilateral or contralateral to each other, the question of metastatic disease versus two independent primary tumors is raised. In this circumstance, routine cervical mediastinoscopy should be performed in order to thoroughly stage the mediastinum. If mediastinal nodal disease is documented, the two pulmonary lesions are more likely to represent metastases than two separate primaries. The radiographic appearance of the lesions needs to be taken into account as well. If both lesions are irregular and stellate, they are more likely to represent two separate primary tumors as opposed to one irregular lesion and one smooth-bordered lesion (Figure 5–12). Finally, if the smaller lesion is amenable to thoracoscopic wedge resection, documentation of carcinoma in situ histologically also implies the presence

of a primary tumor and not a metastatic lesion.[24] Some recently published studies have attempted to evaluate the use of molecular methods evaluating similarities in oncogene and tumor supressor gene mutations as an attempt to answer this question.[25]

In summary, the distinction between two separate primary lung tumors and metastatic disease tends to be difficult, and requires both experience and judgment. However, despite attempts at meticulous staging, in many cases this important question may never be answered with absolute certainty. In the situation where multiple primary tumors are documented, the patient is assigned the clinical and pathologic stage of the most advanced lesion.

Diagnosis of the Solitary Pulmonary Nodule

The management of a solitary pulmonary nodule in a patient with no other evidence of malignant disease, though conceptually simple, remains somewhat controversial and depends on not only the clinician's judgment but also patient preference. Figure 5–13 represents a practical algorithm for the investigation of the solitary pulmonary nodule. Work-up begins by obtaining an accurate history from the

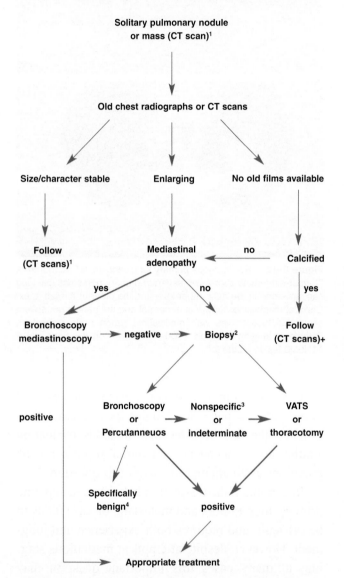

Figure 5–13. Work-up of the solitary pulmonary nodule or mass. [1]Given the speed, resolution, and availability of modern CT scanners, it is the author's belief that virtually all pulmonary nodules or masses seen on chest radiograph should be characterized using CT scannning. [2]The biopsy technique needs to be individualized for each patient. It is not infrequent to go straight to VATS or even thoracotomy in a more elderly patient with a long smoking history and a suspicious-appearing mass on CT scan, while a transthoracic FNA may be a wiser choice in a younger nonsmoker in whom the suspicion for primary lung cancer is lower. [3]A nonspecific or indeterminate FNA usually consists of non-granulomatous inflammation and/or normal pneumocytes, or an unsatisfactory specimen. [4]Specific benign diagnoses usually include benign tumors such as hamartomas, or clear granulomatous inflammation.

patient, including travel or residence in regions known to be endemic for the pulmonary mycoses as well as tobacco use. Certainly, when comparison to old radiographs indicates that a lesion is new or growing in size, aggressive investigation including biopsy is mandated. Patient preference comes into play when deciding on the technique of biopsy. While transthoracic fine-needle aspiration has the advantage of being only marginally invasive, many patients feel uncomfortable leaving an abnormality in their chest despite a negative cytologic diagnosis and insist on its removal via thoracoscopy.

Pleural Effusions

The accumulation of pleural fluid in a patient with NSCLC may indicate spread of the tumor to the visceral and parietal pleurae (T4). However, bulky tumors with associated post-obstructive atelectasis and/or pneumonitis may also result in the formation of a pleural effusion, and it becomes necessary to distinguish between the two possible etiologies. The least invasive approach to these patients is the performance of diagnostic thoracentesis, which can be done at the time of the initial office visit. The pleural fluid is centrifuged, and a cytologic diagnosis is rendered. If the pleural fluid is cytologically benign, the pleural space should be examined directly using thoracoscopy, at which time pleural biopsies may be taken (see Figure 5–11). Thoracoscopy also allows investigation of the primary tumor for such attributes as chest wall or mediastinal invasion, as well as provides an opportunity for pleurodesis should pleural disease be confirmed.

CONCLUSION

Once non-small cell lung cancer is suspected, the diagnosis can presently be confirmed using a variety of minimally invasive procedures. After histology is obtained, it is imperative that the stage of disease is accurately determined, because the treatment of NSCLC is stage-dependent. Every effort should be made by the clinician to stage the patient as efficiently as possible, to avoid the performance of unnecessary procedures. In particular, staging strategies may provide both the diagnosis and stage utilizing only one procedure. Modern day staging procedures are associated with minimal morbidity and mortality in experienced hands.

REFERENCES

1. Ng A, Horack GC. Factors significant to the diagnostic accuracy of lung cytology in bronchial washing and sputum samples. Acta Cytol 1983;27:397.

2. Liang XM. Accuracy of cytologic diagnosis and cytotyping of sputum in primary lung cancer: analysis of 161 cases. J Surg Oncol 1989;40:107.

3. Truong L, Underwood R, Greenberg S, McLarty JW. Diagnosis and typing of lung carcinomas by cytopathologic methods. A review of 108 cases. Acta Cytol 1985;29:379–84.

4. Tockman MS, Mulshine JL, Piantadosi S, et. al. Prospective detection of preclinical lung cancer: results from two studies of heterogeneous nuclear ribonucleoprotein A2B1 overexpression. Clin Cancer Res 1997;3:2237–46.

5. Mao L, Hruban RH, Boyle JO, et al. Detection of oncogene mutations in sputum precedes diagnosis of lung cancer. Cancer Res 1994;54:1634–7.

6. Ikeda N, MacAulay C, Lam S, et al. Malignancy associated changes in bronchial epithelial cells and clinical application as a biomarker. Lung Cancer 1998;19:161–6.

7. Bennett WD, Zeman KL, Foy C, et al. Effect of aerosolized uridine 5'-triphosphate on mucociliary clearance in mild chronic bronchitis. Am J Respir Crit Care Med 2001; 164:302–6.

8. Schenk DA, Bryan CL, Bower JH, Myers DL. Transbronchial needle aspiration in the diagnosis of bronchogenic carcinoma. Chest 1987;92:83–5.

9. Cox JE, Chiles C, McManus CM, et al. Transthoracic needle aspiration biopsy: variables that affect risk of pneumothorax. Radiology 1999;212:165–8.

10. Wescott JL. Direct percutaneous needle aspiration of localized pulmonary lesions: results of 422 patients. Radiology 1980;137:31.

11. Sobin LH, Wittekind CH. International Union Against Cancer (UICC): TNM classification of malignant tumors. 5th ed. New York (NY): Wiley-Liss; 1997. p. 93–7.

12. Tanaka K, Kubota K, Kodama T, et al. Extrathoracic staging is not necessary for non-small cell lung cancer with clinical stage T1-2 N0. Ann Thorac Surg 1999;68:1039–42.

13. Quinn DL, Ostrow LB, Porter DK, et al. Staging of non-small cell bronchogenic carcinoma. Relationship of the clinical evaluation to organ scans. Chest 1986;89:270–5.

14. Carlens E. Mediastinoscopy: a method for inspection and tissue biopsy in the superior mediastinum. Dis Chest 1959;36:343.

15. Hammoud ZT, Anderson RC, Meyers BF, et al. The current role of mediastinoscopy in the evaluation of thoracic disease. J Thorac Cardiovasc Surg 1999;118:894–9.

16. Korst RJ, Thayer JO, Brown L. Cervical mediastinoscopy: routinely indicated in the community hospital setting? Contemp Surg 1993;43:345–52.

17. Ginsberg RJ. Extended cervical mediastinoscopy: a single staging procedure for bronchogenic carcinoma of the left upper lobe. J Thorac Cardiovasc Surg 1987;94:673.

18. Patterson GA, Piazza D, Pearson FG, et al. Significance of metastatic disease in subaortic lymph nodes. Ann Thorac Surg 1987;43:155–9.

19. Landreneau RJ, Hazelrigg SR, Mack MJ, et al. Thoracoscopic mediastinal lymph node sampling: useful for mediastinal lymph node stations inaccessable by cervical mediastinoscopy. J Thorac Cardiovasc Surg 1993;106:554–8.

20. Lee JD, Ginsberg RJ. Lung cancer staging: the value of ipsilateral scalene lymph node biopsy performed at mediastinoscopy. Ann Thorac Surg 1996;62:338–41.

21. Pagani JJ. Non-small cell lung carcinoma adrenal metastases: computed tomography and percutaneous needle biopsy in their diagnosis. Cancer 1984;53:1058.

22. Schwartz LH, Panicek DM, Koutcher JA, et al. Echoplanar MR imaging for characterization of adrenal masses in patients with malignant neoplasms: preliminary evaluation of calculated T2 relaxation values. Am J Roentgenol 1995;164:911–5.

23. McNicholas MM, Lee MJ, Mayo-Smith WW, et al. An imaging algorithm for the differential diagnosis of adrenal adenomas and metastases. Am J Roentgenol 1995;165:1453–9.

24. Martini N, Melamed MR. Multiple primary lung cancers. J Thorac Cardiovasc Surg 1975;70:606–12.

25. Matsuzoe D, Hideshima T, Ohshima K, et al. Discrimination of double primary lung cancer from intrapulmonary metastasis by p53 gene mutation. Br J Cancer 1999;79:1549–52.

6

Imaging Work-Up of Lung Cancer: Utility and Comparison of Computed Tomography and FDG Positron Emission Tomography

TIM AKHURST, MBBS
ROBERT HEELAN, MD

PLAIN FILM CHEST RADIOGRAPHY

The properties of x-rays, in particular their ability to pass through human body parts and display an image of internal structures of the body based on relative density (atomic number), were first described by Roengten in 1895: for this work he received the Nobel prize. It became immediately clear that one of the important applications of this revolutionary modality was in the diagnosis of chest disease.

For 75 years, until the advent of computed tomography, plain chest radiography remained the standard of noninvasive thoracic imaging. The natural contrast provided by the gas density within lung parenchyma, the tracheal and bronchial tree, with the soft tissues and osseous structures of the thorax, provided unique visualization of an internal organ in a living being. Tumors could be diagnosed, as could various inflammatory conditions including pneumonia. A sophisticated system of analysis of normal and abnormal mediastinal and chest wall contours allowed probable diagnosis of a variety of other conditions such as mediastinal and chest wall masses, as well as pleural masses and fluid. Positional changes (eg, oblique projections, decubitus views) provided additional diagnostic information such as localization of nodules in lung, presence and characteristics of pleural fluid/masses. Linear and complex motion tomography provided further refinements for visual-izing air and soft-tissue structures in the lung and tracheobronchial tree.

As with all imaging modalities, however, limitations soon became apparent: plain chest radiography represents a two-dimensional depiction of a three-dimensional organism. Consequently, there was frequent confusion when various anatomic structures and pathologic processes were situated directly in front of one another, as, for example, with the development of infiltrates behind the heart in the left lower lung field. This limitation is only partially offset by the availability of lateral, in addition to the standard posteroanterior (PA), view. Overlying ribs or other anatomic structures within the chest such as the heart, hilar structures, and aortic arch frequently hid potentially important small abnormalities, for example, lung cancers.

In the 1960s through the early 1980s, attempts were made to use chest radiography to detect early lung cancer in studies throughout the world. The results of the NCI-sponsored study involving several centers in the United States indicated that while chest radiography was effective in diagnosing 40 percent of tumors at stage I, no difference in mortality could be demonstrated between the screened and unscreened group. A strong recommendation was made that chest radiography screening was of no value in the early detection of lung cancer. This conclusion may have only been partially justified, as a real benefit may have been hidden in the well-described statistical "noise" of the comparative study. Nevertheless, at the time when the strengths of computed tomography (CT) in depicting thoracic anatomy with a sophistication and subtlety not available to chest radiography were becoming obvious, this recommendation was a death knell for the utility of chest radiography in the evaluation of thoracic disease. With the increasing sophistication of CT, especially with improved spatial resolution and diminishing scan times, the superiority of CT in demonstrating thoracic, and especially lung, anatomy was becoming apparent. The use of intravenous contrast, as well as the development of high-resolution CT further added to the marked discrepancy between the abilities of computed tomography and plain chest radiography.

Nevertheless, in clinical practice, plain chest radiography maintains considerable utility. This is especially true in evaluation of the presence or absence of inflammatory disease in clinical practice, follow-up exams for pneumonias to demonstrate complete resolution, as well as a basic screening procedure in patients who are undergoing medical or surgical procedures (pre-admission radiographs) although these pre-admission chest radiographs probably should be reserved for patients who are to undergo major surgical procedures, or for preoperative patients who have chest symptoms. Chest radiography is also useful in the evaluation of congestive heart failure (CHF), as well as pulmonary edema and pleural effusions frequently associated with CHF. However, beyond the scope of these routine examinations, demonstration of a radiographic abnormality of the chest, not representing a routine pneumonia which completely resolves with appropriate antibiotic treatment, almost always requires follow-up computed tomography. CT has become the standard examination for anatomic evaluation of the thorax. Its utility includes staging evaluation of neoplastic diseases, as well as sophisticated evaluation of the lung parenchyma (with high-resolution CT), chest wall, and mediastinum. The recent availability of multi-detector helical technology allows accurate evaluation of the presence of pulmonary embolization to a segmental and possibly even to a sub-segmental level.

Traditionally, from the earliest days of radiology, chest radiographs were obtained by placing photo-graphic film within a light-proof cassette. The incident x-ray photons, having passed through the patient, result in potential chemical changes in the radiographic film inside the cassette. This x-ray film would then be developed in a manner very similar to photographic film, in later decades by means of automatic film processors. The automatic film processor would produce a black-and-white radiographic image of chest anatomy.

In recent years, new developments have affected the production of all plain-film radiography including chest radiographs. Initially, combinations of analog and digital technology were common, in which an analog rare-earth screen that was exposed to the x-ray beam replaced the film in the cassette. The transfer from analog to digital information would occur within the x-ray "developing" machine in which the analog information on the rare-earth cassette material would be "read" by a laser light and stored digitally. The digital information could be used to either produce an x-ray film or transfer to a PACS-based television monitor image work station. More recently, all digital systems have become available. With these systems, which include flat panel technology, the entire process consists of digital acquisition of raw data with the potential to produce a radiographic film image, but more commonly results in transfer of the digital information to a PACS work station for image interpretation.

COMPUTED TOMOGRAPHY OF THE CHEST

Chest radiographs have been used to diagnose and stage lung cancer for a number of years, but as experience was gained, its deficiencies became apparent: smaller tumors were frequently missed—obscured by ribs or by hilar structures or by the heart, and any spread to the hilar regions and mediastinum, unless quite massive, was usually not diagnosed. Another deficiency of chest radiography was also partially the result of its format, a two-dimensional representation of the three-dimensional object, ie, the human body: disease overlying the heart, or the hilar regions, or even the mediastinum could not be diagnosed. Screening modalities for the detection of early lung cancer demonstrated analogous deficiencies: smaller tumors (under a centimeter) were usually not picked up. Large-scale screening programs demonstrated downstaging of lung cancer and increased survival, without an attendant decrease in mortality from the disease.

The introduction of computed tomography in the mid 1970s provided a partial solution to this problem: the axial tomographic technique allowed one to separate structures behind the heart and similarly to depict anatomy both anterior and posterior to the hilar regions. The frequent diagnosis of enlarged lymph nodes in the mediastinum and hilar regions in patients with known lung cancer resulted in optimistic early reports of the ability of CT to accurately stage lung cancer and other thoracic neoplasms. Continued technical improvements in the ensuing years resulted in exquisite depiction of both lung and mediastinal anatomy. CT, however, being an anatomic representation rather than a functional one, was not capable of diagnosing the presence of metastatic disease in normal-sized lymph nodes in either the hilar region or mediastinum. Conversely, enlarged lymph nodes not containing tumor were frequently mistakenly diagnosed on CT as malignant. A meta-analysis of a large number of scientific papers evaluating CT in diagnosing mediastinal adenopathy demonstrated an overall accuracy of approximately 0.79 percent. Some large, blinded studies found accuracies even lower than this figure.

Clearly, computed tomography, although extremely useful, does not represent the noninvasive "holy grail" of accurate staging of lung cancer within the thorax. As Dales pointed out, accurate staging of lung cancer in the mediastinum would depend upon a new modality capable of differentiating tumor cells from non-tumor cells by means of functional imaging, ie, a modality dependent not upon morphologic change in the lymph nodes as a result of metastatic disease, but upon functional changes in the lymph nodes resulting from the presence of the altered metabolism of tumor disease.

POSITRON EMISSION TOMOGRAPHY SCANNING

It appears that positron emission tomography (PET) fulfills this need in several important respects: fluo-

rodeoxyglucose is preferentially taken up in tumor cells (as well as in some inflammatory cells) and hence provides an anatomic focus of increased activity that may be detected by the PET scanner. In several series, PET scanning has proved significantly more accurate than CT in local and regional staging of lung neoplasms. There is considerable optimism that PET will be able to stage lung cancer accurately and save patients with advanced disease needless surgical interventions. However, PET's improved accuracy in the staging of lung cancer (and other tumors) is accompanied by a number of relative deficiencies: it is relatively expensive both to purchase and to maintain. The radionuclides must be generated in a cyclotron, further adding to cost. Detection of tumor is size-dependent: lesions smaller than 1 cm are frequently missed. Some lung neoplasms, for example carcinoid and bronchoalveolar cancer are either not positive or only weakly positive on PET scanning. PET is frequently positive in the presence of inflammatory disease, making differentiation from neoplasm difficult. Lastly, because of poor spatial resolution of PET, it may be difficult to localize the precise anatomic location of abnormal fluorodeoxyglucose (FDG) uptake. Despite these relative deficiencies, most observers consider FDG-PET scanning to have significantly contributed to improved accuracy of staging (and, potentially, follow-up after treatment) of lung cancer prior to treatment. In fact it appears that the roles of the two modalities (CT and PET) are probably complimentary, with CT providing accurate anatomical location of the presence, local/regional extent of the primary tumor, and with PET detecting foci of regional (hilum, mediastinum) and distant (bone, liver, adrenal, distant lymph nodes) spread of disease. CT would have the added role of providing anatomic correlation of the correct location of PET-detected abnormal foci of tumor involvement.

LUNG CANCER STAGING

The exact work-up to be performed in a patient depends on the pre-test likelihood of finding additional disease. In a study of 29 patients with greater than T1N0M0 lung cancer, without evidence of mediastinal invasion or intra-abdominal metastases reported by Earnest and colleagues, 28 percent of patients had occult disease to the bone or brain demonstrated by a pretreatment MRI or bone scan. In a study by Ichinose and colleagues of 309 non–small cell lung cancer (NSCLC) patients who were clinically stage 1 or 2 by CBC, blood chemistry—including liver function tests and serum calcium, chest CT and CXR, 30 had symptoms suggestive of stage 4 disease. Of these, 22 of 30 (73%) had M1 disease discovered by scintigraphy or CT (chest or brain). In those patients with no clinical evidence of M1 disease, only 1 of 472 scans (0.2%) demonstrated occult disease, suggesting that routine bone scanning and brain CT are not cost-effective in early T-stage tumors that are asymptomatic.

In staging lung cancer, the following illustrations will serve to indicate both the relative strengths and weaknesses of imaging modalities, particularly CT and PET scanning in the staging of lung cancer.

Case 1: Recurrent Lung Cancer with Cerebral Metastasis

This 58-year-old man with a left lower-lobe lung cancer, previously resected, was referred for follow-up CXR. This revealed a new >1.5-cm mass in the lower left lung field (see arrows in Figures 6–1A and B), suspicious for recurrent disease. The chest CT demonstrated the lesion in the left lung without mediastinal adenopathy (not shown). The patient complained of visual disturbance and an MRI of the

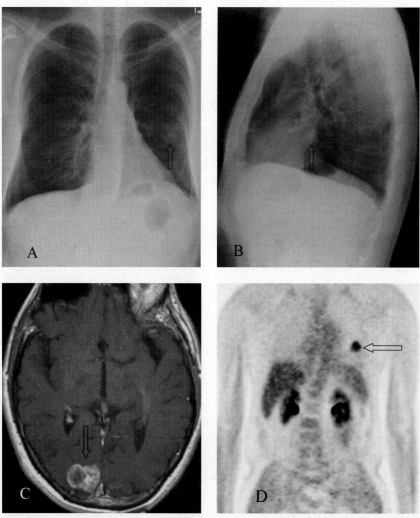

Figure 6–1. A 58-year-old man with previously resected left lower-lobe lung cancer. *A* and *B,* Chest radiography revealed a new >105-cm mass in the lower left lung field (*arrows*). *C,* Magnetic resonance imaging of the brain revealed an enhancing lesion in the occipital lobe, consistent with a metastatic deposit (*arrow*). *D,* The FDG-PET scan revealed only the left lung lesion.

brain was performed which revealed an enhancing lesion in the occipital lobe consistent with a metastatic deposit (Figure 6–1C, arrow). The FDG-PET scan revealed only the left lung lesion (Figure 6–1D). The patient underwent a craniotomy for his symptomatic metastasis.

Case 2: Extensive Disease

This 67-year-old woman presented with right shoulder pain while exercising. A CXR revealed an apical, right upper-lobe mass (Figure 6–2A and B, arrows). The extent of tumor invasion of the mediastinum and lower neck is not accurately assessed by CXR. A CT of the chest revealed a 4.5-cm mass in the right upper lobe with extension to the right upper mediastinum (Figure 6–2C and D) and associated mediastinal lymphadenopathy (not shown) and abdominal lymphadenopathy (Figure 6–2E). A subsequent PET scan, the coronal slices of which are displayed in Figure 6–2F revealed the large, right upper-lobe mass, left supraclavicular lymphadenopathy, as well as extensive intra-abdominal lymphadenopathy (arrows). Biopsy of the lung mass revealed poorly-differentiated non-small cell lung cancer, with the same findings found at laparoscopic biopsy of the peripancreatic lesions. This

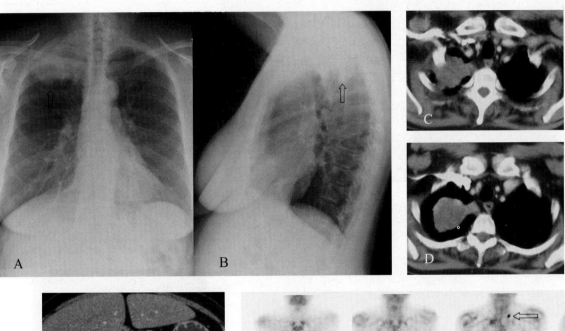

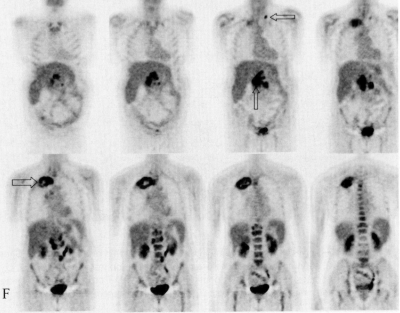

Figure 6–2. A 67-year-old woman with right shoulder pain. *A* and *B,* Chest radiography revealed an apical, right upper-lobe mass (*arrows*). Computed tomography of the chest revealed a 4.5-cm mass in the right upper lobe with extension to the right mediastinum (*C, D*), associated mediastinal lymphadenopathy (not shown), and abdominal lymphadenopathy (*E*). *F,* A PET scan revealed a large, right upper-lobe mass, left supraclavicular lymphadenopathy, and extensive intra-abdominal lymphadenopathy (*arrows*).

patient is undergoing chemotherapy. In those patients with symptoms related to lung cancer, an extensive work-up is required to document the full extent of disease.

Case 3: Extensive Disease

This 81-year-old woman with adenocarcinoma of the right lung was referred for staging; the initial CXR revealed a large, right mid-lung lesion (Figure 6–3A) seen projected under the arch of the aorta on the lateral view (Figure 6–3B). Note the compression fracture in the thoracic spine that was thought to be benign on CXR. The CT in Figure 6–3C reveals the large, right mid-zone mass, consistent with a primary lung cancer. The coronal FDG-PET images in Figure 6–3D reveal the large, right lung mass, as well as multiple skeletal metastases (arrows), including a lesion in the lower thoracic spine. MRI of the right arm (Figure 6–3E) confirmed the metastases in the right humerus (arrows).

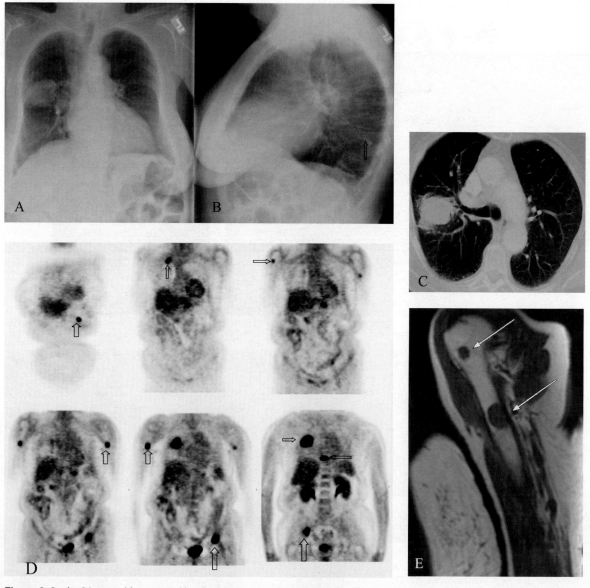

Figure 6–3. An 81-year-old woman with adenocarcinoma of the right lung. Chest radiography revealed a large, right mid-lung lesion (*A*), seen projected under the arch of the aorta on the lateral view (*B*). *C,* Computed tomography revealed a large, right med-zone mass, consistent with primary lung cancer. *D,* Coronal FDG-PET images revealed a large, right lung mass and multiple skeletal metastases (*arrows*). *E,* Magnetic resonance imaging of the right arm confirmed the metastases in the right humerus (*arrows*).

Case 4: PET Demonstration of M Disease

T2N2M0 on FDG-PET and T4N2M0 on CT, but additional positive nodes on FDG-PET, CT, and PET images of an 83-year-old patient with biopsy-proven adenocarcinoma of the right lung. This case was staged as T2N2M0 on FDG-PET and T4N2M0 on CT. Figure 6–4A reveals a large, lobulated mass, adjacent to and invading the right hilum (see arrows). Figure 6–4B reveals multiple lung nodules that appear separate from the main tumor but within the same lobe (see arrow), indicating T4 disease. Figure 6–4C, a large right subcarinal (level 7) lymph node is present (arrow). Figure 6–4D, a coronal PET scan shows a perihilar mass, right hilar lymphadenopathy and a subcarinal lymph node. Figure 6–4E shows an FDG-avid focus in the anterior mediastinum that was negative on CT. Figure 6–4F, a CT through the upper mediastinum demonstrates a normal-sized lymph node.

This case illustrates the sensitivity of CT scan in defining the primary tumor mass as well as the presence of satellite nodules, either in the same lobe

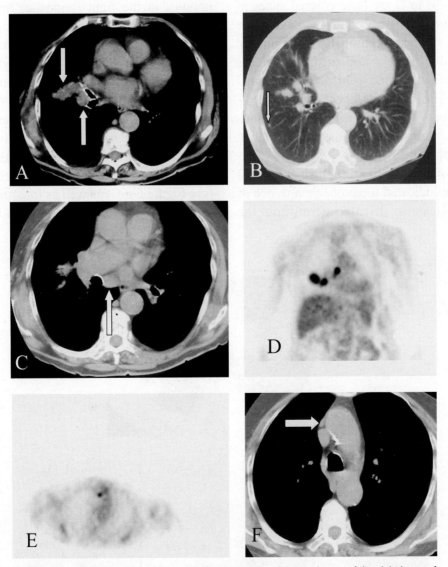

Figure 6–4. An 83-year-old patient with biopsy-proven adenocarcinoma of the right lungs. *A* shows a large, lobulated mass adjacent to and invading the right hilum (*arrows*). *B* shows multiple lung nodules that appear separate from the main tumor but within the same lobe (*arrow*), indicating T4 disease. The arrow in *C* points to a large right subcarinal lymph node. *D,* A coronal PET scan shows a perihilar mass, right hilar lymphadenopathy, and a subcarinal lymph node. *E* shows an FDG-avid focus in the anterior mediastinum. *F,* Computed tomography through the upper mediastinum demonstrates a normal-sized lymph node.

(T4) or in an adjacent lobe (M1). The PET scan demonstrated more extensive N disease in the anterior mediastinum than was apparent on CT scan. This patient received chemotherapy.

Case 5: PET with No Evidence of Distant Disease (M0)

Figure 6–5A, a CT of the chest, shows an approximately 3-cm-wide spiculate mass in the left upper posterolateral lung. Soft-tissue windows showed no associated hilar or mediastinal lymph node enlargement. Figures 6–5B to D are three coronal slices of an FDG-PET scan with increased FDG uptake in the solitary nodule, indicating probable malignancy. Scans of the hilar regions and mediastinum are FDG-negative, indicating no evidence of regional spread of tumor. The left lower lobectomy and mediastinal lymph node dissection revealed squamous cell cancer in the primary tumor mass and negative mediastinal lymph nodes.

The absence of abnormal FDG uptake in the thorax and abdomen indicated the probable absence of macroscopic metastatic disease, permitting the

patient to undergo resective surgery with the intention of cure. Six-month follow-up reveals no evidence of recurrence. FDG-PET has been consistently shown to be more accurate than CT in the detection of tumor in mediastinal lymph nodes.

Case 6: Other Nodules in the Lung

Figure 6–6A demonstrates a mass in the left upper posterior lung, which has a lobulated and slightly spiculate appearance that is highly suspicious for primary lung cancer. Figure 6–6B shows two small nodules in the right (opposite) lung (see arrows). Other CT scan images with lung windows also demonstrated at least two other small nodules. The possibility of metastases to the right lung from the large left primary lung tumor cannot be excluded on the basis of this CT scan. Figure 6–6C to F represent a series of coronal FDG-PET scan tomographic images of the chest and upper two-thirds of the abdomen. Normal findings demonstrated include increased uptake in the left ventricular myocardium (see Figure 6–6C) as well as low-grade uptake in the liver (see Figure 6–6D, arrow) and gastric mucosa

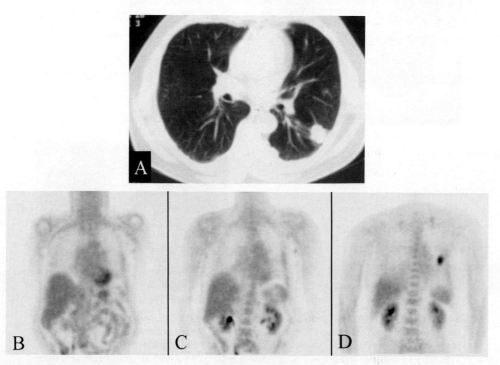

Figure 6–5. *A,* Computed tomography of the chest shows an approximately 3-cm-wide spiculate mass in the left upper posterolateral lung. *B* to *D,* Three coronal slices of an FDG-PET scan with increased FDG uptake in the solitary nodule, indication probable malignancy.

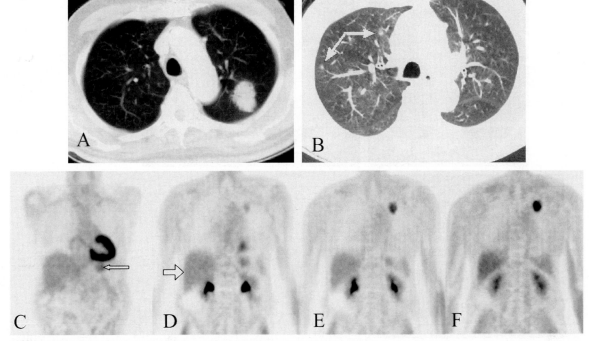

Figure 6–6. *A* shows a mass in the left upper posterior lung that is highly suspicious for primary lung cancer, whereas *B* shows two small nodules in the right lung (*arrows*). *C* to *F,* Coronal FDG-PET images.

(see Figure 6–6C, arrow). Increased uptake is also seen in the renal collecting systems that selectively clear FDG from the body. Note the absence of FDG uptake in the right lung.

At surgery, the patient was found to have a large adenocarcinoma of the left upper lung. Mediastinal lymph node dissection revealed no evidence of local nodal spread. The presence of small nodules in the opposite lung on CT is disturbing; however, the negative FDG-PET scan of the right lung permits some confidence that the nodules seen on CT are benign and not related to the patient's lung cancer. In addition, the PET scan provides additional evidence that there is no metastatic disease elsewhere in the thorax or upper abdomen. Very small nodules may be falsely negative on FDG-PET (no current diagnostic imaging test is able to detect very small volume disease). If these small, right-lung lesions had been hypermetabolic on FDG-PET, it would have indicated inoperable lung cancer.

The performance of an FDG-PET scan as part of the preoperative work-up in candidates of surgery may well detect previously unsuspected foci of regional or distant disease, thus sparing patients unnecessary surgery.

Case 7: PET in Mediastinal Staging

Figure 6–7A demonstrates a mass in the right lower lobe encasing the lower bronchus intermedius. Figure 6–7B shows peripheral atelectasis distal to the tumor mass resulting from bronchial stenosis or occlusion (arrow). The scans of the upper abdomen (Figure 6–7C) demonstrate moderate prominence of the left adrenal gland (see arrow). Density readings through this adrenal gland showed 12 Hounsfield units, indicating that this most probably represents a benign adrenal adenoma or localized hyperplasia of the adrenal gland.

FDG-PET scan demonstrated increased uptake in the region of the tumor. In addition, mildly increased uptake was present posteroinferior to the tumor, corresponding to the region of atelectasis seen on CT scan (Figure 6–7D and E: the open arrow indicates tumor while the closed arrow indicates atelectasis.) In addition, the PET scan demonstrated no uptake in the mediastinum to suggest the presence of mediastinal lymphadenopathy. The patient's tumor was resected and the mediastinal nodes were negative at pathologic examination.

This case illustrates the importance of PET scan-

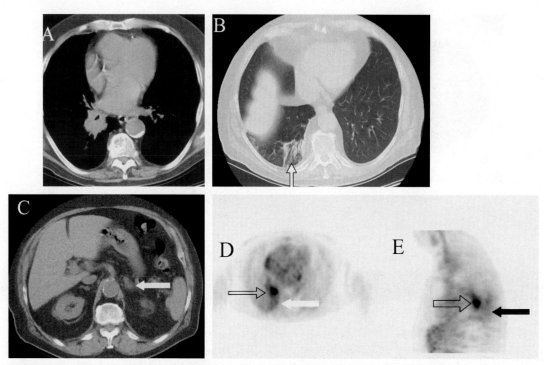

Figure 6–7. *A* shows a mass in the right lower lobe encasing the lower bronchus intermedius, whereas *B* shows peripheral atelectasis distal to the tumor mass resulting from bronchial stenosis or occlusion (*arrow*). *C,* Scans of the upper abdomen demonstrate moderate prominence of the left adrenal gland (*arrow*). *D* and *E,* The open arrow indicates tumor, whereas the closed arrow indicates atelectasis.

ning in staging: a negative PET scan of an enlarged adrenal gland indicates that the enlargement is almost certainly caused by a benign process, especially when the primary tumor is FDG-avid. In addition, a negative mediastinal FDG-PET is a more accurate staging modality than a negative CT.

This patient has small cell lung cancer treated with chemotherapy and radiation therapy to the mediastinum and right hilum. The initial CXR, obtained shortly after radiation therapy, demonstrates an acute infiltrate in the right upper lobe as well as a residual right hilar mass. The image on the right was acquired 8 months later and demonstrates the findings of radiation fibrosis, with loss of lung volume, retraction of the right hilum and elevation of the hemidiaphragm. The increased density of the right upper zone is due to fibrosis of the right upper lobe. The right hilar mass is no longer present. The CT prior to therapy (see Figure 6–7B) revealed a right mid-zone lesion with small peripheral lesions in the right middle lobe. A repeat CT performed early after the course of radiotherapy revealed a major response in the right mid-zone with a progressive infiltrate in the right upper lobe laterally as

well as the anterior portions of the right and left lung fields. An FDG-PET scan was performed at this time and revealed increased FDG metabolism in the sites of abnormality on the CT scan. No FDG-PET scan was performed at the time of the initial presentation. The treating clinician was then faced with the clinical dilemma of a complete radiologic response in the primary tumor with apparent progression in other sites. A biopsy of one of the lesions seen on FDG-PET and CT revealed reactive changes. Twenty-four-month CXR follow-up reveals no evidence of recurrence, and the patient remains well. This case indicates the pivotal role of repeat biopsy in "atypical" cases. In this case, the progressive CT and FDG-PET findings were due to a combination of radiation fibrosis and infection.

Case 8: Response Assessment

This 55-year-old man was found to have a right paratracheal mass on routine chest radiography, a subsequent CT (not shown) revealed right paratracheal lymphadenopathy with no evidence of an intrapulmonary mass. The patient was investigated with bronchoscopy and washings, as well as mediastinoscopy that showed poorly differentiated metastatic non–small cell adenocarcinoma in the right level 2 and level 4 lymph nodes. Subsequently, a PET scan (Figure 6–8A to D) revealed, in addition to paratracheal lymphadenopathy, foci of abnormal uptake in the right supraclavicular region (small arrows), with no evidence of disease in the contralateral lymph nodes, nor is there any evidence of bone or adrenal metastases. Due to the presence of supraclavicular lymphadenopathy, the patient underwent chemotherapy as well as radiation therapy. Following this therapy, the patient underwent a second PET scan, the coronal images of which are shown in Figure 6–8E to H. These demonstrate an enlarging right supraclavicular lymph node (arrow), as well as extensive bilateral mediastinal lymphadenopathy, including new subcarinal and left paratracheal adenopathy. CT of the chest and the lower neck obtained after chemoradiation therapy is shown in Figure 6–8I to L. This series of images shows adenopathy anterior to the trachea (see Figure 6–8I, arrow), right mainstem bronchus (see Figure 6–8J, arrow) and left paratra-

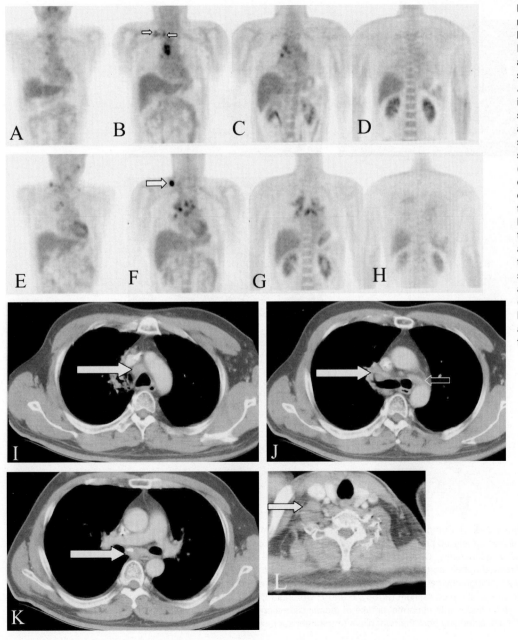

Figure 6–8. A 55-year-old man with right paratracheal lymphadenopathy. *A to D,* A PET scan revealed foci of abnormal uptake in the right supraclavicular region (*small arrows*). *E to H,* Coronal images of a second PET scan following chemotherapy and radiation therapy, demonstrating an enlarging right supraclavicular lymph node (*arrow*) and extensive bilateral mediastinal lymphadenopathy. *I to L,* Computed tomography of the chest and lower neck after chemoradiation therapy demonstrated adenopathy anterior to the trachea (*I, arrow*), right mainstem bronchus (*J, arrow*) and left paratracheal region (*J, open arrow*), subcarinal lymphadenopathy (*K, arrow*), and enlarged lymph node in the right neck (*L, arrow*).

cheal region (see Figure 6–8J, open arrow), sub-carinal lymphadenopathy (see Figure 6–8K, arrow), as well as an enlarged lymph node in the right neck (see Figure 6–8L, arrow). All of these CT abnor-malities are also FDG-avid on PET, indicating residual/recurrent disease activity.

An FDG-PET scan following treatment is useful in demonstrating the extent of response, progres-sion, or new foci of cancer. Moreover, the response or progression on follow-up PET scans can be quan-tified by comparing image-derived measures of local tumor metabolic activity such as the standard-ized uptake value (SUV).

Case 9: N3 Disease in Normal-Sized Lymph Nodes

The CT image in Figure 6–9A shows a bulky mass in the left hilum (arrow). Figure 6–9B, obtained just superior to the left hilar mass, shows soft-tissue prominence in the subcarinal region consistent with level 7 mediastinal adenopathy. The FDG-PET scan—axial view (Figure 6–9C) confirms the CT findings with areas of increased uptake correspond-ing to the left hilum and the subcarinal region. CT at a higher level, above the aortic arch, demonstrates some borderline enlarged lymph nodes on the oppo-

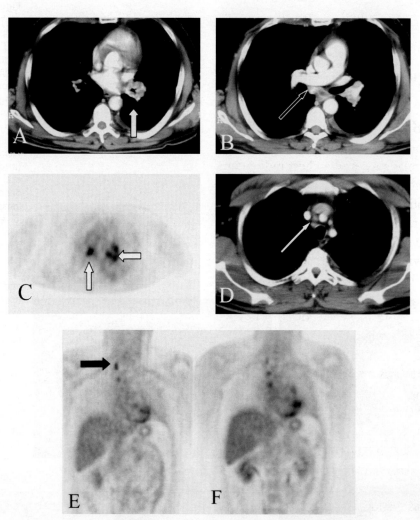

Figure 6–9. *A,* Computed tomography revealed a bulky mass in the left hilum (arrow). *B* shows soft-tissue prominence in the subcarinal region, consistent with level 7 medi-astinal adenopathy. *C,* A FDG-PET scan confirmed the CT findings with areas of increased uptake corresponding to the left hilum and the subcarinal region. *D,* Com-puted tomography demonstrated some borderline enlarged lymph nodes on the oppo-site side of the mediastinum (*arrow*). *E* and *F,* Coronal FDG-PET scans show a chain of lymph nodes with abnormal uptake of radionuclide along the right side of the medi-astinum, extending from the right hilum to the right supraclavicular region (*arrow*).

site side of the mediastinum (Figure 6–9D, arrow). Figure 6–9E and F, coronal FDG-PET scans, show a chain of lymph nodes with abnormal uptake of radionuclide along the right side of the mediastinum, extending from the right hilum to the right supraclavicular region (see arrow). Mediastinoscopy with biopsy showed metastatic non–small cell lung cancer to these N3 lymph nodes.

These scans illustrate the important role of FDG-PET in confirming the presence of N3 (inoperable) malignant lymphadenopathy. Frequently, nodes in these sites are either normal in size or only minimally enlarged on CT. FDG-PET-positive mediastinal lymph nodes on the side opposite the primary lung cancer indicate with a high degree of certainty the presence of inoperable lung cancer.

Case 10: Evaluation of Distant Disease (M Stage)

This 27-year-old nonsmoking female presented with intermittent dry cough and left shoulder pain. She was given muscle relaxants; and a chest radiograph revealed findings consistent with pneumonia. After a course of antibiotics, there was persistence of the changes on chest radiography and a CT was performed, revealing a left upper-lobe mass adjacent to the mediastinum, with peripheral atelectasis (Figure 6–10A). No other foci of disease were detected initially on the CT. Bone scans revealed abnormal uptake in the left glenoid fossa. Following this, the patient underwent a Chamberlain procedure and was found to have malignant involvement of the left level 5 lymph node, as well as a central adenocarcinoma of the left lung. An FDG-PET scan was performed (Figure 6–10B and C, two coronal slices of an FDG PET scan), which revealed pathologic uptake of FDG in the left hilar tumor as well as the left glenoid fossa (arrow). In addition, increased uptake was present in the posterior element of a lower thoracic vertebra (not shown) as well as an upper lumbar vertebra (see Figure 6–10C, arrow). A CT performed at the time of the FDG-PET scan was abnormal in the glenoid fossa (Figure 6–10D, arrow), although the abnormality was not reported. The upper lumbar vertebra at this time was within normal limits on CT scanning (Figure 6–10E, arrow) although subse-

quent CT examinations (performed 3 and 8 months later) through this region clearly revealed metastatic disease (Figure 6–10F and G, arrows). Due to the demonstration of bone lesions on the FDG-PET scan, a pre-surgery induction chemotherapy course was undertaken, and following interval resolution of the disease in the chest, a biopsy of the scapular lesion was performed which revealed residual viable tumor. The patient continues with chemotherapy.

This case illustrates that CT is accurate in establishing the local extent of disease within the chest. The PET scan is able to detect regional chest involvement as well as M1 disease: in this case, five lesions in bone were detected. Retrospective review of the CT demonstrated only three of these, none of which were detected before PET scan correlation (this is, in part, because FDG-PET can image the marrow phase of bone metastases that occurs before bone destruction has occurred).

Case 11: PET in Regional and Distant Disease (CT T3N3M1, PET T3N3M1)

This 51-year-old man initially presented with cough, hoarseness, and left vocal cord paralysis. Chest CT (Figure 6–11A) demonstrates a left para-hilar-mass density (horizontal arrow). A peripheral cavitated pneumonia was also present at the time (vertical arrow). In addition to ipsilateral hilar adenopathy, there was adenopathy involving the opposite right hilum (Figure 6–11B, arrows) that represents N3 disease. Lung windows (Figure 6–11C, arrow) demonstrate a nodule in the right upper anterior lung zone suspicious for representing metastatic disease (M1).

PET scan findings confirm the CT findings, revealing a large left hilar mass, probably centrally necrotic (Figure 6–11D). In addition, there is increased FDG uptake corresponding to the right anterior lung nodule seen on CT, indicating that this probably represents metastatic disease. Figure 6–11D also shows a small focal area of increased uptake in the right side of the lower neck (highest arrow). This focal increased FDG uptake does not, however, represent metastatic disease: axial PET views (Figure 6–11E) at the level of the larynx demonstrate the presence of increased FDG uptake in the right vocal cord muscles that are hyperactive in an attempt to compensate for the paralyzed left cord (which has reduced FDG uptake, small arrow). This is almost certainly due to malignant involvement of the left recurrent laryngeal nerve at the left hilum. Figure 6–11F confirms the CT findings by the presence of increased FDG uptake in the right hilum (smaller arrow).

This case illustrates findings on CT scans with extensive suspected involvement in the opposite hilum (N3) as well as nodularity in the opposite lung (M1 disease). PET scanning confirms these sus-

pected findings and also as reveals a focus of abnormal uptake in the right neck, not seen on CT scan.

Case 12: False-Positive CT

This 64-year-old female underwent a left partial mastectomy with postoperative irradiation for T1 intraductal breast cancer with no evidence of invasion. Subsequent mammography revealed a suspicious finding in the lung beneath the previously excised tumor and a subsequent chest radiograph demonstrated hilar lym-

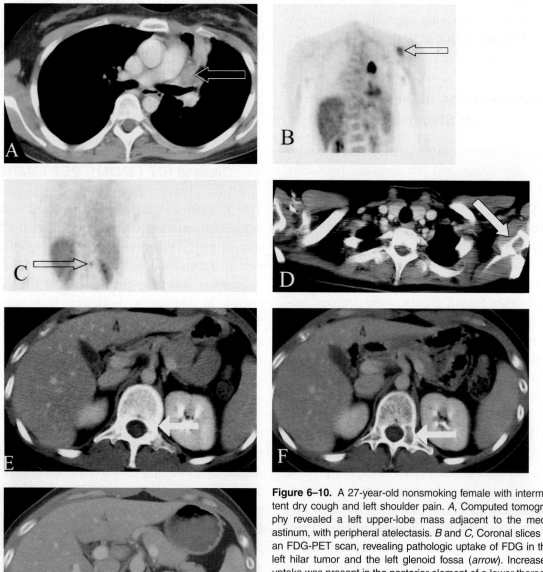

Figure 6–10. A 27-year-old nonsmoking female with intermittent dry cough and left shoulder pain. A, Computed tomography revealed a left upper-lobe mass adjacent to the mediastinum, with peripheral atelectasis. B and C, Coronal slices of an FDG-PET scan, revealing pathologic uptake of FDG in the left hilar tumor and the left glenoid fossa (arrow). Increased uptake was present in the posterior element of a lower thoracic vertebra (not shown) and an upper lumbar vertebra (C, arrow). D, Computed tomography was abnormal in the glenoid fossa (D, arrow). The upper lumbar vertebra was within normal limits on CT scanning (E, arrow), although subsequent CT through this region revealed metastatic disease (F and G, arrows).

phadenopathy. A biopsy revealed non–small cell lung cancer. CT scans were obtained prior to and following administration of chemotherapy (Figure 6–12A and B pre-chemotherapy, Figure 6–12C and D post-chemotherapy). Following chemotherapy a modest response was seen in the size of the spiculate pri-mary tumor in the left lower lung (see Figure 6–12A and C). A partial response was seen in the enlarged subcarinal lymph node (see Figure 6–12B and D). Enlarged lymph nodes were noted on CT scan at the lower left paratracheal region and in the subaortic region both prior to and following chemotherapy.

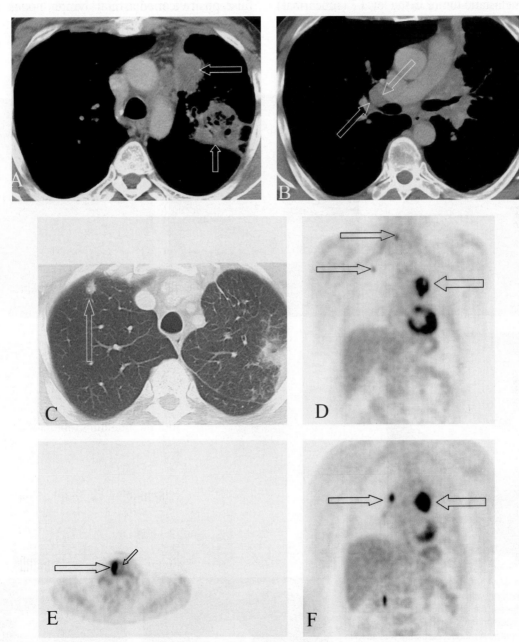

Figure 6–11. A 51-year-old man with cough, hoarseness, and left vocal cord paralysis. *A,* Computed tomogra-phy demonstrated a left parahilar mass density (horizontal arrow). *B* shows adenopathy involving the opposite right hilum (arrows), representing N3 disease. Lung windows (*C, arrow*) demonstrate a nodule in the right upper anterior lung zone suspicious for metastatic disease. *D,* A PET scan revealed a large left hilar mass, probably centrally necrotic, and a small focal area of increased uptake in the right side of the lower neck (highest arrow). *E,* Axial PET views at the level of the larynx demonstrate increased uptake in the right vocal cord muscles that are hyperactive in an attempt to compensate for the paralyzed left cord, which has reduced FDG uptake (*small arrow*). *F* reveals increased FDG uptake in the right hilum (*smaller arrow*).

Following chemotherapy, an FDG-PET scan was performed, which demonstrated low-grade uptake in the primary tumor (Figure 6–12E) as well as avid uptake at the level of the subcarinal region (level 7, Figure 6–12F). The patient underwent left upper lobectomy as well as mediastinal lymph node dissection. The primary site showed persistent viable tumor. There was metastatic tumor in the level 7 (subcarinal) lymph node. Other lymph nodes in the left lower paratracheal region and subaortic region were removed at surgery; both these sites were negative on FDG-PET and at pathologic examination. The enlarged lymph nodes present in the lower paratracheal region and the AP window region both prior to and following chemotherapy (Figure 6–12G and H) were positive on CT but negative on PET and pathology.

This case illustrates the frequent presence of false-positive mediastinal lymph nodes in CT as well as the accuracy of FDG-PET in distinguishing enlarged benign nodes from enlarged malignant

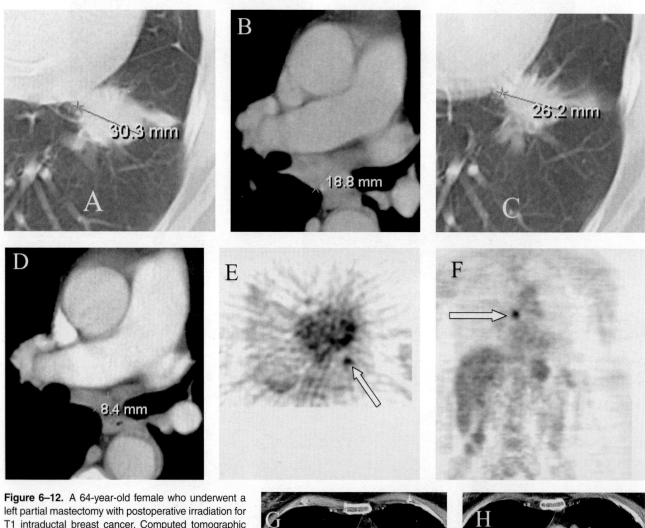

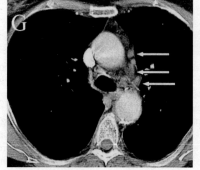

Figure 6–12. A 64-year-old female who underwent a left partial mastectomy with postoperative irradiation for T1 intraductal breast cancer. Computed tomographic scans were obtained prior to (A and B) and following (C and D) chemotherapy. A modest response was seen in the size of the spiculate primary tumor in the left lower lung (A and C), and a partial response was seen in the enlarged subcarinal lymph node (B and D). An FDG-PET scan demonstrated low-grade uptake in the primary tumor (E) and avid uptake at the level of the subcarinal region (F). G and H, Enlarged lymph nodes present in the lower paratracheal region and the AP window region before and after chemotherapy.

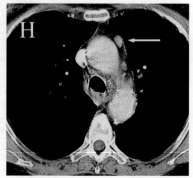

nodes. The persistence of FDG uptake in the mediastinum following chemotherapy is a strong indicator of residual viable regional disease.

Case 13: Synchronous Lung Cancers

This 68-year-old smoker presented with hemoptysis. A chest radiograph revealed a right upper-lobe mass. CT scanning demonstrated a lobulated mass density in the upper portion of the right posterior lung with enlarged ipsilateral mediastinal lymph nodes (Figure 6–13A, arrow). On the same CT scan an infiltrative density measuring approximately 3 cm in maximal dimension was seen in the left upper lung zone (Figure 6–13B, arrow).

A PET scan performed at this time (Figure 6–13C) demonstrated uptake corresponding to the right upper lobe lobular mass, as well as increased uptake in the ipsilateral mediastinum (Figure 6–13D), indicating N2 disease. The region of lung parenchyma corresponding to the left upper lobe infiltrative density was negative.

On the initial PET scan obtained in April 1999 an ill-defined area of equivocal increased uptake was noted corresponding to the right rib cage (see Figure 6–13D, arrow). A follow-up PET scan obtained 2 months later in June demonstrated a positive finding corresponding to the rib (Figure 6–13E, arrow), representing metastatic disease. Initial biopsy of the lobulated lesion in the right upper lobe demonstrated adenocarcinoma. Two months later, a biopsy specimen of the infiltrative density in the left upper lung zone was taken, demonstrating squamous carcinoma. This latter malignant neoplasm of the lung was negative on the PET scan.

This case study indicates that PET scanning, although highly accurate for detection of malignancy and for staging, is not a panacea. For unknown reasons, the squamous cancer in the left upper lung was not FDG-avid. Other lung malignancies such as bronchoalveolar cancer (see Case 14) or carcinoid tumor may be negative or only weakly positive on PET scan. Persistently abnormal findings on CT scan, even if negative on PET, must be further investigated.

Case 14: False-Negative PET Scan

This 50-year-old woman presented with recurrent multifocal bronchoalveolar carcinoma demonstrated on CT. The CT in Figure 6–14A shows a mass in the upper lobe of the right lung with air bronchograms (arrow), which is consistent with recurrent bron-

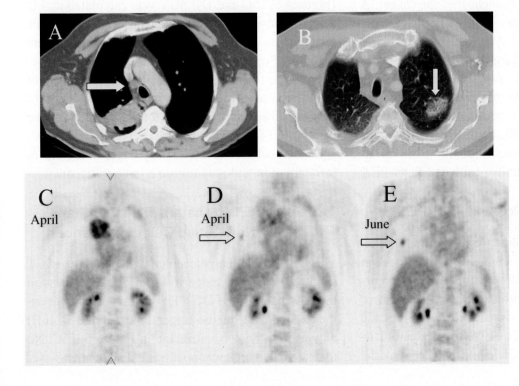

Figure 6–13. A 68-year-old smoker with hemoptysis. *A,* Computed tomography demonstrated a lobulated mass density in the upper portion of the right posterior lung with enlarged mediastinal lymph nodes (*arrow*). *B,* An infiltrative density was seen in the left upper lung zone (*arrow*). A PET scan (*C*) demonstrated uptake corresponding to the right upper lobe lobular mass and increased uptake in the ipsilateral mediastinum (*D*), indicating N2 disease. The initial PET scan revealed increased uptake corresponding to the right rib cage (*D, arrow*), and a follow-up scan revealed a positive finding corresponding to the rib (*E, arrow*), representing metastatic disease.

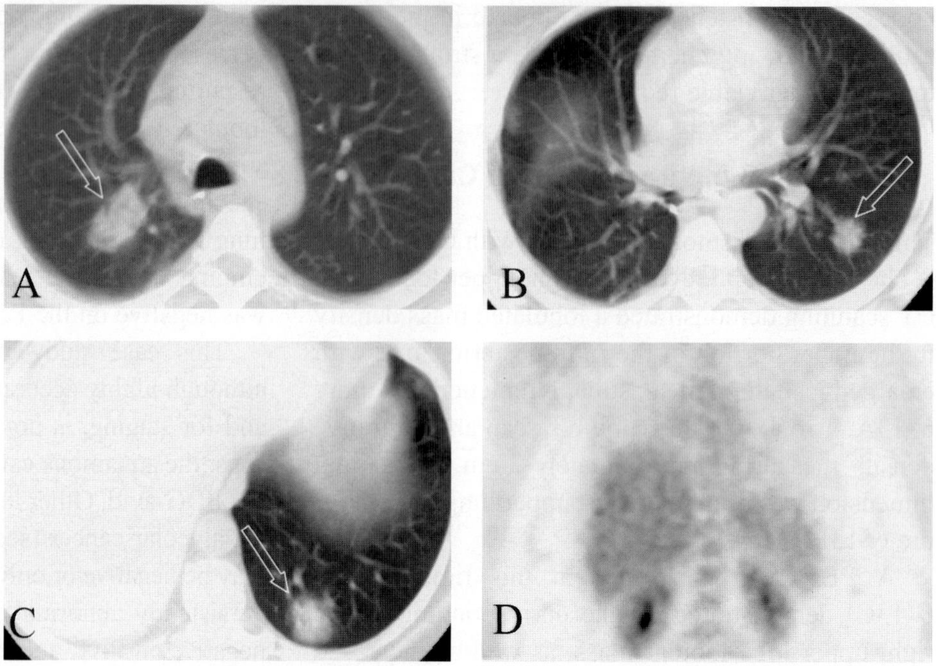

Figure 6–14. A 50-year-old woman with recurrent multifocal bronchoalveolar carcinoma. *A,* Computed tomography revealed a mass in the upper lobe of the right lung with air bronchograms (arrow). *B* shows the typical "bunch of grapes" appearance of bronchoalveolar carcinoma and *C* shows a third focus of recurrent bronchoalveolar carcinoma. *D,* A coronal FDG-PET scan through the posterior lung fields revealed no uptake of FDG at the sites of tumor recurrence on CT.

choalveolar carcinoma. Figure 6–14B demonstrates the typical "bunch of grapes" appearance of bronchoalveolar carcinoma. Figure 6–14C shows a third focus of recurrent bronchoalveolar carcinoma. Figure 6–14D shows a coronal FDG-PET scan slice through the posterior lung fields performed at the same time as the CTs shown reveals no uptake of FDG at the sites of tumor recurrence on CT. FDG-PET is usually negative in patients with bronchoalveolar cancer. A left lower-lobe wedge biopsy revealed bronchoalveolar carcinoma, goblet cell type, well differentiated, and greater than 3 cm in diameter.

A negative FDG-PET scan does not rule out bronchoalveolar carcinoma. Another lung tumor that is often FDG-negative is carcinoid tumor, although the less well-differentiated atypical carcinoid may be FDG-positive. Adenocarcinoma with bronchoalveolar features is usually positive of FDG-PET.

Case 15: False-Positive FDG-PET

This 67-year-old woman completed chemoradiation therapy for limited-stage small cell lung cancer in 1995. She was being followed for possible recurrence of her primary tumor as well as associated paraneoplastic cerebellar dysfunction. A CT of the chest performed in March of 1997 revealed an infiltrative density in the medial lung posterior to the

right hilum (Figure 6–15A, arrow). The patient was followed with CT scans every 6 months until August of 1999. The August 1999 CT revealed an enlarging and more confluent infiltrative density in the same area (Figure 6–15B, arrows). This lesion was thought to be either a recurrent tumor or a second primary cancer. An FDG-PET was performed that showed increased uptake in the same region (Figures 6–15C and D). SUV was calculated at 4.0, a level consistent with malignancy. A fine-needle aspirate was negative for the presence of malignant cells. An operative wedge excision was subsequently performed that revealed the presence of granulomatous inflammation and no evidence of tumor. Subsequent cultures for bacteria, acid-fast bacilli, and fungi were negative.

False-positive FDG-PET may occur in regions of inflammation and may mimic a lung malignancy.

Case 16: PET in Distant Disease (Stage 1 T2N0M0 Non–Small Cell Lung Cancer)

This 65-year-old man presented with hemoptysis. CT (Figure 6–16A) revealed a 4-cm lobulated mass in the left upper lobe; FDG-PET scan revealed a hypermetabolic focus in the upper lobe (Figure 6–16B) and also on the coronal image in Figure 6–16C. No mediastinal lymphadenopathy or distant metastases

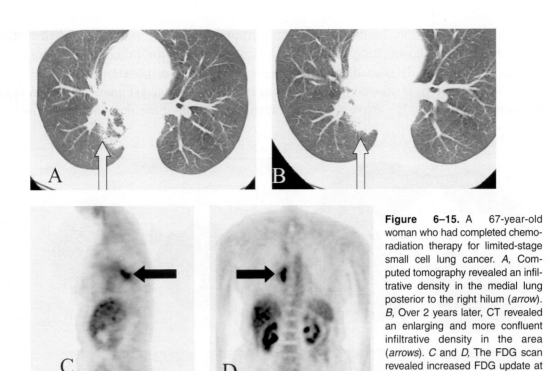

Figure 6–15. A 67-year-old woman who had completed chemoradiation therapy for limited-stage small cell lung cancer. *A,* Computed tomography revealed an infiltrative density in the medial lung posterior to the right hilum (*arrow*). *B,* Over 2 years later, CT revealed an enlarging and more confluent infiltrative density in the area (*arrows*). *C* and *D,* The FDG scan revealed increased FDG update at the site of the CT abnormality.

were seen on the FDG-PET scan. At surgery the tumor was completely resected and the mediastinum was negative for tumor. Subsequent follow-up has revealed no evidence of distant metastatic disease.

FDG-PET is more accurate than CT in detecting regional and distant spread of lung cancer. Therefore, an FDG-PET scan that demonstrates no distant disease provides added confidence that the tumor is a localized process.

Case 17: The Importance of Current Staging Investigations

This 52-year-old female presented with non-small cell lung cancer diagnosed after prior episodes of pneumonia. Figure 6–17A demonstrates a large, partially cavitated mass in the right mid-lung zone extending to the right hilum. Two satellite nodules are present. Since these are in the same lobe as the

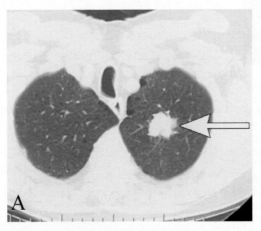

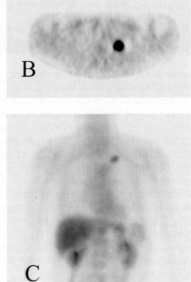

Figure 6–16. A 65-year-old man with hemoptysis. *A,* Computed tomography revealed a 4-cm lobulated mass in the left upper lobe; FDG-PET scan revealed a hypermetabolic focus in the upper lobe (*B*) and on the coronal image (*C*).

primary tumor, this may represent T4 disease. In addition, scans through the upper lung (Figure 6–17B) demonstrate an irregularly shaped satellite nodule. On this CT scan, the right adrenal gland is radiologically normal (Figure 6–17C, arrow).

Approximately 2 months elapsed before the patient presented for initiation of therapy. At this time a PET scan demonstrated increased uptake in the right adrenal gland (Figure 6–17D). A repeat CT scan done at this time demonstrated a mass in the

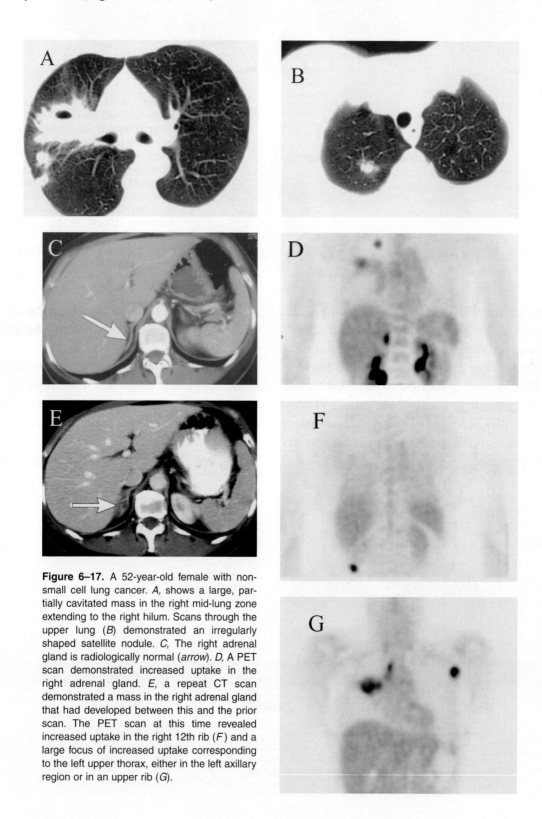

Figure 6–17. A 52-year-old female with non-small cell lung cancer. *A,* shows a large, partially cavitated mass in the right mid-lung zone extending to the right hilum. Scans through the upper lung (*B*) demonstrated an irregularly shaped satellite nodule. *C,* The right adrenal gland is radiologically normal (*arrow*). *D,* A PET scan demonstrated increased uptake in the right adrenal gland. *E,* a repeat CT scan demonstrated a mass in the right adrenal gland that had developed between this and the prior scan. The PET scan at this time revealed increased uptake in the right 12th rib (*F*) and a large focus of increased uptake corresponding to the left upper thorax, either in the left axillary region or in an upper rib (*G*).

right adrenal that had developed in the interval between this and the prior scan (Figure 6–17E).

In addition, the PET scan obtained at this time demonstrated the presence of increased uptake in the right 12th rib (Figure 6–17F) as well as a large focus of increased uptake corresponding to the left upper thorax, either in the left axillary region or in an upper rib (Figure 6–17G). This case illustrates the probable development of right adrenal metastases in the 2-month interval from a presentation CT scan with a normal right adrenal gland. The presence of adrenal metastases is also confirmed on the repeat CT scan obtained 2 months after the initial CT. Furthermore, the PET scan demonstrates two other foci of probable bony distant metastatic disease (M1) that were not seen on the initial or follow-up CT scans.

Untreated lung cancer may progress rapidly. Before initiation of treatment, it is important to have current scans for accurate clinical staging.

Case 18: The Importance of Clinical History

Figure 6–18A, a midline sagittal view from an FDG-PET scan, shows a curved linear area of increased FDG uptake that extends from the skin above the manubrium of the sternum into the mediastinum. The patient had undergone mediastinoscopy with biopsy several days prior to the FDG-PET scan, and this appearance is typical of the inflammatory changes that occur post-mediastinoscopy and should not be confused with malignant mediastinal lymphadenopathy.

Figure 6–18B, a CT scan through the upper mediastinum above the level of the aortic arch, also performed post-mediastinoscopy, shows poorly defined infiltration of the anterior mediastinal structures with obliteration of the normal mediastinal fat planes. The appearance of the CT scan could be misinterpreted as malignant lymphadenopathy if the history of recent mediastinoscopy is not available.

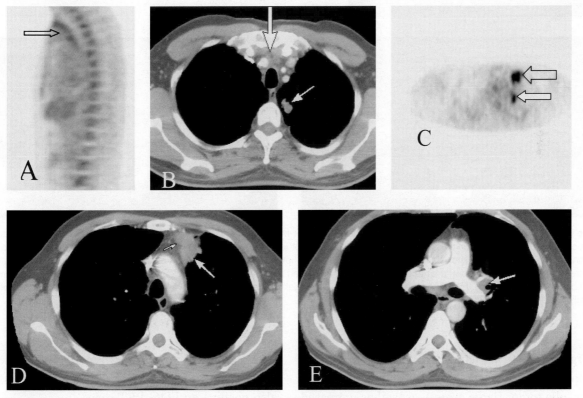

Figure 6–18. *A,* Following mediastinoscopy with biopsy, a midline sagittal view from an FDG-PET scan shows a curved linear area of increased FDG uptake that extends from the skin above the manubrium of the sternum into the mediastinum. *B,* A CT scan through the upper mediastinum above the level of the aortic arch, shows poorly defined infiltration of the anterior mediastinal structures with obliteration of the normal mediastinal fat planes. *C,* An axial FDG-PET scan of the upper thorax revealed increased uptake in the left upper lobe tumor (*large arrow*) and increased uptake corresponding either to left Hilary adenopathy or to a satellite tumor focus seen in the posterior left lung zone on the CT (*B, small arrow*). *D* shows an irregularly shaped mass abutting the anterior mediastinum in the left upper anterior lung zone. *E* demonstrates lymphadenopathy in the hilar region that was also positive on FDG-PET scan.

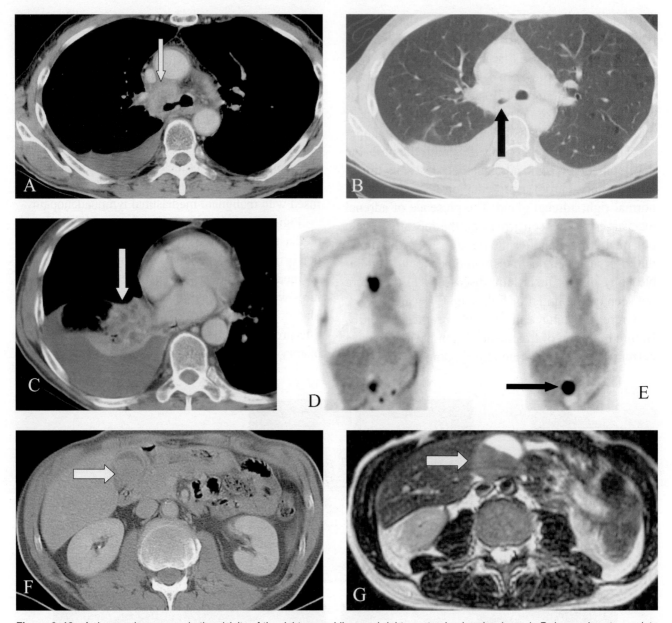

Figure 6–19. *A* shows a large mass in the vicinity of the right upper hilum and right paratracheal region (*arrow*). *B* shows almost complete occlusion of right mainstem bronchus (*arrow*). *C* shows a large, right lower-lung-zone soft-tissue density (*arrow*) with an associated pleural effusion. *D,* An FDG-PET scan shows a large area of increased FDG uptake corresponding to the main tumor mass in the right hilum and right lower paratracheal region. *E* shows a large area of markedly increased metabolism in the right upper quadrant of the abdomen, originating in or just below the liver (*arrow*). *F,* A CT scan showing a mass in the gallbladder (*arrow*). *G,* A T2-weighted MRI scan confirmed the presence of a gallbladder mass (*arrow*).

Figure 6–18C, an axial FDG-PET scan view of the upper thorax shows increased uptake in the left upper lobe tumor (large arrow), as well as increased uptake corresponding either to left hilar adenopathy or to a satellite tumor focus seen in the posterior left lung zone on the CT (see Figure 6–18B, small arrow). Figure 6–18D shows an irregularly shaped mass abutting the anterior mediastinum in the left

upper anterior lung zone. Figure 6–18E demonstrates lymphadenopathy in the hilar region that was also positive on FDG-PET scan.

This case illustrates the importance of an accurate clinical history in the interpretation of both FDG-PET and CT scans: without the history of the recent mediastinoscopy either scan may have incorrectly upstaged the patient due to the soft-tissue changes in the upper mediastinum. Given an accurate clinical history, the scans were correctly interpreted as post-mediastinoscopy change.

Case 19: Lung Cancer: Local Spread and Distant Disease

Figure 6–19A shows a large mass in the vicinity of the right upper hilum and right paratracheal region (arrow). Figure 6–19B, imaged to show the lungs and bronchi, shows almost complete occlusion of the right mainstem bronchus (arrow). Figure 6–19C, a CT image, shows a large, right lower-lung-zone soft-tissue density (arrow) with an associated pleural effusion. Whether this soft-tissue mass represents pneumonia, tumor, or collapse secondary to the proximal right mainstem bronchial occlusion is indeterminate.

Figure 6–19D from an FDG-PET scan shows a large area of increased FDG uptake corresponding to the main tumor mass in the right hilum and right lower paratracheal region. Note that the area of soft-tissue density in the right lower lung seen on CT scan is negative on FDG-PET scan indicating a benign process (consolidation) rather than tumor.

Figure 6–19E shows a large area of markedly increased metabolism in the right upper quadrant of the abdomen, originating in or just below the liver (arrow). Note that the actual site of abnormality is not well localized on this FDG-PET scan. Figure 6–19F, from a CT scan obtained at the same time as the PET, shows a mass in the gallbladder (arrow). Figure 6–19G (a T2-weighted MRI scan), confirms the presence of a gallbladder mass (arrow). Excisional biopsy of this mass demonstrated metastatic lung cancer.

This case illustrates the complimentary nature of CT and FDG-PET scanning. The malignant nature of the large hilar mass is confirmed on the FDG-PET scan. Much of the fine anatomic detail including involvement of the right main bronchus is not well demonstrated on the PET scan. However, FDG-PET was helpful in that it ruled out the presence of tumor in the right lower lobe, as well as detecting a gallbladder metastasis that was initially not recognized on CT.

REFERENCES

1. Fontana RS, Sanderson DR, Miller WE, et al. The Mayo Lung Project: preliminary report of "early cancer detection" phase. Cancer 1972;5:1373–82.

2. Marcus PM, Bergstralh EJ, Fagerstrom RM, et al. Lung cancer mortality in the Mayo Lung Project: impact of extended follow-up. J Natl Cancer Inst 2000;92(16):308–16.

3. Webb WR, Gatsonis C, Zerhouni EA, et al. CT and MR imaging in staging non-small cell bronchogenic carcinoma: report of the Radiologic Diagnostic Oncology Group. Radiology 1991;178:705–13.

4. McLoud TC, Bourgouin PM, Greenberg RW, et al. Bronchogenic carcinoma: analysis of staging in the mediastinum with CT by correlative lymph node mapping and sampling. Radiology 1992;182:319–23.

5. Lewis JW Jr, Pearlberg JL, Beute GH, et al. Can computed tomography of the chest stage lung cancer? Yes and no. Ann Thorac Surg 1990;49:591–5 (discussion 595–6).

6. Musset D, Grenier P, Carette MF, et al. Primary lung cancer staging: prospective comparative study of MR imaging with CT. Radiology 1986;160:607–11.

7. Poon PY, Bronskill MJ, Henkelman RM, et al. Mediastinal lymph node metastases from bronchogenic carcinoma: detection with MR imaging and CT. Radiology 1987;162:651–6.

8. Grenier P, Dubray B, Carette MF, et al. Preoperative thoracic staging of lung cancer: CT and MR evaluation. Diagn Intervent Radiol 1989;1:23–8.

9. Dales RE, Stark RM, Ramon S. Computed tomography to stage lung cancer: approaching a controversy using meta-analysis. Am Rev Respir Dis 1990;141:1096–101.

10. Larson SM, Weiden PL, Grunbaum Z, et al. Positron imaging feasibility studies. II. Characteristic of deoxyglucose uptake in rodent and canine neoplasms: concise communication. J Nucl Med 1981;22:875–9.

11. Wahl RL, Hutchins G, Buchsbaum D, et al. ^{18}F-2-deoxy-2-fluoro-D-glucose (FDG) uptake in human tumor xenografts: feasibility studies for cancer imaging with PET. Cancer 1991;67:1544–50.

12. Nolop KB, Rhodes CG, Brudin LH, et al. Glucose utilization in vivo by human pulmonary neoplasms. Cancer 1987;60:2686–9.

13. Kubota K, Matsuzawa T, Fujiwara T, et al. Differential diagnosis of lung tumor with positron emission tomography: a prospective study. J Nucl Med 1990;31:1927–33.

14. Gupta NC, Frank AR, Dewan NA, et al. Solitary pulmonary nodules: detection of malignancy with PET with 2-[F-18]-fluoro-2-deoxy-D-glucose. Radiology 1992;184:441–4.

15. Patz EF Jr, Lowe VJ, Hoffman JM, et al. Focal pulmonary abnormalities: evaluation with F-18 fluorodeoxyglucose PET scanning. Radiology 1993;188:487–90.

16. Wahl RL, Kaminski MS, Ethier SP, Hutchins GD. The potential of 2-deoxy-2[18F]fluoro-D-glucose for the detection of tumor involvement in lymph nodes. J Nucl Med 1990;31:1831–5.

17. Wahl RL, Cody R, Hutchins G, Mudgett E. Positron emission tomographic (PET) scanning of primary and metastatic breast carcinoma with the radiolabeled glucose analog 2-[18F]-fluoro-deoxy-2-D-glucose (FDG): initial clinical evaluation. Radiology 1991;179:765–70.

18. Malenka DJ, Colice GL, Beck JR. Does the mediastinum of patients with non-small cell lung cancer require histologic staging? Further standards for computed tomography. Am Rev Respir Dis 1991;144:1134–9.

7

In Situ and Occult Lung Cancer

TRACEY L. WEIGEL, MD
JOHN R. PELLETT, MD
NAEL MARTINI, MD

Occult lung carcinomas are lesions that are not evident on routine chest roentgenography or computed tomography (CT) of the chest. These lesions are often suspected because of abnormal sputum cytology. Nearly 30 percent of patients with positive sputum cytology without roentgenographically detectable lung lesions will, however, be found to have primary cancers of the head and neck region.[1] Flexible bronchoscopy is frequently performed in an attempt to localize occult lesions. If a lesion is visualized on bronchoscopy or if bronchial brushings of a segment or sub-segment obtained on two separate examinations reveal malignant cells on both sets of brushings, the lesion is considered to have been definitively localized. Localization can be difficult—the interval between abnormal sputum cytology and bronchoscopic localization ranged from 1 to 1,014 days, with a median of 70 days, in one large series.[1] Recently, 50 patients with positive sputum cytology were screened with the white-light and autofluorescence bronchoscopy using the Xillix LIFE-Lung™ system.[2] Autofluorescence bronchoscopy increased the sensitivity of detection from 85 to 94 percent, and the number of lesions localized with the Xillix LIFE-Lung™ system was higher than historical studies employing systematic brushing of all bronchi (Figure 7–1). Surveillance using conventional white-light bronchoscopy can identify 69 percent of microinvasive endobronchial tumors, but only 29 percent of carcinomas in situ.[3] The Xillix LIFE-lung™ system has been shown to be nearly six times as sensitive as white-light bronchoscopy for identifying intraepithe-lial neoplasias including moderate or severe dysplasia or carcinoma in situ[4] (Figure 7–2).

An occult second primary must be distinguished from a local recurrence in patients with prior lung carcinomas. If an endobronchial lesion is located near, or contiguous to, the previous tumor site, it should be of different histology in order to be classified as a new lung primary. Alternatively, if the histology of the second lesion is the same as the original primary, there should be an in situ component and/or no evidence of cancer in their common

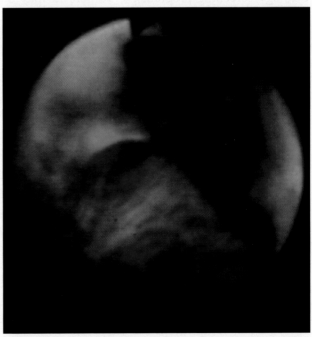

Figure 7–1. LIFE image of an in situ carcinoma (red) at the orifice of the right middle lobe.

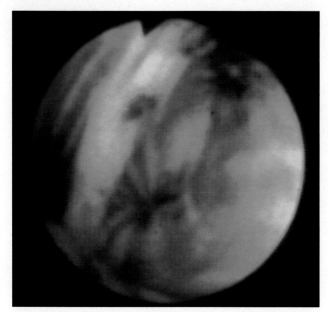

Figure 7–2.   LIFE image of three in situ carcinomas (red).

regional lymphatic drainage for it to be deemed a synchronous primary as opposed to a metastasis.[5]

TUMOR CHARACTERISTICS

Occult lung lesions are often squamous cell carcinomas identified in the context of lung cancer sputum cytology screening programs; > 90 percent may be pathologic stages 0 or I[6] (Figures 7–3 and 7–4). Even if they are of an early stage, occult lesions commonly require major resections to achieve a complete (R0) resection because of their proximal location in the tracheobronchial tree (Figure 7–5A). In addition, the risk of second primaries in patients with occult bronchogenic carcinomas is close to 4 percent per patient per year and complicates their management because patients may eventually require additional surgery. Overall 5-year survival status post-resection of an occult lung carcinoma is as high as 90 percent, but decreases to 59 percent (p < 0.01) in patients with multicentric occult lung primaries.[6]

TREATMENT

Surgical Resection

The treatment of carcinoma in situ remains controversial and varies from observation alone to resec-

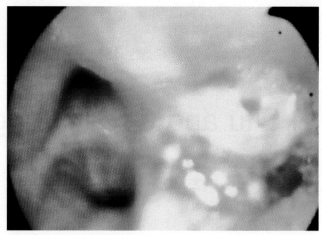

Figure 7–3.   Occult lesion in apical segment of right upper lobe.

tion, because of lack of data on the natural history of this lesion. Resection remains the "gold standard" for the treatment of invasive occult bronchogenic carcinomas based on the favorable results of three major surgical series. The largest series, comprising 127 occult lesions, resulted from a Japanese population-based lung cancer screening program that involved 57,547 person-years of cytologic screening between 1982 and 1988.[5] Ninety-three lobectomies or pneumonectomies and one segmentectomy were performed with an operative mortality of 2.1 percent. Second lung primaries occurred in 16.9 per-

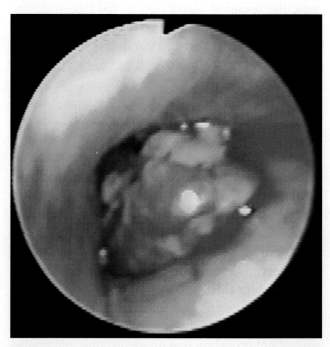

Figure 7–4.   Sputum-positive radiographically occult, right middle lobe lesion.

cent of patients. Overall 5-year survival was 80.4 percent after surgical resection versus 45 percent for patients treated with ablative or medical therapies.

The two U.S. occult lung cancer surgical series were significantly smaller than the Japanese series. Martini reported on 47 occult lung cancers treated at Memorial Sloan-Kettering Cancer Center over the 30-year period from 1947 to 1979.[7] This series began before the introduction of flexible bronchoscopy, and only 27 patients (57%) had stage I disease. Second lung primaries were identified in 15 patients (32%). Investigators at the Mayo Clinic reported on 58 occult bronchogenic carcinomas resected in 54 patients; 27 lesions were detected in the Mayo Lung Project.[1] Most of the lesions (82%) were pathologic stages 0 or I; 83 percent required a lobectomy or bilobectomy, and 17 percent a pneumonectomy; operative mortality was 5.6 percent. Second lung primaries developed in 22 percent at a rate of 5 percent per patient per year of follow-up. Overall 5-year survival after resection was 74 percent in the Mayo series.

Non-Surgical Treatment Options for Occult Non-Small Cell Lung Cancers

Occult lung carcinomas frequently arise in patients with limited pulmonary reserve or other medical comorbidities that make surgical resection prohibitive due to the magnitude of surgical resection commonly required to eradicate even early lesions. Multiple "curative" ablative treatment strategies have thus been attempted. The success of non-resectional approaches is related to the dimensions of the lesion being treated. Endobronchial squamous lesions < 3 mm thick with longitudinal axes ≤ 20 mm are almost uniformly lymph node-negative[8] and may be amenable to endobronchial ablative therapies. Electrocautery, neodymium:yttrium-aluminum-garnet (Nd:YAG) laser, photodynamic therapy, and brachytherapy have all been used to treat endobronchial lesions and will be discussed below.

Electrocautery

In 1998, van Boxem and colleagues[9] reported a prospective study of bronchoscopic electrocautery

to treat 15 occult lung cancers. All lesions were < 1 cm^2 and intraluminal on high-resolution CT. A complete response rate was achieved in 12 lesions (80%), with a median follow-up of 16 months. Two lesions required radical resections after partial response (PR) to electrosurgery, and a third partial responder was treated with photodynamic therapy followed by external beam radiotherapy. Complications were minimal and consisted of two asymptomatic stenotic segmental bronchi. Endobronchial fires[10] and fatal hemorrhage[11] have been reported, however, in patients treated with electrocautery.

Nd:YAG Laser Therapy

The Nd:YAG laser was introduced in 1980 and quickly replaced the CO_2 laser for endobronchial therapy due to its improved tissue penetration and coagulation.[12] The ability to use a flexible fiber and bronchoscope for treatment with Nd:YAG (in contrast to the rigid scope required for CO_2) made Nd:YAG therapy easier on both the patient and the physician. Inability to determine the depth or mucosal extent of occult lesions that extend across a carina or along a sidewall limit the safe use of Nd:YAG laser as a definitive treatment of proximal lesions.[13] Data on Nd:YAG laser therapy have been reported for endobronchial palliation of obstruction or bleeding, however, few prospective data exist on its use for curative therapy for early endobronchial lesions.

Photodynamic therapy

Photodynamic therapy (PDT) involves the administration of a photosensitizer that is relatively selectively retained by malignant cells. When the appropriate wavelength of light illuminates the tumor, the photosensitizer is activated—resulting in the generation of toxic, oxygen free-radicals which result in cell death. Photofrin II® (porfimer sodium) was approved by the FDA for treatment of microinvasive non-small cell lung cancers in 1998. An argon-pumped dye laser is commonly used to deliver 630 nm light, and a 1- or 2.5-cm cylindrical diffusing fiber is passed through the biopsy channel of a fiberoptic bronchoscope and either placed alongside, or used to impale, the lesion (Figure 7–5B). The resultant depth of PDT-induced necrosis is ~ 5 to 8 mm (Figure 7–5C), which is usually débrided bloodlessly with irrigation (Figure 7–5D) and biopsy forceps (Figure 7–5E) the following day at a follow-up bronchoscopy.

In 1993, Japanese investigators reported response rates of 85 to 90 percent for early tracheobronchial lesions treated with PDT.[14,15] The definitive PDT study in the United States for early endobronchial lesions was carried out at the Mayo Clinic. The goal of this study was to determine the efficacy of PDT as an alternative to surgery in patients with early-stage, roentgenographically occult, squamous cell

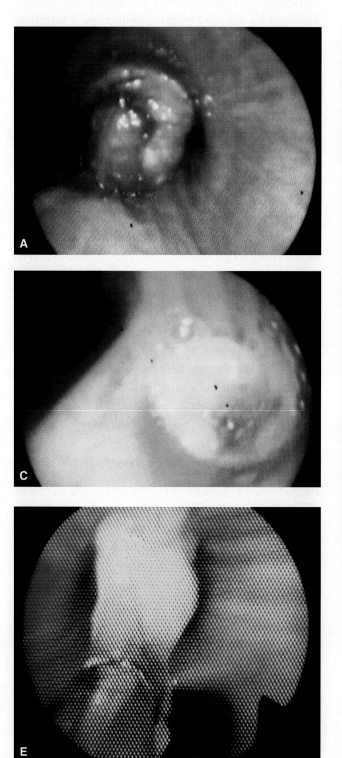

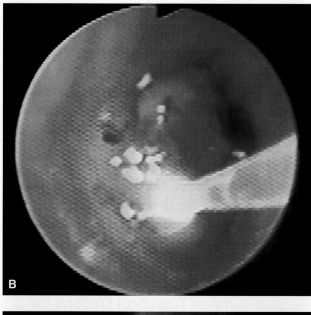

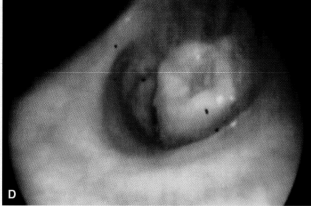

Figure 7–5. *A,* Endobronchial occult carcinoma in left mainstem bronchus (LMSB). *B,* PDT of occult LMSB carcinoma seen in *A.* *C,* Necrotic LMSB lesion, 1 day s/p PDT. *D,* Necrotic LMSB lesion 1 day after PDT and after irrigation. *E,* Bloodless debridement of LMSB lesion, 1 day s/p PDT.

carcinoma of the lung.[16] All patients in this trial were acceptable surgical candidates, and surgical resection was performed if local disease persisted after two sessions of PDT. A total of 23 cancers in 21 patients were treated in the Mayo trial, and a complete response (CR) was seen in 71 percent of patients (15/21) and was maintained longer than 12 months in 73 percent (11/15). Four patients with initial CR to PDT went on to surgical resection for local recurrence, with a 50 percent (2/4) incidence of positive regional nodes on final pathology. Four out of six patients with a partial response to PDT required surgical resection, with one patient having lymph node involvement. Two patients who developed second primaries that required surgery thus, 43 percent (9/21) of patients avoided surgery at a median follow-up of 6 years.

Subsequently, investigators at the University of Pittsburgh treated 7 patients with 10 microinvasive lesions with PDT with curative intent, and observed a complete response rate of 80 percent with no recurrences at 31 months' median follow-up.[17] All patients in this series were considered to be high-risk surgical candidates due to poor pulmonary function or other co-morbidities. Inhomogeneous light delivery and/or insufficient depth of penetration may be responsible for incomplete responses to PDT.[18]

Brachytherapy

Sutedja and colleagues[19] reported the treatment of two patients with severely diminished pulmonary reserve with T1N0 non-small cell lung carcinomas with high-dose rate brachytherapy in 1993. Iridium-192 was used to deliver 3 fractions of 10 Gy at 1 cm from the source axis. One patient died 54 months post-treatment with no evidence of disease and the second patient was disease-free at 25 months post-treatment.

High-dose rate (HDR) brachytherapy was used to treat limited endobronchial non-small cell lung carcinomas by Perol and colleagues.[20] All patients in this study had severe, chronic respiratory failure, prior surgery, or external beam radiation therapy for a previous lung cancer and an endobronchial lesion < 1 cm in diameter. Dose escalation was performed starting with 3 fractions of 7 Gy (at 1 cm from the center of the source) escalating to 5 fractions of 7

Gy. Local control was achieved in 12 out of 16 evaluable patients with 1- and 2-year actuarial survival rates of 78 percent and 58 percent, respectively, with a median survival of 28 months. Asymptomatic stenosis of the treated bronchus occurred in 10 out of 18 patients; 8 out of 12 lesions that received 5 fractions. Two patients treated with 5 fractions (35 Gy) experienced severe necrosis of the bronchial wall and hemoptysis, 4 and 6 months after HDR brachytherapy. Overall, two patients (11%) died of fatal hemoptysis at 12 and 18 months post-HDR brachytherapy. Major complications occurred in 16.5 percent, but four additional deaths of unknown causes occurred during follow-up. After employing applicators with retractable flaps (to prevent contact between the catheter and the bronchial wall), no additional cases of wall necrosis were observed. HDR brachytherapy offers a short, outpatient treatment, however the increased dose rates (compared to low-dose rate brachytherapy) may have a more marked effect on healthy tissue and represent a source of latent complications. Preliminary data suggest that HDR brachytherapy, when used in conjunction with external beam radiotherapy, may be more efficacious than HDR therapy alone.[21]

CONCLUSION

Occult lung cancers are predominantly squamous cell carcinomas that have a high incidence of multicentricity, with second primaries seen in up to 30 percent of patients. Surgical resection, usually lobectomy or pneumonectomy, remains the gold standard for treatment, with 5-year survival of up to 90 percent for early-stage disease. Although relatively uncommon, occult lung carcinomas provide a unique challenge for treatment because of their frequent proximal location, early stage, and intrinsic risk of multicentricity.

REFERENCES

1. Cortese DA, et al. Roentgenographically occult lung cancer. A ten-year experience. J Thorac Cardiovasc Surg 1983; 86:373–80.
2. Sato M, Sakurada A, Sagawa M, et al. Diagnostic results before and after introduction of autofluorescence bronchoscopy in patients suspected of having lung cancer detected by sputum cytology in lung cancer mass screening. Lung Cancer 2001;32(3):247–53.

3. Woolner LB, Fontana RS, Cortese DA, et al. Roentgeno-graphically occult lung cancer: pathologic findings and frequency of multicentricity during a 10-year period. Mayo Clin Proc 1984;59:453–66.

4. Lam S, Kennedy T, Unger M, et al. Localization of bronchial intraepithelial neoplastic lesions by fluorescence bronchoscopy. Chest 1998;113:696–702.

5. Saito Y, Sato M, Sagawa M, et al. Multicentricity in resected occult bronchogenic squamous cell carcinoma. Ann Thorac Surg 1994;57:1200–2.

6. Saito Y, Sato M, Sagawa M, et al. Multicentricity in resected occult bronchogenic squamous cell carcinoma. J Thorac Cardiovasc Surg 1992;104:401–7.

7. Martini N, Melamed M. Occult carcinomas of the lung. Ann Thorac Surg 1980;30:215–23.

8. Nagamato N, Saito Y, Ohta S, et al. Relationship of lymph node metastasis to primary tumor size and microscopic appearance of roentgenographically occult lung cancer. Am J Surg Pathol 1989;14:1009–113.

9. van Boxem TJ, Venmans BJ, Schramel FM, et al. Radiographically occult lung cancer treated with fiberoptic bronchoscopic electrocautery: A pilot study of a simple and inexpensive technique. Eur Respir J 1998;11:169–72.

10. Yankauer S. Two cases of lung tumor treated bronchoscopically. NY Med J 1992:741–2.

11. Sutedja G, van Kralingen K, Schramel F, et al. Fiberoptic bronchoscopy electrosurgery under local anesthesia for rapid palliation in patients with central airway malignancies: A preliminary report. Thorax 1994;49:1243–6.

12. Toty L, Personne C, Colchen A, et al. Bronchoscopic management of tracheal lesions using the neodymium: yttrium-aluminum-garnet laser. Thorax 1981;36:175–8.

13. Lam S. Bronchoscopic, photodynamic, and laser diagnosis and therapy of lung neoplasms. Curr Opin Pulm Med 1996;2:271–6.

14. Hayata Y, Kato H, Konaka C, et al. Photodynamic therapy (PDT) in early stage lung cancer. Lung Cancer 1993; 9:287–94.

15. Furuse K, Fukuoka M, Kato H, et al. A prospective phase II study on photodynamic therapy with photofrin II for centrally located early stage lung cancer. The Japan Lung Cancer Photodynamic Therapy Study Group. J Clin Oncol 1993;11:1852–7.

16. Cortese D, Edell E, Kinsey J. Photodynamic therapy for early stage squamous cell carcinoma of the lung. Mayo Clin Proc 1997;72:595–602.

17. Weigel T, Keenan R, Fernando H, et al. Photodynamic therapy: a curative surgical approach for early non-small cell lung carcinomas in high-risk patients. Proceedings of SPIE 3909:2000.

18. Sutedja T, Lam S, Le Riche Postmus P. Response and pattern of failure after therapy for intraluminal stage I lung cancer. J Bronchol 1994;1:295–8.

19. Sutedja G, Baris G, van Zandwijk N, et al. High-dose rate brachytherapy has a curative potential in patients with intraluminal squamous cell lung cancer. Respiration 1993;61:167–8.

20. Perol M, Caliandro R, Pommier P, et al. Curative irradiation of limited endobronchial carcinomas with high-dose rate brachytherapy: results of a pilot study. Chest 1997;111: 1417–23.

21. Saito M, Yokoyama A, Kurita Y, et al. Treatment of roentgenographically occult endobronchial carcinomas with external beam radiotherapy and intraluminal low-dose rate brachytherapy. Int J Radiat Oncol Biol Phys 1996;34:1029–35.

8

Treatment of Local and Locoregional Non-Small Cell Lung Cancer

SCOTT A. LAURIE, MD

KENNETH K. NG, MD

KENNETH ROSENZWEIG, MD

ROBERT J. GINSBERG, MD

Almost two-thirds of patients with newly diagnosed non-small cell lung cancer (NSCLC) present with local or locoregional disease. Under the 1997 revision of the International Staging System for lung cancer[1] these patients are staged as I, II, IIIA or IIIB. The more advanced locoregional-disease patients will have ipsilateral (N2) or scalene, supraclavicular, or contralateral mediastinal (N3) lymphadenopathy, and/or will present with a primary tumor which invades adjacent structures (for example, chest wall or diaphragm [T3]; esophagus, vertebral body, or heart [T4]).

For early NSCLC (stages I and II), surgery alone can produce a cure in 40 percent (stage II) to 70 percent (stage IA) of patients. In contrast, single modality therapy with either surgery or radiation therapy alone is curative for only a small minority of patients who present with stage III NSCLC. After initial therapy, a majority of patients will suffer disease recurrence; relapses are distant in two-thirds of patients and local in one-third. It has become established that multimodality treatment strategies involving varying combinations of systemic treatment (chemotherapy) with a local treatment (surgery and/or radiation), can lead to improved long-term outcomes for patients with advanced locoregional disease. With these approaches, 5-year survival of 25 percent and 15 percent in stages IIIA and IIIB, respectively, can be expected. Patients with poorer performance status, weight loss, or significant co-morbid illnesses have not been shown to benefit from this multi-

modality approach, and indeed are likely to suffer excessive toxicity. For these patients, the goals of therapy should be palliation and prolongation of life rather than cure. Although classified as stage IIIB, patients with ipsilateral malignant pleural effusions are not considered to be candidates for curative therapy, and are instead managed as patients with stage IV or metastatic disease, with palliative chemotherapy being the mainstay of treatment.

This chapter will review the current therapy of local and locoregional NSCLC. The management of completely resectable (stage I and II), potentially resectable (some patients with IIIA disease), and unresectable patients will be discussed separately. Patients with node-negative T3 tumors (stage IIB), for example with Pancoast's tumors or chest-wall invasion represent a subgroup with a distinct approach to management, and will also be considered independently (Table 8–1).

"LOCAL" DISEASE: STAGE I AND II DISEASE

Stage I and II lung cancer is afforded a reasonably good prognosis with total surgical excision. There is no evidence from randomized trials that adjuvant therapy has any real beneficial effect in this group of patients. When surgical treatment results in complete removal of the primary tumor and involved lymph nodes, there is a reasonable chance for ultimate cure.

Table 8–1. STAGING OF NON-SMALL CELL LUNG CANCER			
Current		**New 1997 Staging**	
STAGE I	T1N0M0	STAGE IA	T1N0M0
	T2N0M0	STAGE IB	T2N0M0
STAGE II	T1N1M0	STAGE IIA	T1N1M0
	T2N1M0	STAGE IIB	T2N1M0
			T3N0M0
STAGE IIIA	T3N0M0	STAGE IIIA	T1–3 N2M0
	T3N1M0		T3N1M0
	T1–3 N2M0		
STAGE IIIB	Any T N3M0	STAGE IIIB	T4 Any N M0
	T4N3M0		Any T N3M0
STAGE IV	Any T Any N M1	STAGE IV	Any T Any N M1

TNM DEFINITIONS
Primary Tumor
TX Positive malignant cell; no lesion seen
T1 < 3 cm diameter
T2 > 3 cm diameter
    Distal atelectasis
T3 Extension to pleura, chest wall diaphragm, or pericardium
    < 2 cm from carina, or total atelectasis
T4 Invasion of mediastinal organs, spine
    Malignant pleural effusion
Regional Lymph Node Involvement
N0 No involvement
N1 Ipsilateral bronchopulmonary or hilar
N2 Ipsilateral or subcarinal mediastinal
N3 Ipsilateral and contralateral supraclavicular nodes
    Contralateral mediastinal or hilar nodes
Metastatic Involvement
M0 None
M1 Metastases present

An adequate surgical resection mandates a complete excision of all disease including all involved lymphatics. Minimum requirements include extensive mediastinal lymph node sampling to identify occult N2 disease or, as we prefer, a mediastinal lymph node dissection for optimum excision and final pathologic staging. An ongoing randomized trial in North America will resolve whether lymphadenectomy is superior to lymph node sampling in these "early stages" of disease.

Despite the apparent local nature of the disease when surgery is offered, following complete resection, two-thirds of all first recurrences will be in distant sites, rather than local or regional. Whether adjuvant radiotherapy or chemotherapy, or both, improves the chances of total cure once surgical excision has been performed is a moot point. In the past 10 years, many phase II and phase III trials have assessed the role of these modalities in improving disease-free survival. Radiotherapy following surgery can improve local control. However, only one trial has ever demonstrated a prolongation of survival using radiotherapy either preoperatively or postoperatively.[2–4] Although newer combination chemotherapy treatments can yield up to a 70 percent response rate in localized non-small cell lung cancer, there have been few trials demonstrating a beneficial survival employing this treatment postoperatively.[4–7] Recent meta-analyses fail to support the use of postoperative adjuvant chemotherapy or radiotherapy.[8,9]

In most instances, the surgical resection of choice is lobectomy. In T1N0 patients, limited resections (wedge resection or segmentectomy) are reserved for compromised patients (Figures 8–1 to 8–3). In stage IB disease, because of tumor size, about 20 percent of patients will require a pneumonectomy.

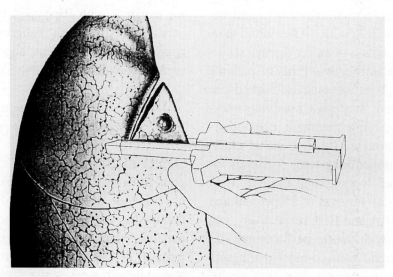

Figure 8–1.   An example of a wedge resection.

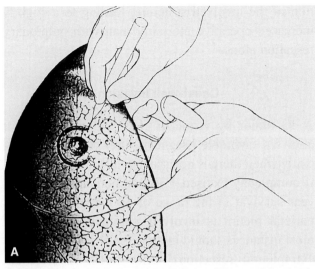
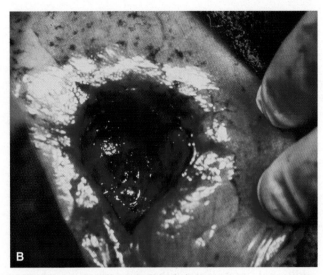

Figure 8–2. *A* and *B*, For deeper lesions, a lesser excision can be performed using a precision cautery technique.

In general, the perioperative mortality and postoperative morbidity in these early-stage tumors is very acceptable (less than 3%), but is higher following extended surgical resections, such as pneumonectomy, that may be required to remove locally advanced tumors (Figure 8–4). Selection of appropriate patients is important prior to embarking upon such operations. A complete, potentially curative resection should be anticipated. Because of the significant potential for occult metastatic disease with clinical stage II tumors, screening for such disease (bone, brain, liver, and adrenals) may be performed prior to considering surgery, although its cost-effectiveness is questionable. It is certainly not cost-effective in stage I disease. We feel that in most patients mediastinoscopy is important for complete preoperative nodal assessment, avoiding preoperatively identified N2 or N3 disease for primary surgical excision.

The indications and results of surgery are best analyzed by isolating the various T and N categories, identifying those cases that can be afforded long-

Figure 8–3. An apical segmentectomy is oncologically a more adequate limited resection.

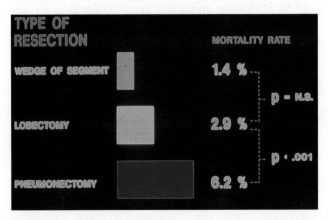

Figure 8–4. The overall mortality for the various surgical procedures as described in 1982 by the Lung Cancer Study Group. These postoperative mortality figures have not changed significantly over the past 20 years.

term survival after surgical resection, and suggesting the current role of multimodality treatment.

Stage I: T1–2 N0 Disease

In this early stage of lung cancer, complete surgical resection, usually by lobectomy, is the treatment of choice. Lesser resections (wedge, segment) yield higher local recurrence rates and are reserved for patients with compromised pulmonary function. As with other stages of resectable disease, mediastinal lymph node sampling or ipsilateral mediastinal lymph node dissection completes the surgical management. There has been no proven advantage for additional treatment—either postoperative chemotherapy or radiotherapy[10]—although randomized trials are ongoing to reexamine the question.

With newer screening techniques (low-dose spiral CT scans), very small (< 1 cm) tumors are being discovered. Studies are underway to assess limited resections for this subset (Figure 8–5).

Stage II: N1 Disease

Intrapulmonary or hilar lymph node involvement does augur a much poorer prognosis than N0 disease. Complete resection remains the treatment of choice, keeping in mind that when "sump nodes" (interlobar) are involved, a larger resection may be required, often pneumonectomy. In all instances, surgeons should attempt a complete resection of the involved lobe or lung as well as a complete ipsilateral mediastinal lymph node dissection (Figures 8–6 and 8–7). As yet, there has been no decided advantage to adjuvant therapy, although the standard practice in North America still often dictates postoperative mediastinal radiotherapy if hilar lymph nodes are involved. Recently, there has been interest in extending induction chemotherapy prior to surgery (see below) with this stage of disease when diagnosed clinically; randomized trials are ongoing to examine this approach.[11]

T3 Tumors

The curability of T3 tumors varies according to the involved site. These tumors require en-bloc resec-

tion of the involved structure, leading to a slightly increased operative mortality than with pulmonary resection alone.

Chest-Wall Invasion

A T3 tumor by virtue of chest-wall invasion still allows a favorable prognosis after resection, especially when there is no associated N1 or N2 disease. If completely excised, T3N0 tumors can yield a 5-year survival in the range of 50 percent. Once the parietal pleura is involved, complete resection in most instances should include the chest wall (versus extrapleural resection). Once nodal involvement occurs, the survival rate is much less favorable. Very few T3N2 tumors, even when completely resected, will be cured. Because of this, it is questionable whether this stage of disease, when identified preoperatively, should be considered for primary resection. A review of 334 patients with NSCLC invading the chest wall who were surgically resected at Memorial Sloan-Kettering Cancer Center revealed that a complete resection is necessary for long-term survival.[12] Five-year survival in the 175 patients who had a complete resection was 32 percent, compared to only 4 percent for those patients who had incomplete resections. In those who were completely resected, survival did decrease with increasing nodal stage: for N0 patients, 5-year survival was 49 percent; N1 patients, 27 percent; and for N2 patients, 15 percent. Independent of nodal status, the depth of invasion of the chest wall was also prognostic, with parietal pleural invasion more favorable than deeper invasion of the soft tissue or bones (Figure 8–8).

Superior Sulcus Tumors

Tumors arising in the superior pulmonary sulcus at the apex of the lung, and which invade locally to cause a syndrome of pain in the shoulder and ulnar distribution of the arm, weakness and atrophy of the intrinsic hand muscles, and ipsilateral Horner's syndrome, are termed Pancoast's tumors. The pain is due to local invasion and destruction of the lower cords of the brachial plexus and of the chest wall and

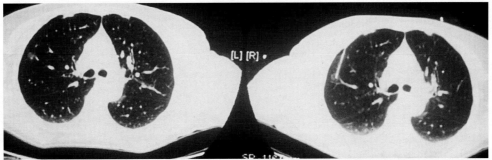

Figure 8–5. A very early lung cancer identified on CT screening (left) and proven on percutaneous needle aspiration biopsy (right). These sub-centimeter lesions may well be adequately treated by limited resections, but this requires further confirmation.

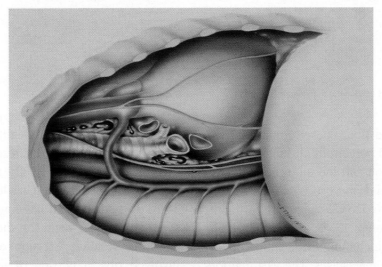

Figure 8–6. The right hemithoracic lymph nodes to be removed with complete ipsilateral mediastinal lymphadenectomy.

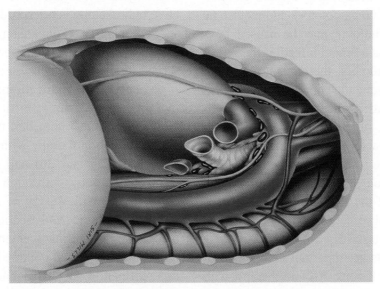

Figure 8–7. The left mediastinal lymph nodes to be removed by complete ipsilateral mediastinal lymphadenectomy.

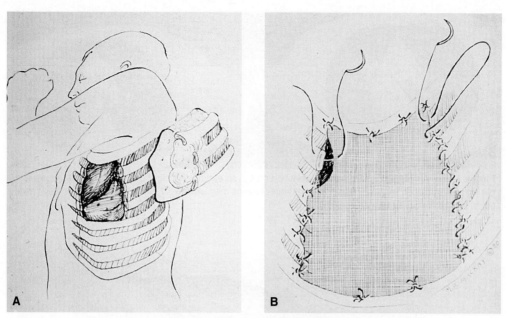

Figure 8–8.   A chest-wall tumor can be adequately excised en bloc, together with the appropriate lobectomy. The resulting chest-wall defect can be replaced by inserting a plastic prosthesis (*A* and *B*).

first, second, and third ribs. These tumors are rare, comprising less than 5 percent of all lung cancers.

Due to their location and the multiple structures (brachial plexus, subclavian vessels) which may be invaded, MRI is preferred to CT scan in assessing the extent of the lesion. Complete staging, as for all lung cancers, is required, including mediastinoscopy to assess for lymph node metastases. The vast majority of Pancoast's tumors are non-small cell lung cancers. However, tissue biopsy, usually via fine-needle aspiration, is mandatory, as occasionally this presentation may be seen in small cell carcinomas and metastatic tumors; rarely, the syndrome may be caused by a benign process, such as a fungal infection.

As these are rare tumors, there are no randomized trials to guide therapeutic choices. Management of patients with Pancoast's tumors requires the cooperation of the surgical, radiation, and medical oncologists. An important factor to determine is whether the patient is felt to be resectable. In general, invasion of the vertebral body, the subclavian artery, and the upper branches of the brachial plexus are contraindications to initial resection, as is the presence of N2 or N3 nodal metastases.

Radiation therapy is an important component of the treatment of these lesions. As sole therapy, with doses of 55 to 70 Gy, 5-year survival of 20 to 25 percent has been reported. More often, radiotherapy is used as part of a multimodality approach. Induction radiotherapy may increase resectability. Preoperative radiotherapy, to 30 to 35 Gy followed 4 to 6 weeks later by en-bloc resection has led to 5-year survival of 30 to 35 percent, and has long been considered the standard management for these tumors.[13] En-bloc resection includes excision of the chest wall and involved ribs, a portion of the lower trunk of the brachial plexus and the stellate ganglion and sympathetic chain, and a lobectomy with complete mediastinal lymph node dissection (Figure 8–9). Postoperative radiotherapy is often added if there are positive surgical margins. Comparison of the results obtained from surgical series with those from radiotherapy series is not possible because of selection bias.

It is becoming more common to use tri-modality therapy in the management of these lesions. A North American Intergroup trial has examined the use of induction therapy with cisplatin (50 mg /m^2, days 1, 8, 29, and 36) and etoposide (50 mg/m^2 intravenously, days 1 through 5 and 29 through 33), concurrently with 45 Gy of standard-fractionation radiotherapy, prior to resection in patients without mediastinal nodal involvement. This study is based on promising results obtained in a phase II trial of this regimen in stage IIIA and IIIB patients, which showed that it was safe and associated with a high response rate and resectability rate.[14] A recent report suggests a high complete-response rate at the time of surgery.[15]

A recent analysis of our own results at MSKCC suggests that a complete en-bloc resection and lobectomy can yield a 60 percent 5-year survival in completely resected patients.

Proximal Airway Involvement

In cases of tumors of the main bronchi within 2 cm of the carina—if such tumors are completely resected—the patient can certainly be afforded long-term survival. Sleeve lobectomy or pneumonectomy for tumors in this location should afford approxi-

mately a 50 percent 5-year survival if no nodal disease is present.

Diaphragmatic and Mediastinal Invasion

Complete resection of T3N0 tumors by virtue of diaphragmatic involvement without associated sub-diaphragmatic organ invasion can be carried out with minimal morbidity. However, in most cases the diaphragmatic involvement is diffuse, and a complete resection cannot be performed. Patients with mediastinal invasion, if completely resected, will be cured in about 40 percent of patients with N0 disease. Nodal disease in this

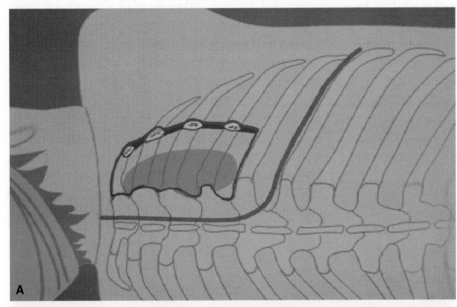

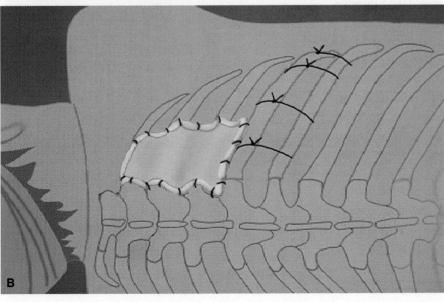

Figure 8–9. Superior sulcus tumors can be surgically removed by en-bloc resection of the involved vertebrae, chest wall, and ipsilateral lung, replacing the chest wall, when necessary, with a plastic prosthesis.

subset confers a similar poor prognosis as with other T3 tumors.

Approximately 5 percent of bronchogenic carcinomas invade the parietal pleura and soft tissues or bones of the chest wall. These tumors are usually peripheral in location, and are less likely to have spread to the hilar or mediastinal lymph nodes. Because of the rarity of this presentation, there are no randomized data regarding the multimodality management of these tumors.

The role of radiotherapy, given either pre- or postoperatively, remains controversial. In the retrospective study described above, there was no difference in outcome between those patients with a complete resection who received radiotherapy and those who did not. While some retrospective studies have suggested an improvement in local control with the addition of radiotherapy, in the absence of randomized trials, radiotherapy should be reserved for patients with positive surgical margins.

There are no data from randomized trials regarding the use of chemotherapy in node-negative patients. Patients with positive mediastinal lymph nodes should be managed with induction chemotherapy, as discussed above.

LOCOREGIONAL DISEASE:
STAGE III DISEASE

Surgery as a Single Therapeutic Modality

Some patients with locoregional (stage IIIA) disease are potential candidates for primary surgical resection; in most series, this represents no more than 20 percent of all patients presenting at this stage. There is controversy as to exactly which stage IIIA patients are resectable. Patients who are stage IIIA based on T3N1 tumors are usually resectable, and these patients have a similar outcome to those who are stage IIIA on the basis of N2 disease (5-year survival of 25 percent versus 23 percent)[1] (Figure 8–10).The results of resection in patients with N2 disease depend on whether the patient had macroscopic, clinically obvious N2 disease (ie, readily apparent mediastinal adenopathy on imaging, at bronchoscopy, or at mediastinoscopy), or if N2 disease was unsuspected and found only at the time of

thoracotomy. For example, a review of 151 patients with completely resected stage IIIA (N2) disease at the Memorial Sloan-Kettering Cancer Center[16] found that for those with subclinical, microscopic N2 disease, the 5-year survival rate approached 30 percent. In contrast, patients with clinical N2 disease had a 5-year survival rate in this series of only 8 percent, despite an apparent "complete" resection. These results are similar to those found in other surgical series of N2 patients. In general, these studies suggest that for patients who have microscopic N2 disease found incidentally at thoracotomy following negative imaging studies and mediastinoscopy, the 5-year survival is in the range of 25 percent following surgery alone. Those with clinically apparent bulky N2 disease (macroscopic disease, or with multi-level nodal involvement) do much less well with primary resection, with 5-year survival of less than 10 percent. The majority of these patients relapse with distant metastatic disease.

As a rule, patients with N3 (stage IIIB) disease do not benefit from surgery. Highly selected patients with T4 tumors, such as those with carinal or vertebral body invasion, may be resectable (Figure 8–11). However, the outcome of resection alone in those with T4 tumors is poor, with series reporting 5-year survivals of only 8 percent[17] and 12 percent.[18]

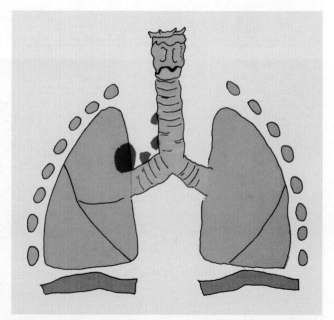

Figure 8–10. Ipsilateral N2 disease. This type of disease can be managed by combined modality therapy, with or without surgery.

Radiation as a Single Therapeutic Modality

Definitive radiotherapy has historically been employed for patients having resectable stage IIIA disease. Long-term results with radiotherapy alone appear worse than those obtained with resection, but this may reflect selection bias: patients with resectable disease who are treated with radiotherapy are often older, with underlying medical co-morbidities, and are therefore less favorable surgical candidates. There has been no head-to-head comparison of definitive radiotherapy and surgery in patients with resectable locally advanced NSCLC. Definitive radiotherapy has also been considered the only potentially curative therapy for patients having unresectable disease or for those patients with stage I and II disease who cannot tolerate a surgical resection because of concurrent medical problems.

Randomized studies have established that both local control and short-term survival are improved by increasing radiation dose, and with continuous rather than split-course treatment. Traditional management is to treat with standard 2 Gy fractions, 5 days per week, to 60 to 65 Gy. While this often results in a transient tumor response and palliation of symptoms, it only rarely leads to long-term cure, with median survival of about 1 year, and 5-year overall survival of less than 10 percent.

Given the poor results obtained with standard radiotherapy, several methods to improve outcome have been investigated. These include the use of three-dimensional conformal radiotherapy (3D-XRT), the use of altered fractionation, and the use of combinations of radiotherapy and chemotherapy. Data suggest that 3D-XRT allows an escalation of radiation dose delivered to the tumor, improving local control while remaining tolerable to normal tissues. A recent randomized trial compared continuous hyperfractionated accelerated radiotherapy (CHART) to standard radiotherapy in NSCLC.[19] The control arm in this trial received 60 Gy in 2 Gy fractions over 6 weeks, while patients assigned to CHART received 36 fractions of 1.5 Gy, given 3 times per day for 12 consecutive days, for a total of 54 Gy. The CHART arm led to an absolute improvement in 2-year survival of 9 percent (29 percent versus 20 percent), which was due to an improvement in local control.

The strategy most investigated has been the use of radiotherapy in combination with cisplatin-based chemotherapy. Studies of the combined-modality treatment have shown improved outcomes when compared to standard radiotherapy alone; this is discussed in greater detail below in the section on unresectable locoregional disease. In the curative therapy of locally advanced NSCLC, radiotherapy as a single modality is no longer considered the standard of care.

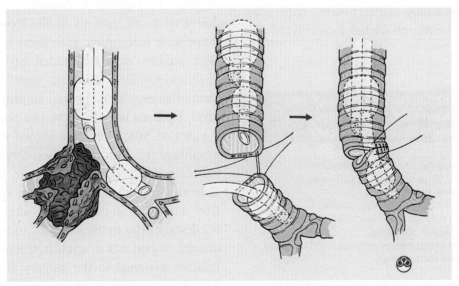

Figure 8–11. A proximal tumor encroaching on the carina which can be managed by sleeve pneumonectomy. (Illustration courtesy Dr. R. Tsuchiya.)

Multimodality Therapy of "Resectable" Disease

Preoperative (Induction) Chemotherapy

Given the poor results seen with surgery alone, a number of strategies designed to increase resectability and cure of clinically apparent N2 disease have been investigated. Of these, the use of preoperative ("induction") chemotherapy has been the most successful. Chemotherapy given before surgery has a number of theoretical advantages; these are summarized in Table 8–2.

Pilot studies of preoperative chemotherapy were developed using cisplatin-based chemotherapeutic regimens with established anti-tumor activity in patients with metastatic NSCLC. Selected phase II trials are listed in Table 8–3.[20–23] The trials listed are those in which all, or almost all, of the enrolled patients underwent surgical staging of the mediastinum to confirm N2 disease prior to the initiation of therapy. CT scanning alone is imperfect in predicting the presence of mediastinal nodal involvement, with a sensitivity and specificity of only 60 to 70 percent.

These trials showed that the response rate to chemotherapy is higher in stage III disease than it is in patients with stage IV disease, in the order of 65 percent to 70 percent. Most patients go on to surgical exploration following chemotherapy, and resectability rates are high. Further, the use of preoperative chemotherapy appears safe, with most series reporting treatment-related mortality of less than 10 percent. One trial[21] had a mortality rate of 18 percent, with four deaths seen in patients with bronchial obstruction and post-obstructive pneumonia, suggesting that caution is required when considering induction chemotherapy for patients having this presentation. Finally, a small minority of patients (roughly 10 to 15 percent) who receive preoperative chemotherapy will have no pathologic evidence of cancer in the resected specimen, and it is these patients who will enjoy the longest survival. Pisters and colleagues[24] retrospectively reviewed the outcomes of 21 patients with clinical N2 disease enrolled in the MSKCC phase II induction chemotherapy protocol 6 who achieved a pathologic complete response (pCR) after receiving mitomycin–vindesine–cisplatin chemotherapy. Patients who achieved a pCR were those who had a major radiographic response. In this group of patients, 5-year overall survival was 54 percent; in contrast, the 5-year survival for all enrolled patients was 17 percent. This highlights the importance of attainment of a pCR for long-term survival.

Two randomized phase III studies[25,26] have shown a survival advantage to the use of induction chemotherapy followed by surgical resection, as compared with resection alone. These trials are summarized in Table 8–4. The trials by Roth[26] and Rosell[25] are similar in design. In each, patients randomized to the experimental arm received three cycles of cisplatin-based chemotherapy before surgery. Postoperative thoracic radiotherapy was delivered to all patients in the Rosell trial, and to those with incomplete resections in the Roth trial. Both studies were terminated early when interim analyses revealed dramatic benefits to induction chemotherapy, with marked improvements in survival. Updated reports of the two positive trials with 7 years of follow-up have shown that the survival advantage to induction chemotherapy has been maintained.[27,28] These studies can be criticized on several points, in addition to their small size. In the Roth study, not all patients had surgically confirmed N2 disease prior to the initiation of therapy, and one-quarter of patients in each trial had T3N1 disease. Patients assigned to the surgery-alone arm on the Rosell trial had much poorer survival than would be expected. Finally, there was an imbalance in the two

Table 8–2. THEORETICAL ADVANTAGES AND DISADVANTAGES OF INDUCTION (PREOPERATIVE) CHEMOTHERAPY

Advantages
  In vivo assessment of the effect of chemotherapy
  Better drug delivery to the primary tumor, because of undisturbed vasculature
  Early treatment of subclinical micrometastases
  Shrinkage of tumor may increase resectability and increase the number of complete resections
  Better tolerability of chemotherapy preoperatively; increased delivery of planned chemotherapy
Disadvantages
  Delay in the definitive therapy if the tumor is chemoresistant
  Increased perioperative complications

Table 8-3. SELECTED PILOT STUDIES OF INDUCTION CHEMOTHERAPY FOLLOWED BY RESECTION IN STAGE IIIA NSCLC

Author	No. of Patients	Chemotherapy	Postop Radiation?	Response Rate (%)	% Surgically Explored	% Complete Resection (of those explored)	pCR Rate (%)	Median Survival (months)	3-year OS (%)	Treatment-Related Deaths (%)
Martini et al	136	MVP or MVbP x 2–3 preop	Yes, some patients	77	72	84	19	19	28	3
Burkes et al	39	MVP x 2 preop and postop	No	64	56	81	8	19	26	18
Sugarbaker et al	74	P / Vb x 2 preop and postop	Yes	88 (PR or SD)	86	37	0	16 (explored patients only)	23	7
Elias et al	34	P / 5 FU/LV x 3 preop	Yes	65	82	75	15	18	33	0

M = mitomycin; V = vindesine; Vb = vinblastine; P = cisplatin; 5FU = 5-fluorouracil; LV = leucovorin; preop = preoperatively; postop = postoperatively; OS = overall survival; PR = partial response; SD = stable disease.

Table 8-4. RANDOMIZED TRIALS OF INDUCTION CHEMOTHERAPY FOLLOWED BY RESECTION VERSUS RESECTION ALONE

Author	No. of Patients	Chemotherapy	Postoperative Radiotherapy	Median Survival (months)	3-year Overall Survival	5-year Overall Survival	P Value
Rosell et al	30	MIP x 3	50 Gy	22	20%	17%	p = 0.005
	30	—	50 Gy	10	5%	0%	
Roth et al	28	CEP x 3	66 Gy (+ margin only)	21	43%	36%	p = 0.048
	32	—	66 Gy (+ margin only)	14	19%	15%	

M = mitomycin; I = ifosfamide; P = cisplatin; E = etoposide; preop = preoperative; postop = postoperative; NR = not reported; NS = not significant.

arms of the Rosell trial in the frequency of the presence of *K RAS* mutations, a possible poor prognosis indicator. Despite these limitations, the results of these randomized trials, combined with the encouraging results from phase II studies, have established that for resectable IIIA patients, induction cisplatin-based chemotherapy for two to three cycles followed by surgery is an approach which is safe, feasible, and appears to improve survival. However, the optimal chemotherapy regimen and number of cycles needed remains unclear.

Postoperative (Adjuvant) Chemotherapy

In contrast to the number of studies examining preoperative chemotherapy, postoperative chemotherapy in locoregional disease has been much less studied. Most trials have only investigated the use of adjuvant chemotherapy in resected early-stage lung cancer. Those trials in which at least a proportion of enrolled patients had locoregional disease that had been completely resected have not shown consistent benefit.[29–31] A recent meta-analysis of 14 trials comparing surgery alone with surgery plus chemotherapy found that the use of cisplatin-containing chemotherapy in conjunction with surgery led to a small improvement in survival at 5 years of only 5 percent (95% CI, −1 to +10%).[32] Compared to induction chemotherapy, disadvantages of adjuvant chemotherapy include the lack of an effective method of monitoring for tumor response, and the decreased patient tolerance of chemotherapy given in the postoperative setting. At the present time, adjuvant chemotherapy following complete resection of locoregional disease is an acceptable strategy, but is not considered standard. For the most part, its use is confined to patients who did not receive induction chemotherapy and are found, incidentally, to have N2 disease at the time of thoracotomy. Most patients with clinical N2 disease should receive at least some of their chemotherapy prior to surgery.

Preoperative or Postoperative Radiotherapy Added to Surgery

The rationale of delivering radiotherapy prior to surgery is that shrinkage of the tumor induced by radiation will facilitate surgical resection and increase resectability rates. Early phase III trials of induction radiotherapy followed by surgery versus resection alone did not reveal any increase in resectability or benefit in terms of local control or overall survival.[33] Two studies of preoperative radiation revealed pCR rates of 5 percent and 14 percent.[33,34] In contrast to the results seen with chemotherapy-induced pCR, in these two trials there was no difference in survival between those patients who obtained a pCR and those who did not. This suggests that the attainment of a pCR by chemotherapy indicates the possibility of eradication of subclinical micrometastatic disease, an outcome that cannot be obtained with radiation, a local therapy. Given the benefit seen with induction chemotherapy, there is no role for single-modality induction radiotherapy in locoregional NSCLC.

Postoperative radiotherapy has been extensively studied. While it may lead to improvements in local control,[35] a meta-analysis of nine randomized, controlled trials comparing surgery alone with surgery followed by radiation therapy found that for the subgroup of patients with completely resected stage III, N2 disease, postoperative radiotherapy was not significantly beneficial with regard to survival.[32] Thus, at the present time, the only defined role for postoperative radiotherapy is in the setting of an incomplete resection and/or positive surgical margins. Despite this, many patients with resected N2 disease do receive postoperative radiotherapy in an attempt to decrease locoregional recurrences.

Induction Chemoradiation for Resectable Locoregional NSCLC

A number of phase II trials have investigated the use of induction chemoradiation followed by surgical resection in stage IIIA disease.[15,36,37] These trials show that the response rate to induction therapy does not appear to be significantly increased with the combined approach compared to preoperative chemotherapy alone. There may be a small increase in pCR rates, to approximately 15 to 20 percent. However, there does not appear to be a significant improvement in rates of resection over that obtained with induction chemotherapy alone, nor is there convincing evidence of improvement in survival. Induction chemoradiotherapy is more toxic than induction chemotherapy alone, with increased incidence of myelosuppression and esophagitis. Randomized, controlled trials of induction chemotherapy alone versus induction chemoradiotherapy are underway; at the current time, tri-modality therapy is not the standard of care outside a clinical trial.

Summary of Multimodality Therapy of Resectable Stage IIIA Disease

To optimize the chance for cure, suitable patients who have N2 disease documented preoperatively and who are felt to be potentially resectable should receive induction chemotherapy with a cisplatin-based regimen. The optimal number of preoperative cycles is unclear, but two to three have been the most popular in the randomized trials and in most phase II studies. An alternative, but unproven, strategy is to continue chemotherapy to maximum response, provided patient tolerance permits it. Currently, there is no clear role for the routine addition of radiotherapy in resectable locally advanced NSCLC; it should be offered postoperatively to patients who were incompletely resected. Adjuvant chemotherapy with a platinum-based regimen is an option for patients who are found to have N2 disease at the time of thoracotomy. Patients with no viable tumor seen in the resected specimen (a pathologic complete response) enjoy the greatest likelihood of long-term survival.

Future research will examine how best to combine the three modalities. Incorporation of newer, more effective chemotherapeutic agents such as docetaxel, paclitaxel, and gemcitabine into induction regimens, with the hope of improving response rates, may lead to improved outcomes. The value of surgery and radiotherapy in the multimodality treatment of resectable locoregional disease is the subject of ongoing clinical trials. Randomized trials are underway comparing preoperative chemotherapy with chemoradiotherapy. A North American Intergroup trial is assessing the value of surgical resection, randomizing patients to surgery or no surgery following induction chemoradiotherapy. A European trial examines the relative benefits of the two methods of local control: following induction chemother-

apy, patients will be randomized to undergo either resection or definitive radiotherapy. These studies will help to define the relative benefits and toxicities of each component of therapy.

Other areas of investigation include the use of altered fractionation radiotherapy, such as CHART, in combination with chemotherapy, and the role of positron emission tomography in staging of the mediastinum. Further, since a majority of patients who are rendered "free of disease" following current multimodality therapy will relapse, new adjuvant therapy strategies, such as use of immunotherapy with vaccines and biology-modifying agents, are being investigated. Tumor markers are also being developed to monitor for "minimal residual disease."

"Unresectable" Locoregional Disease

Combined Chemoradiation: Concepts

The majority of patients who present with locoregional disease are not considered candidates for surgical resection. These include patients with very bulky multi-level N2 disease, most patients with N3 disease, and all but a few selected patients with T4 disease. These patients may be suitable for combined modality treatment with chemotherapy and radiation. Several trials of induction chemotherapy followed by radiotherapy ("sequential" therapy), and of chemotherapy delivered concomitantly with radiotherapy ("concurrent" therapy), have shown improved survival over definitive radiotherapy alone. Just as combining chemotherapy with surgery has several theoretic advantages, so does the use of chemotherapy with radiotherapy (Table 8–5).

Sequential Chemoradiation

Landmark randomized trials of induction chemotherapy followed by standard radiotherapy are summarized in Table 8–6. The first trial to address this issue was published by Dillman and colleagues in 1990.[38] This trial had relatively stringent inclusion criteria, enrolling only those patients with good performance status and weight loss of less than 5 percent of body weight. Patients were randomized to receive induction chemotherapy with cisplatin (100 mg/m^2, weeks

Table 8–5. THEORETICAL ADVANTAGES AND DISADVANTAGES OF SEQUENTIAL AND CONCURRENT CHEMORADIATION

Concurrent Chemoradiation	
Advantages	Disadvantages
When delivered concurrently, chemotherapy may sensitize the tumor cells to radiation, thus improving local control There is no delay in the treatment of the primary tumor site	Increased overlapping toxicities of both modalities may preclude the use of full doses of either, thus leading to less than optimal dosing
Sequential Chemoradiation	
Advantages	Disadvantages
When delivered sequentially, chemotherapy offers early treatment of metastatic disease, and may de-bulk the tumor, increasing the effectiveness of radiation and decreasing the radiation target volume Avoidance of direct overlapping toxicities	Lack of radiosensitizing effects of chemotherapy

1 and 5) and vinblastine (5 mg/m^2, weeks 1 through 5), followed by standard radiotherapy (60 Gy in 2 Gy fractions), or to standard radiotherapy alone. A total of 155 patients were enrolled before an interim analysis led to early closure of the trial. A survival advantage to combination therapy was detected. Seven-year follow-up data[39] confirm the improvement in outcome with combined therapy: both median survival (13.7 versus 9.6 months) and 5-year overall survival (17% versus 6%) were in favor of the combined modality approach. Toxicity, such as weight loss and vomiting, while increased with the combined therapy, was manageable. A confirmatory trial performed by the Radiation Therapy Oncology Group (RTOG 88-

08)[40] has reported very similar results. This trial also had a third treatment arm of hyperfractionated radiotherapy alone that led to results that were intermediate to those obtained with dual modality therapy or with radiation alone. A trial from France[41] also showed a survival benefit to the use of chemotherapy with radiation. In this study, while the incidence of distant metastasis was significantly decreased with the use of chemotherapy, local failure occurred equally and in the vast majority of patients in both arms of the trial, thus accounting for the limited survival benefit to combined-modality therapy.

There have been trials of cisplatin-based sequential chemoradiation which have not shown an advan-

Table 8–6. SELECTED RANDOMIZED TRIALS OF SEQUENTIAL PLATINUM-BASED CHEMORADIATION VERSUS RADIOTHERAPY ALONE

Author	No. of Patients	Chemotherapy	Radiotherapy	Median Survival (months)	2-year OS (%)	5-year OS (%)	P Value	Comments
Dillman et al	78	Vb/ P x 2	60 Gy	13.8	26	17	p = 0.012	Vomiting, infections and weight loss more common with combined therapy; no deaths due to treatment in either arm
	77	—	60 Gy	9.7	13	6		
Sause et al	151	Vb/ P x 2	60 Gy	13.8	31	8	p = 0.04 (CT / RT versus RT alone)	4 deaths on CT/RT arm were felt to be due to treatment Severe esophagitis more likely with BID RT
	149	—	60 Gy	11.4	20	5		
	152	—	69.6 Gy (1.2 Gy BID)	12.3	24	6		
Le Chevalier et al	176	VCyPC x 3 pre- and post-RT	65 Gy	12	21	6	p = 0.02	Distant metastases rate decreased in combined arm: 67 vs. 45% (p < 0.001) Local control at 1 year: 17% and 15%
	177	—	65 Gy	10	14	3		

Vb = vinblastine; P = cisplatin; V = vindesine; Cy = cyclophosphamide; C = CCNU; CT = chemotherapy; RT = radiotherapy; OS = overall survival.

tage to combined-modality therapy. For the most part, these trials have been small, enrolling less than 100 patients, and may have lacked the statistical power to detect a difference in outcome between the two arms.

Concurrent Chemoradiation

Selected randomized trials of concurrent chemoradiation are summarized in Table 8–7. In most of these studies, chemotherapy consisted of a platinum compound given as a single agent. The most widely quoted is that of Schaake-Koning and colleagues,[42] who reported a three-arm trial comparing 55 Gy of split-course radiotherapy alone, with the same radiation administered concurrently with the same total dose of cisplatin given either weekly or daily. A significant improvement in survival was seen in the daily, concurrent chemoradiation arm compared with the radiation-alone arm, with 3-year survival rates of 16 percent versus 2 percent. Local control was improved in the combined-modality arm, but there was no difference in the rate of development of distant metastases. Toxicity, mainly nausea and vomiting, was increased in the concurrent arm, but was tolerable. However, as can be seen in Table 8–7, other trials of single-agent cisplatin or carboplatin given concurrently with radiotherapy did not show a survival benefit.[43–46]

Trials of both sequential and concurrent chemoradiation have led to conflicting results regarding the benefits of combining chemotherapy and radiotherapy. However, meta-analyses of trials comparing radiation alone to cisplatin-based chemoradiation for locoregional disease have confirmed the survival benefit of combined modality therapy. The Non-Small Cell Lung Cancer Cooperative Group analyzed 11 randomized trials using cisplatin-based chemotherapy and found a 13 percent reduction in the risk of death, corresponding to an absolute improvement in overall survival at 5 years of 2 percent.[20] The second meta-analysis found that the addition of chemotherapy to radiation increased the median survival duration of these patients by 2 months.[47] The importance of radiotherapy was confirmed in a Japanese trial that randomized patients to platinum-based combination chemotherapy with or without conventional thoracic radiation.[48] Three-year survival was 29 percent in the combined-modality group, but only 3 percent in the chemotherapy-only arm, underscoring that radiotherapy is a necessary component of the management of locally advanced NSCLC.

The preferred strategy of combining chemotherapy with radiotherapy remains unresolved. It seems that the two approaches may lead to improvements in outcome through different mechanisms. Induction

Author	No. of Patients	Chemotherapy	Radiotherapy	Median Survival (months)	2-year OS (%)	5-year OS (%)	P Value	Comments
Schaake-Koning et al	108	—	55 Gy, split	NR	13	2	p = 0.009	Increased nausea and
	98	P weekly on RT	55 Gy, split	NR	19	13	(RT vs RT	vomiting in those
	102	P daily on RT	55 Gy, split	NR	26	16	with daily P)	assigned chemotherapy
						(3-yr)		
Blanke et al	111	—	60–65 Gy	10.6	13	2	p = NS	Increased nausea and vomiting,
	104	P x 3 (q 3 weeks)	60–65 Gy	9.9	18	5		leukopenia, and esophagitis in the combined therapy arm
Trovo et al	83	—	45 Gy	10.3	17	NR	p = NS	Increased nausea and vomiting,
	84	P daily on RT	45 Gy	10	20	NR		and severity of esophagitis in the combined therapy arm
Soresi et al	50	—	50 Gy	11	6	2	p = 0.02 (3-year)	Decreased local relapse in the combined arm: 27 vs. 46%;
	45	P weekly on RT	50 Gy	16	24 (3-year)	11	p = 0.07 (5-year)	p < 0.04
Clamon et al	120	Induction P/Vb	60 Gy	13.5	26	10	p = NS	Increased hematologic toxicity
	130	Induction P/Vb; C weekly on RT	60 Gy	13.4	29	13 (4-yr)		in concurrent therapy arm; other toxicities similar

Table 8–7. SELECTED TRIALS OF CONCURRENT CISPLATIN-BASED CHEMORADIATION VERSUS RADIOTHERAPY ALONE

P = cisplatin; Vb = vinblastine; C = carboplatin; OS = overall survival; RT = radiotherapy; NS = not significant; NR = not reported.

chemotherapy, through administration of full doses of active agents, leads to a reduction in distant metastases. Concurrent chemoradiation results in improved local control, due to the radiosensitizing effects of low-dose chemotherapy, but no decrease in the rates of distant failure. The meta-analyses discussed above could not detect a variation in outcome with the two different approaches. One recently published trial from Japan has addressed this issue.[49] A total of 314 patients were randomized to receive two cycles of chemotherapy with mitomycin, vindesine, and cisplatin, with either sequential or concurrent radiotherapy. The radiotherapy dose was 56 Gy in each arm, but was given in the concurrent arm as a split course, in order to minimize the potential toxicities of full doses of chemotherapy and radiation given concurrently. This study found that the response rate was increased in the concurrent arm, and there was also a 3-month improvement in median survival (16.5 months versus 13.3 months, $p = 0.04$). Five-year survival was likewise increased: 16 percent versus 9 percent. The concurrent strategy resulted in more myelosuppression, but was otherwise no more toxic than sequential administration. In this trial, there were no differences in sites of recurrence. This trial suggests that the administration of full-dose chemotherapy concurrent with thoracic irradiation may be the strategy that leads to the best outcome. Further trials of this approach are underway.

Some may argue that the survival benefit of combined chemoradiation (2% at 5 years) is too modest to justify the added toxicity and expense. However, because NSCLC is so common, even small improvements in survival will impact large numbers of patients. In the United States in 1998, approximately 140,000 cases of NSCLC were diagnosed, of which 40,000 cases were stage IIIA or IIIB. A 2 percent increase in survival means an additional 800 people will be alive 5 years from the time of their diagnosis. Further, an economic analysis of combined-modality therapy has suggested that it is cost-effective.[50]

Summary of Therapy for Unresectable Locoregional Disease

Medically suitable patients with unresectable locally advanced NSCLC should receive platinum-based

combination chemotherapy combined with definitive thoracic radiotherapy. There is a greater body of published evidence that sequential chemoradiation leads to superior outcomes over radiation alone. Ongoing trials will help to determine whether concurrent therapy leads to superior outcomes compared with induction chemotherapy followed by radiation. At the present time, either strategy is acceptable, although concurrent therapy is obviously more toxic.

A logical step in the evolution of therapy of unresectable locally advanced NSCLC is to combine the sequential and concurrent approaches. This involves giving two or more cycles of induction chemotherapy, followed by further cycles of the same agents given at lower doses concurrently with radiotherapy. This, theoretically, would combine the benefits of the two treatment strategies, both attacking distant metastases and leading to improvements in local control. Studies of this approach are underway.

Ongoing studies are incorporating newer chemotherapeutic agents into the induction regimens, while others are examining the use of those newer agents that possess radiosensitizing properties, such as the taxanes, concurrent with radiotherapy. Several trials are comparing various platinum-based induction regimens, to assess for differences in effectiveness and toxicity. Given the results of RTOG 88-08, which reported that hyperfractionated radiotherapy alone led to results which were intermediate to those obtained with standard radiotherapy and chemoradiation, trials are evaluating the role of altered fractionation radiotherapy in combined modality treatment. For example, one cooperative group is performing a randomized trial of induction chemotherapy with carboplatin and paclitaxel followed by either standard thoracic radiotherapy or hyperfractionated radiotherapy of 57.6 Gy in 16 days. These and other trials will help to determine the optimal method of combining these two modalities of therapy.

CONCLUSION

In local (stage I and II) disease, complete surgical resection is the treatment of choice. Adjuvant therapies have been disappointing. Induction chemotherapy is being investigated in all but T1N0 tumors. In

T3N0 tumors, the role of combined modality therapy continues to be investigated. With modern techniques, the postoperative morbidity and mortality from surgical resection is quite acceptable (see Figure 8–11).

Combined-modality therapy has led to improved outcomes for patients with locoregional NSCLC. These patients can represent a therapeutic challenge for physicians. Close cooperation between surgical, radiation, and medical oncologists is necessary for optimal management. A major issue to be determined early in the assessment is whether the patient is medically suitable for an attempt at curative therapy. Age alone is not a contraindication to an aggressive approach; rather it is the patient's performance status and the presence or absence of co-morbid illnesses which will determine suitability. Initial workup of these patients requires careful staging, with particular attention paid to the status of the mediastinal lymph nodes. For those in whom curative therapy is the goal, surgical assessment of the mediastinum should be undertaken. CT scanning alone should not be relied upon to decide on nodal status, as it has known limitations; it remains to be determined whether PET scanning will be sufficiently sensitive and specific to replace mediastinoscopy.

For fit patients, the most important distinction is whether the disease is potentially resectable, a decision which should be made by the surgeon. Resectable patients with N2 disease should receive induction platinum-based chemotherapy with or without radiotherapy followed by resection. If resection is incomplete or if surgical margins are positive, then postoperative radiotherapy should be given. Patients who are deemed unresectable should receive cisplatin-based chemoradiation: either the sequential or concurrent strategy is equally acceptable at the present time. Patients who are not suitable for a combined-modality approach, because of poor performance status or underlying co-morbid illnesses, are usually treated with definitive radiotherapy as a sole modality.

Whenever possible, these patients should be enrolled in clinical trials. Trials of newer chemotherapeutic agents and new radiation techniques will help lead to treatment approaches which may improve outcome. For those who complete definitive therapy, trials of strategies to decrease recurrence, such as vaccine therapies or new biology-modifying agents, are anticipated. In this group of patients, smoking cessation is mandatory. In those who are fortunate to be cured, careful surveillance for the development of other smoking-related malignancies is indicated. A common cause of death in those who survive one NSCLC is the development of a second lung cancer. Chemoprevention agents are needed in this population; trials of differentiating agents are ongoing.

REFERENCES

1. Mountain CF. Revisions in the International System for Staging Lung Cancer. Chest 1997;111:1710–7.
2. The Lung Cancer Study Group. Effects of postoperative mediastinal radiation on completely resected stage II and stage III epidermoid cancer of the lung. N Engl J Med 1986;315:1377–81.
3. Ladd T, Rubinstein L, and Sadeghi A. The Lung Cancer Study Group. The benefit of adjuvant treatment for resected local advanced non-small cell lung cancer. J Clin Oncol 1988;6:9–17.
4. Postoperative therapy in non-small cell lung cancer: systematic review and meta-analysis of individual patient data from nine randomized controlled trials. PORT meta-analysis Trialists Group. Lancet 1998;352:257–63.
5. The Ludwig Lung Cancer Study Group. Patterns of failure in patients with resected stage I and II non-small cell carcinoma of lung. Ann Surg 1987;205:67–71.
6. Feld R, Rubinstein L, Thomas PA. The Lung Cancer Study Group. Adjuvant chemotherapy with cyclophosphamide, doxorubicin and cisplatin in patients with completely resected stage I non-small cell lung cancer. J Natl Cancer Inst 1993;85:2990–306.
7. Holmes EC, Gail M. The Lung Cancer Study Group. Surgical adjuvant therapy for stage II and stage III adenocarcinoma and large-cell undifferentiated carcinoma. J Clin Oncol 1986;4:710–5.
8. Non-Small Cell Lung Cancer Collaborative Group. Chemotherapy in non-small cell lung cancer: a meta-analysis using updated data on individual patients from 52 randomized clinical trials. BMJ 1995;311:899–909.
9. VanHoutte P. Postoperative radiotherapy for lung cancer. Lung Cancer 1991;7:57–64.
10. Ginsberg RJ, Rubinstein LV. Lung Cancer Study Group. Randomized trial of lobectomy versus limited resection for T1 N0 non-small cell lung cancer. Ann Thorac Surg 1995;60:615–23.
11. Pisters KMW, Ginsberg RJ, Bunn PA, et al (for the Bimodality Lung Oncology Team [BLOT]). Induction chemotherapy prior to surgery for early stage lung cancer—a novel approach. J Thorac Cardiovasc Surg 2000;119:429–39.
12. Downey RJ, Martini N, Rusch VW, et al. Extent of chest wall invasion and survival in patients with lung cancer. Ann Thorac Surg 1999;68:188–93.
13. Shaw RR, Paulson DL, Kee JL. Treatment of the superior sul-

cus tumor by irradiation followed by resection. Ann Surg 1961;154:29–40.

14. Albain KS, Rusch VW, Crowley JJ, et al. Concurrent cis-platin/etoposide plus chest radiotherapy followed by surgery for stages IIIA(N2) and IIIB non-small cell lung cancer: Mature results of southwest oncology group phase II study 8805. J Clin Oncol 1995;13:1880–92.

15. Rusch VW, Giroux DJ, Kraut MJ, et al. Induction chemoradiation and surgical resection for non-small cell lung carcinomas of the superior sulcus: initial results of Southwest Oncology Group Trial 9416 (Intergroup Trial 0160).

16. Martini N, Flehinger B, Zaman M, Beattie E. Results of resection in non-oat cell carcinoma of the lung with mediastinal lymph node metastases. Ann Surg 1983;198:386–97.

17. Naruke T, Goya T, Tsuchiya R, Suemasu K. Prognosis and survival in resected lung carcinoma based on the new international staging system. J Thorac Cardiovasc Surg 1988;96:440–7.

18. Martini N, Yellin A, Ginsberg RJ, et al. Management of non-small cell lung cancer with direct mediastinal involvement. Ann Thorac Surg 1994;58:1447–51.

19. Saunders M, Dische S, Barrett A, et al. Continuous hyper-fractionated accelerated radiotherapy (CHART) versus conventional radiotherapy in non-small cell lung cancer: a randomised multicentre trial. Lancet 1997;350:161–5.

20. Martini N, Kris MG, Flehinger BJ, et al. Preoperative chemotherapy for stage IIIa (N2) lung cancer: the Memorial Sloan-Kettering experience with 136 patients. Ann Thorac Surg 1993;55:1365–74.

21. Burkes RL, Ginsberg RJ, Shepherd FA, et al. Induction chemotherapy with mitomycin, vindesine, and cisplatin for stage III unresectable non-small cell lung cancer: results of the Toronto phase II trial. J Clin Oncol 1992;10:580–6.

22. Sugarbaker DJ, Herndon J, Kohman LJ, et al. Results of Cancer and Leukemia Group B Protocol 8935. A multiinstitutional phase II trimodality trial for stage IIA (N2) non-small cell lung cancer. Cancer and Leukemia Group B Thoracic Surgery Group. J Thorac Cardiovasc Surg 1995; 109:473–83.

23. Elias A, Skarin A, Leong T, et al. Neoadjuvant therapy for surgically staged IIIA N2 non-small cell lung cancer. Lung Cancer 1997;17:147.

24. Pisters KMP, Kris MG, Gralla RJ, et al. Pathologic complete response in advanced non-small cell lung cancer following preoperative chemotherapy: implications for the design of future non-small cell lung cancer combined modality trials. J Clin Oncol 1993;11:1757–62.

25. Rosell R, Gomez-Codina J, Camps C, et al. A randomized trial comparing preoperative chemotherapy plus surgery with surgery alone in patients with non-small cell lung cancer. N Engl J Med 1994;330:153–8.

26. Roth JA, Fosella F, Komaki R, et al. A randomized trial comparing perioperative chemotherapy and surgery with surgery alone in resectable stage IIIa non-small cell lung cancer. J Natl Cancer Inst 1994;86:673–80.

27. Roth JA, Neely Atkinson E, Fossella F, et al. Long-term follow-up of patients enrolled in a randomized trial comparing perioperative chemotherapy and surgery with surgery alone in resectable stage IIIA non-small cell lung cancer. Lung Cancer 1998;21:1–6.

28. Rosell R, Gomez-Codina J, Camps C, et al. Preresectional chemotherapy in stage IIIA non-small cell lung cancer: a 7-year assessment of a randomized controlled trial. Lung Cancer 1999;47:7–14.

29. Pisters KMW, Kris MG, Hilaris B, et al. Randomized trial of postoperative vindesine and cisplatin in patients with stage III (T1-3N2M0) non-small cell lung cancer. In: Salmon SE, ed. Adjuvant Therapy of Cancer VII. 1993. p.118–24.

30. Holmes EC, Gail M, Group TLCS. Surgical adjuvant therapy for stage II and stage III adenocarcinoma and large cell undifferentiated carcinoma. J Clin Oncol 1986;4:710–5.

31. Ohta M, Tsuchiya R, Shimoyama M, et al. Adjuvant chemotherapy for completely resected stage III non-small cell lung cancer. J Thorac Cardiovasc Surg 1993;106:703–8.

32. Non-Small Cell Lung Cancer Collaborative Group. Chemotherapy in non-small cell lung cancer: a meta-analysis using updated data on individual patients from randomised clinical trials. BMJ 1995;311:899–909.

33. Shields TW, Higgins GA, Lawton R, et al. Preoperative X-ray therapy as an adjuvant in the treatment of bronchogenic carcinoma. J Thorac Cardiovasc Surg 1970;59:49–61.

34. Bromley LL, Szur L. Combined radiotherapy and resection for carcinoma of the bronchus. Lancet 1955:937–41.

35. Weisenburger TH, Gail M, Group LCS. Effects of postoperative mediastinal irradiation on completely resected stage II and stage III epidermoid cancer of the lung. N Engl J Med 1986;315:1377–81.

36. Strauss GM, Herndon JE, Sherman DD, et al. Neoadjuvant chemotherapy and radiotherapy followed by surgery in stage IIIA non-small cell carcinoma of the lung: report of a Cancer and Leukemia Group B phase II study. J Clin Oncol 1992;10:1237–44.

37. Faber LP, Kittle CF, Warren WH, et al. Preoperative chemotherapy and irradiation for stage III non-small cell lung cancer. Ann Thorac Surg 1989;47:669–77.

38. Dillman R, Seagren S, Propert K, et al. A randomized trial of induction chemotherapy plus high-dose radiation versus radiation alone in stage III non-small cell lung cancer. N Engl J Med 1990;323:940–5.

39. Dillman RO, Herndon J, Seagren SL, et al. Improved survival in stage III non-small cell lung cancer: seven-year follow-up Cancer and Leukemia Group B (CALGB) 8433 trial. J Natl Cancer Inst 1996;88:1210–5.

40. Sause WT, Scott C, Taylor S, et al. Radiation Therapy Oncology Group (RTOG) 88-08 and Eastern Cooperative Oncology group (ECOG) 4588: Preliminary results of a phase III trial in regionally advanced, unresectable non-small cell lung cancer. J Natl Cancer Inst 1995;87:3.

41. Le Chevalier T, Arriagada R, Quoix E, et al. Radiotherapy alone versus combined chemotherapy and radiotherapy in nonresectable non-small cell lung cancer: first analysis of a randomized trial in 353 patients. J Natl Cancer Inst 1991;83:417–23.

42. Schaake-Koning C, Van Den Bogaert W, Dalesio O, et al. Effects of concomitant cisplatin and radiotherapy on inoperable non-small cell lung cancer. N Engl J Med 1992;326:524–30.

43. Soresi E, Clerici M, Grilli R, et al. A randomized clinical trial comparing radiation therapy v. radiation therapy plus CIS-dichlorodiammine platinum (II) in the treatment of

locally advanced non-small cell lung cancer. Semin Oncol 1988;15(Suppl 7):20–5.

44. Clamon G, Herndon J, Copper R, et al. Radiosensitization with carboplatin for patients with unresectable stage III non-small cell lung cancer: a phase III trial of the Cancer and Leukemia Group B and the Eastern Cooperative Oncology Group. J Clin Oncol 1999;17:4–11.

45. Trovo MG, Minatel E, Franchin G, et al. Radiotherapy versus radiotherapy enhanced by cisplatin in stage III non-small cell lung cancer. Int J Radiat Oncol Biol Phys 1992;24: 11–5.

46. Blanke C, Ansari R, Mantravadi R, et al. Phase III trial of thoracic irradiation with or without cisplatin for locally advanced unresectable non-small cell lung cancer: a Hoosier Oncology Group protocol. J Clin Oncol 1995;13:1425–9.

47. Pritchard RS, Anthony SP. Chemotherapy plus radiotherapy compared with radiotherapy alone in the treatment of locally advanced, unresectable, non-small cell lung cancer. A meta-analysis. Ann Intern Med 1996;125:723–9.

48. Kubota K, Furuse K, Kawahara M, et al. Role of radiotherapy in combined modality treatment of locally advanced non-small cell lung cancer. J Clin Oncol 1994;12:8.

49. Furuse K, Fukuoka M, Kawahara M, et al. Phase III study of concurrent versus sequential thoracic radiotherapy in combination with mitomycin, vindesine and cisplatin in unresectable stage III non-small cell lung cancer. J Clin Oncol 1999;17:2692–9.

50. Evans WK, Will BP, Berthelot J-M, Earle CC. The cost of combined modality interventions for stage III non-small cell lung cancer. J Clin Oncol 1997;15.

9

Follow-Up After
Lung Cancer Resection

ROBERT J. DOWNEY, MD

The treatment of choice for localized non-small cell carcinoma is complete resection, with or without chemoradiation therapy. Unfortunately, even after an apparently complete resection, a substantial number of patients will suffer recurrences (Figures 9–1 to 9–10). Careful follow-up may allow for earlier detection and hence earlier, and possibly more effective, management of recurrent disease. Close postoperative follow-up may also provide other benefits

to both patient and doctor, for example, allowing early detection of second primary malignancies in a population at risk, or by enabling better management of non-malignant medical problems often coexisting in this patient population, as well as providing physicians with feedback on the effectiveness and complications of their therapies (Figures 9–11 to 9–21). In this chapter, we will review the types and patterns of recurrence, the methods available to detect recurrence, and review the debate over the benefits that may be possible of ongoing surveillance by close follow-up after apparently curative lung cancer resection.

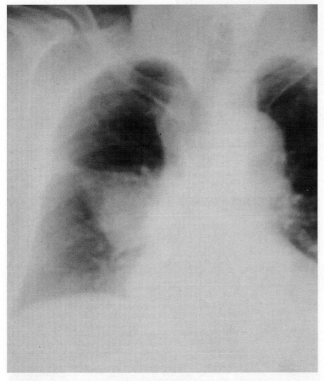

Figure 9–1. Patient A: Chest radiograph of a primary lung cancer (T2N1) in an 82-year-old female, apparently completely resected by lobectomy.

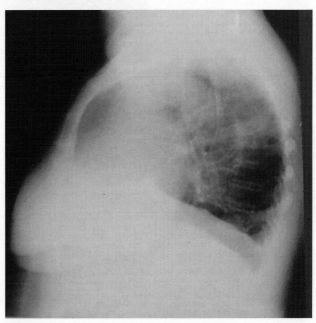

Figure 9–2. Patient A: Lateral chest radiograph 24 months after resection without evidence for disease.

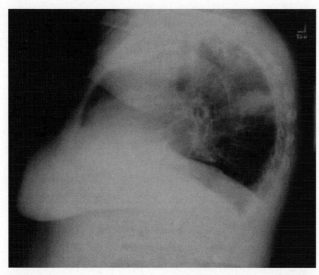

Figure 9–3. Patient A: Lateral chest radiograph 30 months after resection with new posterior mass.

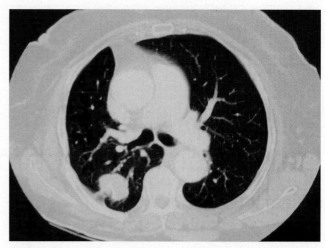

Figure 9–4. Patient A: Thoracic CT scan demonstrating mass enveloping staple line, representing locoregional recurrence. Mass was resected in continuity with chest wall, and patient is without evidence of disease.

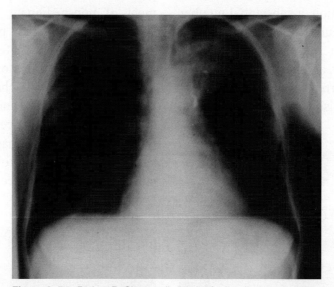

Figure 9–5. Patient B: Chest radiograph of a locally recurrent lung cancer after apparent complete resection by left upper lobectomy.

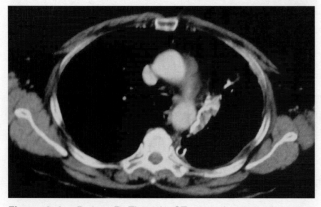

Figure 9–6. Patient B: Thoracic CT scan demonstrating mass enveloping staple line, representing locoregional recurrence.

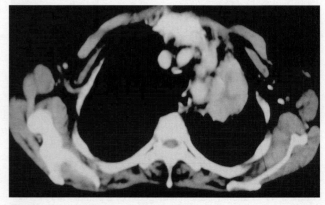

Figure 9–7. Patient B: Thoracic CT scan demonstrating superior extent of mass, abutting aorta and other great vessels.

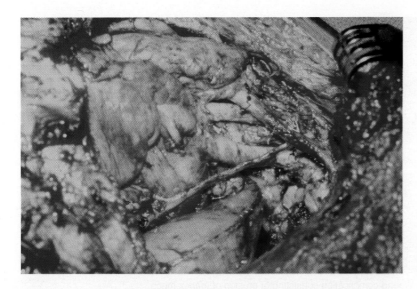

Figure 9–8. Patient B: Operative photograph after apparent complete resection of mass from mediastinal structures, including arch of aorta and great vessels.

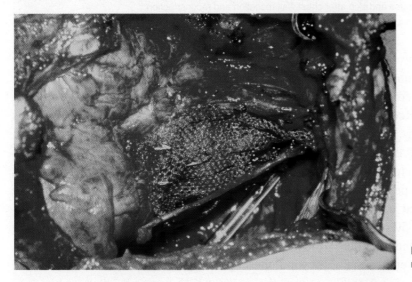

Figure 9–9. Patient B: Operative photograph after resection and placement of brachytherapy seeds.

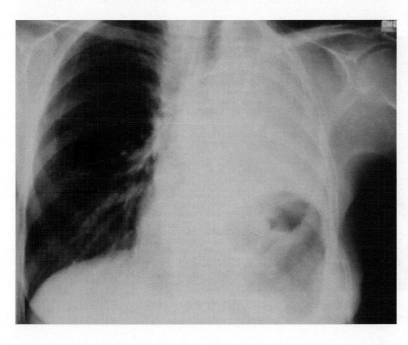

Figure 9–10. Patient B: Follow-up chest radiograph 2 years after resection of locoregional recurrence.

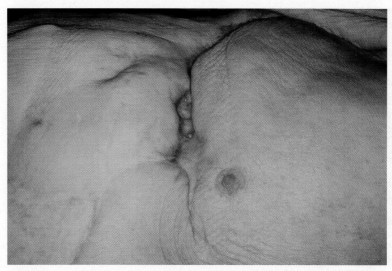

Figure 9–11. Patient C: Wound complication consisting of erosion of marlex mesh through subcutaneous tissues and skin after chest wall resection and reconstruction.

Currently, each year, approximately 170,000 patients will be diagnosed with primary lung cancer in the United States,[1] of who only 25 percent will undergo resection with curative intent. Recurrence after an apparently complete resection may be either locoregional, distant, or both, and will develop over the following 5 years in approximately 20 to 30 percent of patients with stage I disease, 50 percent of those with stage II, and 70 to 80 percent of those with stage III disease.[2] It is estimated that 50 percent of recurrences will occur in the first and second postoperative year, and 90 percent by the end of the fifth year; subsequently, patients are at risk for the development of new primary lung malignancies, which occur at rates of 1 to 3 percent per year. Once recurrent lung cancer is diagnosed, prognosis is poor, with 2-year survival estimates for stage I, II, and III lung cancer of 37 percent, 20 percent, and 14 percent, respectively. Local recurrence is defined as recurrence within the soft tissues of the same hemithorax or the bronchial stump; regional recurrence occurs in the draining lymphatics involving the mediastinum and neck, and distant disease is that beyond these confines. The rate of isolated local

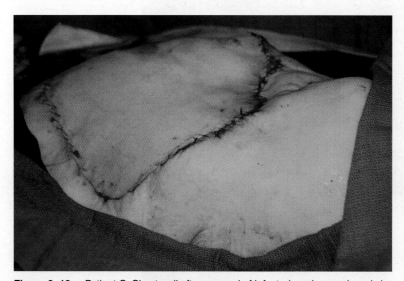

Figure 9–12. Patient C: Chest wall after removal of infected marlex mesh and closure of chest wall defect with rotation skin flaps.

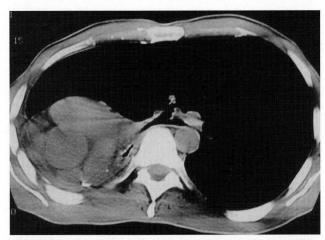

Figure 9–13. Patient D: Following right pneumonectomy, rotation of mediastinal structures into the empty right pleural cavity led to compression of the left main bronchus over the vertebral bodies and respiratory insufficiency.

recurrence for completely resected stage I tumors is 10 to 30 percent over 3 to 5 years,[3,4,5] for stage II, 30 percent, and for stage III, 40 percent.[4] For all stages, approximately two-thirds of patients will recur first in distant sites (most commonly the brain, bone, liver, and adrenal glands).

There is, unfortunately, little published information available to guide us in setting up a schedule for monitoring the completely resected patient. Ideally,

a plan would allow follow-up that is both sensitive and specific in detecting recurrent disease while minimizing costs, and not overly burdensome for either medical personnel or patients. In the Division of Thoracic Surgery at Memorial Sloan-Kettering Cancer Center[6] our practice of following patients after resection of a primary lung malignancy has evolved without either prospective or retrospective evaluation as to effectiveness, and is as follows: After postoperative recovery, and if the patient does not develop subsequent problems, an office visit is scheduled every 3 months for the first year, every 4 months for the second, every 6 months for the third and fourth, and yearly thereafter. At each office visit, a careful interval history is obtained. The patient is queried about the presence or absence of symptoms suggestive of recurrent or new malignant lung disease, including new or recurrent chest wall pain, new persistent cough (generally present for 4 weeks without signs or symptoms associated with infection), hemoptysis, new wheezing, new hoarseness, weight loss and/or anorexia (suspicious for liver metastases), new neurologic symptoms such as unsteadiness, speech disorders, or seizures, or unrelenting and progressive skeletal pain suggestive of osseous metastases. Physical examination is

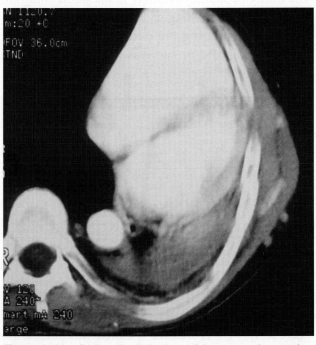

Figure 9–14. Patient E: Following left-lung resection, patient developed symptomatic left-lung herniation into the left chest wall.

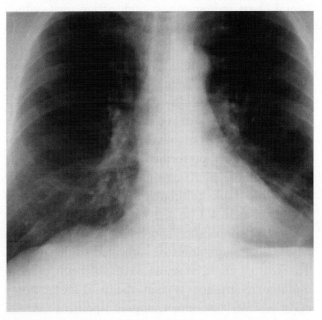

Figure 9–15. Patient F: Following left pneumonectomy for bronchoalveolar carcinoma, patient developed multiple nodules within the subcutaneous tissues of the chest wall due to malignant implants in the incision.

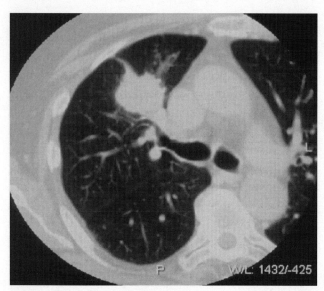

Figure 9–16. Patient G: Right upper lobe mass suspicious for primary lung carcinoma.

directed at probable sites of recurrence, specifically, palpation for adenopathy in the supraclavicular fossae, auscultation of the lung, to detect any changes (especially localized wheezing), palpation of the upper abdomen (primarily to assess the liver), and inspection of the wound. Further examination is guided by symptoms elicited by the history.

Radiologic surveillance for the asymptomatic patient is currently limited to a posteroanterior and lateral chest radiograph at each office visit, which has proven reliable in detecting locoregional recurrences with an almost 80 percent sensitivity rate.[7,8] The ordering of additional imaging studies, such as thoracic CT scans, bone scans, brain imaging, or PET scans, is guided by changes in the chest radiograph, physical exam, or symptoms.

As yet not investigated is the use of serial thoracic CT scans performed on the asymptomatic patient without significant changes on postoperative chest radiographs (although it must be noted that a single thoracic CT in the asymptomatic patient 6 months or more after surgery is very useful as a baseline should studies be indicated in the future). The reason that CT scans have not been used to monitor recurrence is that the post-thoracotomy chest always has abnormalities apparent on CT scans that could be interpreted as recurrence, but that most often can only be definitively established as such by reoperative thoracotomy. Abnormalities

that rise to the level of detection on chest radiographs have been far more likely to warrant further investigation, most often by some combination of thoracic CT imaging or PET scans, followed by tissue confirmation, most often by a radiographically guided needle biopsy. The recent report from the Early Lung Cancer Action Project[9] suggests that low-radiation-dose spiral CT may be able to detect lung cancer at an early stage in patients without a prior history of malignancy but at risk for developing lung cancer. It remains to be seen whether a modification of such a protocol could be used to improve monitoring of patients after an apparently complete lung cancer resection.

Blood tests such as serum calcium, alkaline phosphatase, and serum glutamic oxalate transaminase, among others, can be elevated in patients with recurrences in the bone or liver. The physicians at Memorial Sloan-Kettering Cancer Center have not found these tests helpful, but their utility has not been explored systematically. Measurement of carcinoembryonic antigen (CEA) has been of use in following for recurrence—if the test was elevated prior to surgery, and then returned to normal after resection. Otherwise, no consistent marker for non-small cell lung carcinoma has been found.

Sputum cytologies are not routinely obtained. The utility of sputum cytology in mass screenings of patients at risk for lung cancer was explored in the United States during the period of 1974 to 1984, without a significant survival benefit being found

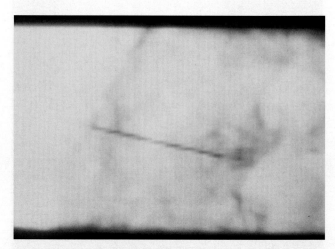

Figure 9–17. Patient G: Fine-needle aspiration of right upper lobe mass diagnosed adenocarcinoma of the lung; patient underwent a complete resection by right upper lobectomy.

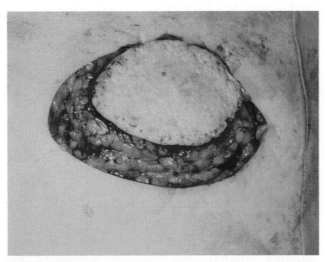

Figure 9–18. Patient G: Three months after lobectomy, a mass developed at the site of the needle biopsy, and was resected.

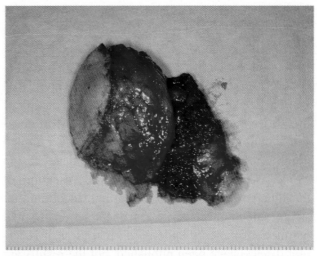

Figure 9–20. Patient G: Pathology specimen of the full-thickness chest wall resection specimen for needle-track implant.

for patients with "early" detection of disease. Currently, a multicenter trial, utilizing more recently developed antibodies that may act to improve the accuracy of cytologic examination of expectorated sputum, is underway under the auspices of the Lung Cancer Early Detection Working Group with accrual-to-date of over 50 percent of the target. There is no proven utility of the use of sputum cytology to detect recurrence, with the possible exception of the ability to detect second primary cancers in patients who presented with their first malignancy with hemoptysis, who presented with squamous cell carcinoma detected on bronchoscopy, or who had radiographically occult carcinomas.[10]

Serial bronchoscopy in the asymptomatic patient does not appear to be indicated. Surveillance bronchoscopy is generally reserved for those patients with tumors resected close to a bronchial margin (eg, sleeve resections), for patients known to have bronchial mucosa with either severe dysplasia or carcinoma in situ, and, possibly, for patients with multiple prior aerodigestive squamous cell malignancies. Bronchoscopy is indicated for the patient with a new persistent cough (after the postoperative period) or a persistent local wheeze, or any patient with hemoptysis.

This pattern of follow-up is similar to those at other major institutions,[11,12] but is considerably less

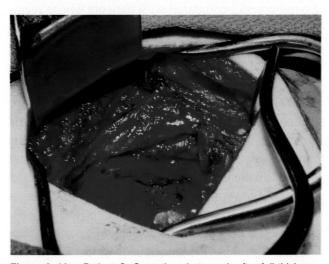

Figure 9–19. Patient G: Operative photograph after full-thickness resection of needle-track implant.

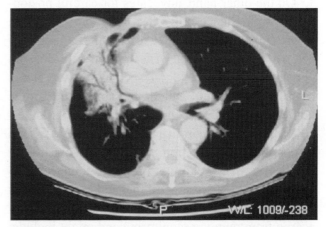

Figure 9–21. Patient G: Thoracic CT after full-thickness chest wall resection for needle-track implant and postoperative radiation. Patient remained without evidence for recurrent disease in the right lung and chest wall, but subsequently died of distant metastases.

intensive than that practiced by others, most notably in Japan.[13] American physicians do follow patients closely after resection, less because of a belief in the likelihood of curative resection of recurrent disease,[14] than for a desire to "please patients, avoid malpractice suits, and [to] improve patient quality of life."[15] Reoperation for recurrence is only an occasional option, but one likely to benefit only a limited number of patients. Beattie and colleagues, in 1954,[16] reported the first successful resection of locally recurrent disease, by a carinal resection after a right pneumonectomy. Subsequent series of small numbers of patients undergoing resection of recurrent disease have been published, but the results are not encouraging. Dartevelle and Khalife[17] and Kulka and colleagues[18] report a total of 46 patients with a median survival of only 12 months after apparent complete resections of recurrent disease. Conversely, series examining the percentage of patients with recurrences that are amenable to reoperation suggest that the number is limited. Walsh and colleagues[7] retrospectively reviewed 358 consecutive patients undergoing apparent complete lung cancer resections at M.D. Anderson Cancer Center over 14 years; 135 patients developed recurrences, of which 40 received treatment with curative intent (resection or radiation therapy > 50 cGy). In this study, detection of asymptomatic recurrences did not appear to improve survival. Similarly, Varela and colleagues[19] suggested that of 27 patients with recurrences detected during careful follow-up, only one underwent surgery with curative intent.

On the other hand, advocates for careful postoperative surveillance programs argue that a program of careful surveillance after resection of a lung cancer may have other benefits beyond affording an opportunity for curative re-resection of locoregional disease. These could include the ability to institute non-curative medical therapies, such as chemotherapy, or potentially curative radiation therapy as soon as possible post-resection, to either prolong life, or sustain a level of quality of life for as long as possible (or both). Others suggest that additional benefits not directly related to the original malignancy may accrue from ongoing monitoring and might include: improved management of non-oncologic medical problems; detection of new primary malignancies in

a population at heightened risk; the opportunity to allay fears about symptoms or physical findings wrongly interpreted by the patient or family as suggesting recurrent disease; and provision to the surgeon with feedback on the effectiveness of surgical management.

In their paper, *Follow-up in lung cancer,* Younes and colleagues[20] provide a retrospective analysis of 130 patients with apparent complete resection of non-small cell lung cancer followed by either a "strict" protocol (consisting of a schedule of office visits, imaging studies, and blood tests—even if the patient is asymptomatic) or clinical visits and radiographic studies, not formally scheduled but arranged only the basis of the patient detecting either worrisome symptoms or new physical findings ("symptom" group). The regimen that the "strict" group was asked to follow consisted of clinical interviews and physical exams with chest radiographs every 2 months for 6 months, then interviews and exams every 3 months for the next 18 months with chest radiographs and thoracic CT scans alternately being obtained. The authors found no statistical significance in median survival following diagnosis of recurrent disease between the two groups. This study can be criticized for such problems as the lack of explanation as to how these non-randomized patients were assigned to the "strict" and "symptom" groups. As well, the authors assessed only follow-up performed within the first 2 years after resection. The paper does not provide information on the survival of patients with recurrences detected and treated while asymptomatic, compared with patients whose recurrences were detected by the onset of symptoms. In contrast, the study by Walsh and colleagues[7] suggested that the median survival of patients with recurrences treated while asymptomatic was 34 months, while the survival of patients treated when symptomatic was 19 months. However, Younes and colleagues[20] made the important discovery that the "strict" surveillance group appeared to have better overall medical care with fewer emergency room visits, and fewer inpatient days required for management of their non-oncologic medical problems, raising questions as to whether benefits other than potentially curative management of recurrent disease may arise from close management of a group of patients who often have co-morbidities, such as COPD or atherosclerotic disease. In the era of cost-containment, this will require testing in well-designed prospective studies.

CONCLUSION

In the absence of better published data, a clinician setting up a follow-up program for a patient with a completely resected lung cancer can tailor the program to the available resources of the institution, the capabilities of the various physicians following the patient, and the patient's desires. No program can, at this time, be demonstrated as superior. However, even if the likelihood of detecting a recurrence at a time when it is likely to be surgically resectable is low, and the benefits of initiating medical therapies when the patient is asymptomatic are unclear, other than for cost implications, it is difficult to argue against interval clinical interviews, physical exams, and chest radiographs, rather than no follow-up at all, given probable benefits of improved medical care in a group of patients likely to have significant medical co-morbidities, and the psychological needs of patients at risk for recurrent disease. In the current environment of cost-containment, there is clearly a need for well-designed prospective trials investigating the benefits of follow-up after surgical management of lung cancer.

REFERENCES

1. Greenlee RT, Hill-Harmon MB, Murray T, Thun M. Cancer Statistics. 2001. CA Cancer J Clin 2001;51:15–36.
2. Martini N. Surgical treatment of non-small cell lung cancer by stage. Semin Surg Oncol 1990;6:248–54.
3. Martini N, Bains MS, Burt ME, et al. Incidence of local recurrence and secondary primary tumors in resected stage I lung cancer. J Thorac Cardiovasc Surg 1995;109:120–9.
4. Feld R, Rubinstein LV, Weisenberger TM. The Lung Cancer Study Group. Sites of recurrence in resected stage I non-small cell lung cancer: a guide for future studies. J Clin Oncol 1984;2:1352–8.
5. The Ludwig Lung Cancer Study Group. Patterns of failure in patients with resected stage I or II non-small cell carcinoma of the lung. Ann Surg 1987;205:67–71.
6. Downey RJ, Martini N, Ginsberg RJ. Bronchogenic carcinoma. In: Johnson FE, Virgo KS, editors. Cancer patient follow-up. St. Louis: Mosby; 1997. p. 226–30.
7. Walsh GL, O'Connor M, Willis KM, et al. Is follow-up of lung cancer patients following resection medically indicated and effective? Ann Thorac Surg 1996;60:1563–72.
8. Gorich J, Beyer-Enke SA, Flentje M, et al. Evaluation of recurrent bronchogenic carcinoma by computed tomography. Clin Imaging 1990;13:131–7.
9. Henschke CI, McCauley DI, Yankelevitz DF, et al. Early Lung Cancer Action Project: overall design and findings from baseline screening. Lancet 1999;354:99–105.
10. Tockman MS, Erozan YS, Gupta P, et al. The early detection of second primary lung cancers by sputum immunostaining. LCEWDG Investigators. Lung Cancer Early Detection Group. Chest 1994;106(6 Suppl):385S–90S.
11. Johnkoski JA, Wood DE. Bronchogenic carcinoma: University of Washington Medical Center counterpoint. In: Johnson FE, Virgo KS, editors. Cancer patient follow-up. St. Louis: Mosby; 1997. p. 233–7.
12. Urshel JD. Bronchogenic carcinoma: Roswell Park Cancer Institute counterpoint. In: Johnson FE, Virgo KS, editors. Cancer patient follow-up. St. Louis: Mosby; 1997. p. 232.
13. Ichinose Y. Bronchogenic carcinoma: National Kyushu Cancer Center counterpoint. In: Johnson FE, Virgo KS, editors. Cancer patient follow-up. St. Louis: Mosby; 1997. p. 230–2.
14. Virgo KS, Naunheim KS, Coplin MA, Johnson FE. Lung cancer follow-up: motivation of thoracic surgeons. Chest 1998;114:1519–34.
15. Naunheim KS, Virgo KS, Coplin MA, Johnson FE. Clinical surveillance testing after lung cancer surgery. Ann Thorac Surg 1995;60:1612–6.
16. Beattie EJ Jr, Davis C Jr, O'Kane C, Friedberg SA. Surgical intervention in recurrent bronchogenic carcinoma. JAMA 1954;155:835–7.
17. Dartevelle P, Khalife J. Surgical approach to local recurrence and the secondary primary lesion. In: Delarue NC, Eschapanese H, editors. International trends in general thoracic surgery. Vol 1. Philadelphia: WB Saunders Company; 1985. p. 156–63.
18. Kulka F, Kostic S. Surgical alternatives in episilateral recurrence of bronchogenic carcinoma. Eur J Cardiothorac Surg 1988;2:430–2.
19. Varela G, Jiminez M, Hernandez-Mezquita M. Follow-up patients with non-small cell pulmonary cancer undergoing complete resection. Should surgeons be in charge? Arch Bronchopneumonol 1998;34:14–6.
20. Younes RN, Gross JL, Deheinzelin D. Follow-up in lung cancer: how often and for what purpose? Chest 1999;115:1494–9.

10

Advances in the Treatment of Metastatic Non-Small Cell Lung Cancer

VINCENT A. MILLER, MD
CHRISTOPHER G. AZZOLI, MD

BACKGROUND

Lung cancer continues to be the most lethal malignant tumor, annually killing more women than breast, ovary, and uterine cancer combined, and taking nearly four times as many lives as prostate cancer in men. Over 160,000 cases of lung cancer are diagnosed in the United States each year. Of these, three-quarters will be of the non-small cell lung carcinoma (NSCLC) phenotype, and about 60 percent of these patients have advanced disease, incurable with surgery or radiation.[1] Recent meta-analyses have shown that cisplatin-based, combination chemotherapy for patients with advanced NSCLC improves median survival by 2 months and 1-year survival proportion by 10 to 15 percent.[2] Similarly, such chemotherapy has been shown to improve quality of life and to be cost-effective.[3] Systemic chemotherapy is now considered to have an important role in the treatment of advanced NSCLC, so long as the patient is functionally independent, and has no critical metastases. If the patient has critical metastases, we follow the algorithm displayed in Figure 10–1.

Historically, cisplatin was combined with etoposide, ifosfamide, mitomycin, vinblastine or vindesine in the treatment of NSCLC. Triplet combinations of these older drugs achieved response rates as high as 40 percent in phase III trials, with median survivals centering around 7 months, and reaching as high as 9 months.[4] In the past decade, a number of new agents—docetaxel, gemcitabine, irinotecan, paclitaxel, tirapazamine, and vinorelbine—have been identified as useful in this disease. The availability of these new drugs not only increases the potential for monotherapy, but also allows for approximately 70 new two-drug, and more than one hundred new three-drug combinations which could be studied in NSCLC, not considering variations in drug dosing and scheduling (Table 10–1). As the list of potential chemotherapeutic alternatives grows, it is becoming more important to incorporate cost-effectiveness and quality-of-life assessments into trials in order to provide additional criteria to distinguish between the various therapies. When considering which combinations to study, an investigator must weigh whether the combination is likely to improve at least one of a number of study endpoints when compared to a standard therapy (Table 10–2).

FIRST LINE CHEMOTHERAPY— SINGLE AGENTS

Of the new agents, docetaxel, gemcitabine, paclitaxel, and vinorelbine are considered active as single agents, based on the results of completed phase II and phase III clinical trials powered to detect a response rate of 20 percent with a type I error of 5 percent.[5] A number of recent randomized trials have compared these drugs as single agents to best supportive care with promising results (Table 10–3). Despite this, the use of single-agent chemotherapy in the treatment of advanced NSCLC is discouraged,

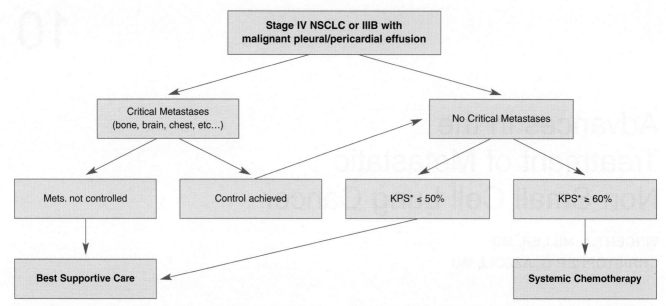

Figure 10–1. Algorithm for the treatment of advanced NSCLC. Mets. = metastases. KPS* = Karnofsky performance status: ≤ 50%: "Patient requires considerable assistance and frequent medical care." ≥ 60%: "Patient requires occasional assistance, but is able to care for most of his needs." (Karnofsky, 1948.)

due to the higher response rates and survival times observed with combination regimens.

Docetaxel (Taxotere®) is a semisynthetic taxane derived from the precursor 10-deacetylbaccatin III. Its mechanism of action is similar to that of its sister drug, paclitaxel, namely the promotion of microtubule assembly and inhibition of the depolymerization of tubulin, which stabilizes microtubules. However, subtle differences in mechanism of action exist and may explain some clinical differences observed between the taxanes (Table 10–4). The dose-limiting toxicity of docetaxel is neutropenia. Non-hematologic side effects include mucositis, asthenia, rash, alope-

cia, infusion-related reactions, and peripheral neuropathy. Notably, longer infusions were associated with an increased incidence of mucositis. Based on phase I trials, the recommended phase II dose was 100 mg/m² given as a 1-hour infusion every 3 weeks. Dexamethasone is given orally, 8 mg every 12 hours for 5 doses, beginning 24 hours prior to administration of the chemotherapy, to prevent allergic reactions to the drug and minimize side effects such as nausea, asthenia, or edema. In phase II trials, a pooled major objective response rate of 26 percent was observed with a median survival of 10 months for this single agent (Table 10–5). Observed response rates were slightly lower at lower doses, 60 and 75 mg/m², with no apparent difference in survival. A recent phase III study randomized 207 patients with advanced disease to receive docetaxel (100 mg/m²) versus best supportive care. The response rate to chemotherapy was

Table 10–1. POSSIBLE COMBINATIONS OF ACTIVE AGENTS FOR THE TREATMENT OF ADVANCED NSCLC*

42	2-drug platinum-containing combinations
70	3-drug platinum-containing combinations
30	2-drug non-platinum-containing combinations
40	3-drug non-platinum-containing combinations

*Assuming no combination will contain 2 members of the same drug class:

2	Platinum analogues:	carboplatin, cisplatin
1	Antineoplastic antibiotic:	mitomycin
1	Alkylating agent:	ifosfamide
1	Bioreductive agent:	tirapazamine
1	Pyrimidine analogue:	gemcitabine
2	Taxanes:	paclitaxel, docetaxel
1	Topoisomerase I inhibitor:	irinotecan
3	Vinca alkaloids:	vindesine, vinblastine, vinorelbine

Table 10–2. STUDY ENDPOINTS TO CONSIDER WHEN EVALUATING NEW CHEMOTHERAPY REGIMENS

Potential Benefit	Likelihood of Demonstrable Benefit		
Efficacy	High	Intermediate	Low
Toxicity	High	Intermediate	Low
Quality of life	High	Intermediate	Low
Tolerability	High	Intermediate	Low
Ease of administration	High	Intermediate	Low
Cost	High	Intermediate	Low

Table 10–3. RECENT RANDOMIZED TRIALS OF SINGLE-AGENT CHEMOTHERAPY VERSUS BEST SUPPORTIVE CARE IN ADVANCED NSCLC				
Investigator	Drug (dose, mg/m^2)	N	RR (%)	Median Survival (mos.)
Anderson, 1997[67]	Gemcitabine (1000, d 1,8,15; q28 d.)	299	17	5.6 vs. 5.9 (NS)
ELVIS*, 1999[16]	Vinorelbine (30, d 1,8; q21 d.)	154	20	7.0 vs. 5.2 (p = 0.03)
Roszkowski, 2000[6]	Docetaxel (100; q21 d.)	207	13	6.0 vs. 5.7 (p = 0.03)
Ranson, 2000[14]	Paclitaxel (200 / 3 hrs.; q21 d.)	157	16	6.8 vs. 4.8 (p=0.04)

*Elderly Lung Cancer Vinorelbine Italian Study Group.
N = number of patients; RR = response rate.

around 13 percent. The docetaxel-treated patients lived longer (2-year survival of 12% versus 0%) and also enjoyed a quality-of-life benefit.[6]

Gemcitabine (Gemzar®) (2'2'difluorodeoxycytidine) is a fluorine-substituted cytarabine (ara-C) analogue. Like cytarabine, it is a pro-drug requiring intracellular phosphorylation. But unlike cytarabine, gemcitabine has greater membrane permeability and enzyme affinity. The incorporation of the phosphorylated gemcitabine into DNA appears to be the major mechanism by which gemcitabine causes cell death. Gemcitabine also acts both as an inhibitor of ribonucleotide reductase and as a chain terminator. Because of gemcitabine's inherent ability to inhibit DNA replication and repair, this drug is an attractive candidate for combination with drugs that damage DNA.

Data from phase I trials demonstrate important schedule-dependent differences in gemcitabine toxicity.[7,8] Studies employing frequent drug administration (daily x 5 or twice weekly) led to a higher incidence of non-hematologic side effects including flu-like symptoms (fever, malaise, headache).[9] The most commonly employed dose and schedule in NSCLC patients in phase II trials has been a weekly 30-minute infusion of 800 to 1,250 mg/m^2 for 3 weeks, followed by a 1-week rest period (see Table 10–5). Side effects such as peripheral edema, asthenia, and malaise are mild and easily managed with this schedule. Grade 4 hematologic side effects occur in less than 1 percent of patients. Rarely, pulmonary toxicity and microangiopathic hemolytic anemia are seen.[10,11] A randomized phase II study compared single-agent gemcitabine at the 1,000 mg/m^2 weekly dose with standard cisplatin/etoposide combination chemotherapy in 147 chemotherapy-naïve patients

and documented equivalent activity; there were fewer side effects with the single agent (response rate 17.9% and 15.3%, median survival time 6.6 and 7.6 months, respectively [p = NS]).[12]

Given the mild adverse side-effect profile, dose escalation studies in chemotherapy-naïve NSCLC patients sought to better define the phase II single-agent dose on the weekly schedule. Weekly doses up to 2,400 mg/m^2 were safely given with a response rate of 25 percent in 32 assessable patients, and a projected median survival of 12 months.[13] Dose-limiting toxicities were reversible transaminase elevation and myelosuppression. In general, however, use of this higher dose is not recommended, due to a lack of reproducible clinical benefit.

Paclitaxel (Taxol®) is a plant-derived antineoplastic agent initially isolated from the bark of the Pacific yew tree, *Taxus brevifolia*. Paclitaxel entered clinical trials in the early 1980s and the dose-limiting toxicity was determined to be neutropenia. Other toxicities included infusion-related reactions, alopecia, peripheral neuropathy, mucositis, and myalgias/arthralgias. The recommended dose of paclitaxel for phase II

Table 10–4. MECHANISM OF ACTION—DOCETAXEL VERSUS PACLITAXEL		
Parameter	Docetaxel	Paclitaxel
Relative binding affinity for β-tubulin	1.9	1.0
Binding sites for β-tubulin	τ	N-terminal, 31 amino acids
Relative depolymerization inhibition	2.0	1.0
Mitotic structure affected	Centrosome	Mitotic spindle
Changes in protofilament numbers	none	12, rather than 13
Cell cycle specificity	S-phase	G$_2$/M phase

Table 10–5. REPRESENTATIVE PHASE II/III TRIALS OF SINGLE AGENT CHEMOTHERAPY IN ADVANCED NSCLC

Drug	No. Trials (Ph. II/III)	Dose Range (mg/m²)	N (total)	Pooled RR (%)	Median Survival (mos.)
Docetaxel[6,53,68–72]	7 (6/1)	60–100/1–3 hrs q3w	376	21	7
Gemcitabine[73–76]	4 (4/0)	800–1250 d1,8,15 q4w	393	20	8
Vinorelbine[46,77–80]	5 (3/2)	25–30 qw	697	20	8
Paclitaxel[14,81–87]	7 (6/1)	135–250/1–24hrs	313	21	8
Irinotecan[19,88–91]	5 (5/0)	100–350 qw	242	26	8

N = number of patients; RR = response rate.

study ranged from 135 to 250 mg/m² with infusion duration ranging from 3 to 24 hours every 3 weeks. A number of phase II trials of paclitaxel have been conducted in previously untreated NSCLC patients, the results of which are summarized in Table 10–5. These trials provide no definite conclusions regarding the optimal length of infusion. Shorter infusion times result in more neurotoxicity, but less neutropenia. There is a suggestion that doses < 200 mg/m² over 3 hours may be associated with lower response rates. A recently published, randomized phase III trial compared paclitaxel versus best supportive care in 157 patients with advanced NSCLC.[14] Paclitaxel was administered at a dose of 200 mg/m² intravenously over 3 hours every 3 weeks with dexamethasone premedication (20 mg orally 12 and 6 hours prior to paclitaxel), as well as cimetidine (300 mg) and diphenhydramine (50 mg) premedications. Patients treated with paclitaxel showed improvements in survival (6.8 versus 4.8 months, p = 0.037) and functional activity score, justifying its use as a single agent in the first-line therapy of advanced disease.

Vinorelbine (Navelbine®) is a semi-synthetic vinca alkaloid approved in the United States as a single agent, or in combination with cisplatin, for the treatment of NSCLC. The compound was created by a modification in the catharanthine (rather than the vindoline) ring which appears to be responsible for a favorable toxicity and activity profile. Neutropenia is the most frequent toxic effect of vinorelbine and is dose-limiting, occurring more frequently than with vinblastine or vindesine.[15] Cumulative neurotoxicity may limit its use, especially in patients with a pre-existing neuropathy. Phase II studies have generally employed a schedule of 30 mg/m² weekly as intravenous push given over 6 to 10 minutes. Response rates range from 12 to 29 percent with median survival times of 7 to 9 months (see Table 10–5).

Recently, a randomized trial in elderly patients with NSCLC demonstrated a survival benefit of single-agent vinorelbine over best supportive care.[16]

Irinotecan (Camptosar®, CPT-11) is a semi-synthetic derivative of the plant product, camptothecin, which inhibits the enzyme topoisomerase I. Topoisomerase I causes reversible, single-strand breaks in DNA, allowing the helical molecule to rotate open and participate in DNA replication. Thus, irinotecan effectively blocks DNA replication by inhibiting the activity of this enzyme. Phase I trials revealed the dose-limiting toxicities to be leukopenia and diarrhea, and the recommended phase II dose was 100 mg/m² weekly.[17] Several phase II trials have documented response rates ranging between 13 and 32 percent.[18] One such trial treated 73 patients with inoperable or metastatic NSCLC with 100 mg/m² weekly with dose adjustment based on the leukocyte count on the day of re-treatment.[19] Twenty-three of 72 evaluable patients achieved a partial response (32%); no complete responses were observed. Grade 3 or 4 leukopenia was seen in 25 percent and grade 3 or 4 diarrhea occurred in 21 percent. The incidence and severity of diarrhea did not correlate with the total dose administered and loperamide was not routinely employed. The median response duration was 15 weeks and the median survival was 42 weeks. Results of several phase II trials (see Table 10–5) justify randomized studies of irinotecan as a single agent as well as in combination therapy.

Tirapazamine (Tirazone, WIN 59075; SR 4233; 3-amino-1,2,4-benzotriazine-1, 4-dioxide) is the lead compound in a new class of bio-reductive anticancer drugs, the benzotriazine di-N-oxides, characterized by their preferential cytotoxicity for hypoxic cells. Human solid tumors are commonly composed of a significant proportion of cells with low oxygen levels. While this decreases the efficacy of DNA alkylating agents such as cisplatin, the hypoxic conditions allow tirapazamine to undergo one-electron reduction and conversion into a free radical species that produces lethal DNA strand breaks. Tirapazamine is synergistic with cisplatin both in vitro and in vivo. Preclinical studies have also demonstrated that tirapazamine may enhance the cytotoxicity of radiation.[20,21]

The initial phase I trial of single-agent tirapazamine in patients with advanced solid tumors defined the dose-limiting toxicity to be acute, reversible tinnitus and hearing loss at 450 mg/m^2.[22] Muscle cramping and vomiting were also noted. Following phase I trials of the combination of tirapazamine and cisplatin, a phase II/III dose of tirapazamine = 390 mg/m^2, and cisplatin = 75 mg/m^2 (every 3 weeks), was selected because of higher incidences of nausea/vomiting and renal insufficiency observed with the cisplatin dose of 100 mg/m^2. The phase II trials demonstrated response rates ranging from 23 percent to 26 percent.[23–25] The toxicity of the combination was not substantially increased over cisplatin alone, and little myelosuppression occurred. A phase III, multicenter trial comparing the cisplatin/tirapazamine combination to cisplatin alone demonstrated a significantly higher response rate and longer median survival for patients receiving the combination, thus confirming the advantage of the combination.[26] A pilot trial with the addition of paclitaxel to the combination has been completed, and a three-drug regimen (carboplatin, paclitaxel, tirapazamine) will be studied in a phase III trial in the Southwest Oncology Group (SWOG).

FIRST LINE CHEMOTHERAPY— COMBINATIONS

With the availability of new, somewhat less toxic agents with diverse mechanisms of action, the opportunity to develop novel, more tolerable and effective combinations is intriguing. Historically, combination chemotherapy with traditional agents improves response rate at the expense of increased toxicity, and commonly without improving survival.[27–31] To date, this has also proven to be the case with the newer drugs in platinum-containing combinations. Nevertheless, many new regimens are now available for first-line therapy, with efficacy comparable to the best results achieved by traditional chemotherapy, increasing the number of viable treatment options for

patients with advanced disease. The most widely tested regimens are discussed below.

Platinum-Taxane Combinations

Phase I trials combining cisplatin (75 mg/m^2) with paclitaxel as a 24-hour infusion found neutropenia to be dose-limiting. With the routine use of filgrastim (G-CSF), the paclitaxel dose could be increased to 250 mg/m^2, at which point neurotoxicity became dose-limiting.[32,33] Phase III trials comparing cisplatin plus paclitaxel (3 and 24-hour infusions) with standard chemotherapy regimens have, on occasion, demonstrated improved response rates and survival (Figure 10–2).[34] No appreciable difference in efficacy was seen between two paclitaxel dose levels (135 and 250 mg/m^2). A survival benefit has not been universally demonstrable with this combination, probably due to the usefulness of second-line chemotherapy after progression of disease. However, in quality-of-life analysis, the patients receiving the paclitaxel frequently fared better.[35]

Paclitaxel has also been explored in combination with **carboplatin** because of a decreased risk of renal and neurologic toxicity and ototoxicity, and ease of administration of this analogue compared to cisplatin. In one of the first trials to combine carboplatin with paclitaxel, Langer and colleagues administered paclitaxel as a 24-hour infusion, 135 to 215 mg/m^2, on day 1, followed by carboplatin with an area under the concentration x time curve (AUC) of 7.5.[36] At a paclitaxel dose of 135 mg/m^2, neutropenia was dose-limiting without growth factor use. However, with prophylactic filgrastim, paclitaxel doses were successfully escalated to 215 mg/m^2. In this trial, a 62 percent major response rate and 1-year survival of 54 percent were observed in 53 patients. An alternative schedule using paclitaxel as a 3-hour infusion followed by carboplatin at an AUC of 6 has also been evaluated extensively.[37] Paclitaxel doses were escalated in successive cohorts of patients from 150 to 250 mg/m^2. At this highest dose level, neurotoxicity proved dose-limiting, and a paclitaxel dose of 225 mg/m^2 was recommended for further study. Major responses were reported in 20 of 32 patients (63%) including two complete responses. A third trial employed an analogous schedule to that of Langer and used paclitaxel (135 or 175 mg/m²) and carboplatin (300 mg/m² or AUC of 6) and treatment was given once every 4 weeks.[38] Fourteen responses were seen in 51 patients (27%) with a median survival of 8.8 months and a 1-year survival of 32 percent. A suggestion of higher response rates at the higher dose of paclitaxel was noted.

Phase III trials studying the carboplatin/paclitaxel combination are detailed in Figure 10–2. Similar to many other regimens, when subjected to phase III testing, the earlier results were difficult to duplicate. In these trials, response rates for carboplatin/paclitaxel range from 15 to 29 percent and median survivals range from 8 to 11 months.

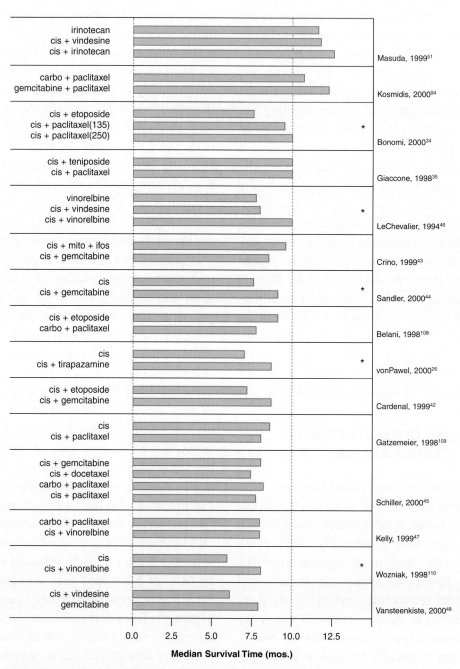

Figure 10–2.   Recent Phase III trials in NSCLC.
cis = cisplatin, carbo = carboplatin, mito = mitomycin, ifos = ifosfamide.
*Indicates the difference in median survival time observed between the treatment groups was statistically significant, p ≤ 0.05.

Platinum-Gemcitabine Combinations

Gemcitabine in combination with cisplatin is highly active against NSCLC in vitro.[39,40] A number of phase II trials of gemcitabine and cisplatin have been conducted in patients with advanced NSCLC. These trials report a pooled response rate of 44 percent and promising median and 1-year survival rates. Gemcitabine is typically administered at doses between 1,000 and 1,250 mg/m^2 on days 1, 8 and 15, with cisplatin 100 mg/m^2 on day 1, repeated every 28 days. A phase II trial comparing gemcitabine/cisplatin combination, with or without day 15 gemcitabine on a 4 or 3-week cycle, respectively, shows a better toxicity profile on the 3-week schedule despite the higher dose intensity, with similar or better response rate.[41] The cisplatin dose was reduced to 70 mg/m^2 in this trial to accommodate the 3-week schedule.

Results of phase III studies testing the gemcitabine/cisplatin combination are summarized in Figure 10–2. The combination frequently demonstrates superior response rates and improvement in time-to-disease-progression compared with traditional cisplatin-based combinations, but similar overall survival.[42,43] One trial has shown a statistically significant improvement in overall survival with gemcitabine/cisplatin versus cisplatin alone (9.1 months versus 7.6 months).[44] A four-armed randomized trial conducted by ECOG failed to show a survival benefit regardless of which drug was combined with cisplatin or carboplatin, however the paclitaxel/carboplatin combination appears to be marginally less toxic, and gemcitabine/cisplatin was associated with a modest improvement in time-to-disease-progression.[45]

Platinum-Vinca Alkaloid Combinations

Phase III trials have compared vinorelbine plus cisplatin to single-agent vinca alkaloids and other vinca alkaloid combinations, and have demonstrated improved response rate and survival with the vinorelbine/cisplatin combination (see Figure 10–2). Neutropenia was significantly higher in the vinorelbine/cisplatin-treated patients, but neurotoxicity occurred more frequently with vindesine/cisplatin.[46] In a head-to-head comparison, vinorelbine/cisplatin was comparable to carboplatin/paclitaxel in terms of response rate, survival, and quality-of-life benefit.

However, vinorelbine/cisplatin appeared to be a more cost-effective drug regimen ($18,000 versus $35,000 treatment cost per patient).[47] Vindesine/cisplatin combination has been compared with single-agent gemcitabine with results showing similar response rate and survival, but significantly better and longer lasting symptom control and less toxicity were obtained with gemcitabine monotherapy.[48]

Platinum–Irinotecan Combinations

Following phase I trials, a phase II study of combination irinotecan and cisplatin was conducted with irinotecan delivered on 3 consecutive weeks (60 mg/m^2), with cisplatin (80 mg/m^2) on the first day of each 4-week treatment cycle. The response rate was 29 percent with a 10-month median survival, and 37 percent 1-year survival proportion. The majority of the patients (60%) required dose reduction of the irinotecan at some point during the trial in order to limit toxicities, which included nausea, vomiting, diarrhea, and neutropenia.[49] Another phase II study from Japan used the same doses in both chemotherapy-naïve and pretreated patients. Response rates were 48 percent in the group with no prior chemotherapy, and 25 percent in the salvage group.[50] The survival outcome of a recent phase III trial of cisplatin/irinotecan is included in Figure 10–2. Response rates were superior, but survival was equivalent compared to both single-agent irinotecan and the cisplatin/vindesine combination.[51]

Non-Platinum Combinations

Many patients with advanced NSCLC are not good candidates to receive platinum chemotherapy due to renal insufficiency, hearing loss, borderline functional status, pre-existing sensory neuropathy, diabetes mellitus, or coronary artery disease. Combination chemotherapy regimens using newer agents may provide effective alternatives to platinum as first-line therapy, but with a more favorable or individualized toxicity profile. In the last 3 years there have been numerous phase II trials of these novel combinations, the best studied and most promising of which are summarized in Table 10–6. Gemcitabine/paclitaxel is the first non-platinum containing regimen to be included in a randomized phase III trial, currently being compared with cisplatin/paclitaxel and cisplatin/gemcitabine by the European Organization for Research and Treatment of Cancer (EORTC).

CHEMOTHERAPY FOR PLATINUM-REFRACTORY DISEASE

Historically, patients with disease progression after initial chemotherapy for advanced NSCLC were either treated with best supportive care or referred for trials of phase I agents. This practice was well founded, as the median survivals reported with active agents used in the second-line setting were 5 months or less, and major objective response rates were routinely < 10%.[52] Recent trials now indicate that several of the new agents, primarily docetaxel, but also gemcitabine, are useful in this situation (Table 10–7).

In the phase II trials testing **docetaxel** as second-line therapy, response rates ranged between 15 and 25 percent.[53–56] These unparalleled results led to phase III trials, which have established docetaxel as the first chemotherapeutic agent with proven benefit for patients with platinum-refractory disease. The TAX 320 trial randomized 373 patients whose disease was progressing on platinum chemotherapy to receive either docetaxel (arm 1 = 100 mg/m², arm 2 = 75 mg/m²), versus "traditional" salvage chemotherapy (arm 3 = vinorelbine or ifosfamide (V/I) at standard doses).[57] Patients were stratified by performance status and best response to previous platinum therapy. Patients who had received prior paclitaxel therapy were included in this trial, and composed about 40 percent of patients in each arm. Overall response rates were 11 percent with D100, and 7 percent with D75—both significantly higher than the response rate with V/I which was only 1 percent. Although overall survival was not significantly different between the

groups (around 6 months), patients treated with D75 enjoyed an improvement in 1-year survival proportion (32% versus 19%) in comparison with patients treated with V/I. However, investigators noted that about 30 percent of patients in the control group eventually went on to receive docetaxel. When survival analysis was censored at the time of administration of additional post-study chemotherapy, 1-year survival rates were significantly greater for docetaxel-treated patients (32% versus 10%, p < 0.01). Overall, patients treated with D100 and D75 also enjoyed a quality-of-life benefit as measured by the Lung Cancer Symptom Scale (LCSS) questionnaire.[58] Interestingly, prior exposure to paclitaxel did not decrease the likelihood of response to docetaxel, nor did it impact on survival.

In another phase III trial, Shepherd and colleagues randomized 204 patients, similarly stratified by performance status and best response to prior chemotherapy, to receive either salvage docetaxel (100 mg/m²) or best supportive care.[59] Patients who had received prior paclitaxel therapy were excluded from this trial. Interim analysis identified a significant increase in toxicity in the treatment arm, requiring dose reduction to 75 mg/m² in the second half of the trial. At final analysis, the objective response rate of patients with measurable disease was 7 percent, similar to that observed in the TAX 320 trial. Treated patients enjoyed statistically significant improvement in time-to-progression (11 weeks versus 7 weeks), median survival (7 months versus 5 months), as well as quality of life as measured by the lung cancer symptom scale (LCSS) questionnaire.[60] The authors attributed the increased toxicity of D100 in this trial to the unusually poor functional status of participating patients.

Although the response rates to salvage chemother-

Table 10–6. SELECTED PHASE II/III TRIALS WITH NON-PLATINUM-CONTAINING COMBINATION CHEMOTHERAPY IN PREVIOUSLY UNTREATED PATIENTS*				
Investigator	Drug (dose, mg/m²)	N	RR (%)	Med. (mos.) / 1-yr. Surv. (%)
Georgoulias, 1999[92]	Docetaxel (100) d8 + Gemcitabine (900) d1,8	51	37	13/51
Frasci, 2000[93]	Gemcitabine (1200) + Vinorelbine(30) d1,8 q3w	120	22	7/—
	versus			
	Vinorelbine(30) d1,8 q3w		15	4/—
Kosmidis, 2000[94]	Gemcitabine (1000) d1,8 + Paclitaxel (200/3h); q3w	164	36	12/51
Miller, 2000[95]	Docetaxel (60) + Vinorelbine (45); q2w	35	51	14/60
Rebattu, 2000[96]	Docetaxel (85) d8 + Gemcitabine (1000) d1,8	36	30	—/35

*This table includes only non-platinum-containing arms of randomized trials.
Chemotherapy given with granulocyte colony-stimulating factor (G-CSF) support.

Table 10–7. PHASE II/III TRIALS OF CHEMOTHERAPY FOR PLATINUM-REFRACTORY ADVANCED NSCLC

Drug (Trial Phase)	No. Trials	Dose Range (mg/m²)	N (total)	Pooled RR (%)	Median Survival (mos.)
Docetaxel (II)[53,55,56,97–99]	6	60–100 q3w	285	20	8
Docetaxel (III)[57,59]	2	75–100 q3w	343	8	6
Paclitaxel (II)[83,84,100–102]	5	135–250/1-96 hrs.	83	11	4
Gemcitabine (II)[62,63,103–107]	7	1000d1,8,(15)–3500 q2w	279	15	7

N = number of patients; RR = response rate.

apy with docetaxel remain low in the phase III trials, the observed benefit in quality of life and 1-year survival for treated patients justify its use as therapy for platinum-refractory disease. The optimal dose in this patient population is 75 mg/m², infused over 1 hour, every 3 weeks. Phase II trials testing docetaxel in this setting using weekly schedules are ongoing.[61]

Similar to docetaxel, **gemcitabine** has been tested as a second-line agent in the treatment of advanced NSCLC refractory to platinum-based chemotherapy. A phase II trial by Crino and colleagues tested gemcitabine at a dose of 1,000 mg/m² once a week for 3 weeks, every 28 days, in this patient population.[62] The results were promising, with a 19 percent observed-response rate, a median duration of response of 29 weeks, and tolerable toxicity levels. However, only one of the 16 observed responses occurred in a patient with progression of disease as best response to platinum. Other phase II trials have had response rates varying between 6 percent and 20 percent for salvage gemcitabine (see Table 10–7).[63,64] Further investigations of gemcitabine for use in this setting are warranted. Gemcitabine has yet to be tested in a phase III trial.

Trials of **paclitaxel** in second-line therapy have also been reported (see Table 10–7). Unlike docetaxel, there is less evidence for paclitaxel to be an active agent in second-line therapy, especially at doses under 200 mg/m². Available data show little activity for vinorelbine or irinotecan in previously-treated patients, and thus these agents are unlikely to be useful for salvage therapy, even in combination regimens.

CLINICAL PRACTICE GUIDELINES FOR ADVANCED NSCLC

The Thoracic Oncology Service at Memorial Sloan-Kettering Cancer Center (MSKCC) has developed clinical practice guidelines for the treatment of patients with advanced NSCLC. As current chemotherapy offers only palliation of symptoms and modest prolongation of life, it is vitally important to determine that the patient truly has stage IV disease, or stage IIIB with a malignant pleural or pericardial effusion, and is therefore not a candidate for treatment with curative intent. Confirmation of advanced disease typically involves pathologic or cytologic documentation of a malignant pleural or pericardial effusion, biopsy-proven metastatic (M1) disease, or strong radiologic evidence of metastatic disease, such as highly suspicious lesions visible on a plain radiograph or computed tomography (CT) scanning which are also metabolically active on bone scan or positron emission tomography (PET) scanning. If even a remote possibility exists that a probable site of metastatic disease is not such, biopsy at this area should be pursued (eg, increased uptake on PET scan in a patient from an area known to have a high rate of granulomatous disease). In very rare instances, patients with a solitary metastatic site of disease can be cured with surgery or combined modality therapy.[65,66]

Once the clinician is convinced the patient's disease is incurable, initiation of systemic chemotherapy is indicated. However, chemotherapy should be delayed pending control of critical metastases which may present an immediate threat to the patient (see Figure 10–1). Furthermore, a patient requires a minimum performance status (≥ 60% on the Karnofsky scale) in order to be likely to benefit from systemic chemotherapy. Therefore, chemotherapy may also be delayed or withheld while the patient is afforded the best supportive medical care for their cancer and/or co-morbid illnesses.

Once control of critical metastases has been achieved, and the patient has demonstrated adequate performance status, a chemotherapy regimen should be chosen based on the immediate goal of therapy. If the patient is highly symptomatic from his or her lung cancer, the initial goal of chemotherapy is rapid palliation of symptoms. A drug regimen is chosen which has a high expected-response rate, with less immediate concern for the toxicity of the chemotherapy in a risk-benefit analysis. Thus, for symptomatic patients, a cisplatin-containing regimen may be appropriate. If, however, the patient is relatively asymptomatic from his or her disease, the immediate goal of chemotherapy is to improve overall survival with less treatment-related toxicity. In this situation, it is appropriate to avoid the added toxicity of cisplatin, and pursue combination chemotherapy with carboplatin, or even avoid platinum analogues altogether. A third scenario involves patients with borderline performance status who may not be able to tolerate a platinum-based regimen. Platinum-free combinations or even monotherapy with gemcitabine or a taxane is reasonable in some patients with a low (60%) performance status and minimal burden of disease. Given the shortcomings of all current chemotherapy for advanced NSCLC, it is appropriate to enroll eligible patients in an investigational protocol whenever possible during the course of their treatment, including at presentation.

Once a chemotherapy regimen is selected, investigational or otherwise, the MSKCC practice guideline is to treat to best response. Baseline radiologic studies are performed, based on the location of evaluable disease, with chest radiographs or physical exam assessments preferred as simple methods of evaluating disease response. However, most patients require baseline CT scan, followed by serial CT scanning every 2 to 3 months, in order to follow the response of their disease to therapy. If the tumor shrinks in size or is stabilized by chemotherapy, the drugs are continued indefinitely, as tolerated. Given the limited utility of available drugs, it is important not to abandon a chemotherapy regimen too early. Patients must demonstrate incontrovertible evidence of progression before discontinuing an agent or combination for lack of efficacy.

If a patient's disease is refractory to, or progresses on, first-line therapy, salvage chemotherapy is appropriate. Selection of a second-line drug is based, in part, on the drugs included in the initial chemotherapy regimen. If the patient is taxane-naïve, docetaxel is clearly the appropriate choice, re-

inforced by the recent phase III data.[57,59] In patients with borderline functional status, docetaxel can be administered on a weekly schedule at a dose of 36 mg/m^2 to minimize myelosuppression and neuropathy.[61] If the patient has received paclitaxel up front, gemcitabine is typically used in the second line, although the results of the TAX 320 trial support the use of docetaxel, even in patients who have failed paclitaxel. The MSKCC treatment guidelines are presented in a schematic form in Figure 10–3.

CONCLUSIONS AND FUTURE DIRECTIONS

Over the last decade, the use of new chemotherapeutic agents, either alone or in combination, appears to have made a clear improvement in the survival of advanced NSCLC patients. Median survival times in recent phase III trials with new agents consistently improve upon survival times achieved with the older platinum-containing combinations, and 1-year survival proportions are consistently 30 to 40 percent, compared to 20 to 30 percent with older regimens such as cisplatin/etoposide. Recent trials have changed the reference regimens for most major cooperative groups in the United States.

The increasing number of available single-agent and combination drug regimens afford patients more viable treatment options. Although platinum-containing combinations remain the standard of care, there are now proven therapies for platinum-refractory disease, and promising alternatives to platinum in first-line therapy. Although increased response rates can be expected with novel combinations of cytotoxic chemotherapy, these programs will continue to be limited by increased hematologic and non-hematologic toxicities. The comparable survival times achieved in recent phase III trials suggest that a new therapeutic plateau may have been reached.

As knowledge about the molecular biology of NSCLC improves, new targets for therapy are being uncovered, and new agents identified, which may provide alternatives or adjuncts to cytotoxic chemotherapy. Monoclonal antibodies which block growth factor receptors, tyrosine kinase inhibitors which block signal transduction, angiogenesis inhibitors, anti-metastatic agents, and immunotherapy pro-

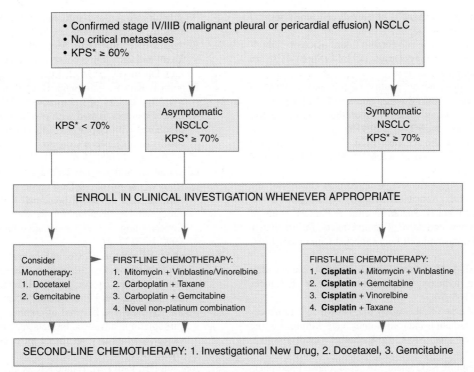

Figure 10–3.   MSKCC guidelines for the treatment of patients with advanced NSCLC. *Karnofsky performance status: 60%: "Patient requires occasional assistance, but is able to care for most of his needs." 70%: "Patient cares for self." (Karnofsky, 1948.)

grams are all currently being tested in phase I and II trials, either alone or in combination with cytotoxic chemotherapy. The next decade will hopefully see rational integration of the best targeted therapies with cytotoxic agents or, in some cases, as monotherapy, and should result in appreciably better outcomes for advanced NSCLC.

REFERENCES

1. Greenlee RT, Murray T, Bolden S, Wingo PA. Cancer Statistics, 2000. CA Cancer J Clin 2000;50:7–33.
2. Chemotherapy in non-small cell lung cancer: a meta-analysis using updated data on individual patients from 52 randomised clinical trials. Non-small Cell Lung Cancer Collaborative Group. BMJ 1995;311:899–909.
3. Goodwin PJ, Shepherd FA. Economic issues in lung cancer: a review. J Clin Oncol 1998;16:3900–12.
4. Crino L, Clerici M, Figoli F, et al. Chemotherapy of advanced non-small-cell lung cancer: a comparison of three active regimens. A randomized trial of the Italian Oncology Group for Clinical Research (G.O.I.R.C.). Ann Oncol 1995;6:347–53.
5. Meert AP, Berghmans T, Branle F, et al. Phase II and III studies with new drugs for non-small cell lung cancer: a systematic review of the literature with a methodology quality assessment. Anticancer Res 1999;19:4379–90.
6. Roszkowski K, Pluzanska A, Krzakowski M, et al. A multicenter, randomized, phase III study of docetaxel plus best

7. supportive care versus best supportive care in chemotherapy-naïve patients with metastatic or non-resectable localized non-small cell lung cancer (NSCLC). Lung Cancer 2000;27:145–57.
7. Richards F, White D, Muss H, et al. Phase I trial of gemcitabine (2',2'-difluorodeoxycytidine) (G) over 30 minutes in patients (PTS) with non-small cell lung cancer (NSCLC). Proc Am Soc Clin Oncol 1994;13:344.
8. Abbruzzese J, Grunewald R, Weeks E, et al. A phase I clinical, plasma, and cellular pharmacology study of gemcitabine. J Clin Oncol 1991;90:491–8.
9. Poplin EA, Corbett T, Flaherty L, et al. Difluorodeoxycytidine (dFdC)-gemcitabine: A phase I study. Invest New Drugs 1992;10:165–70.
10. Vander Els NJ, Miller V. Successful treatment of gemcitabine toxicity with a brief course of oral corticosteroid therapy. Chest 1998;114:1779–81.
11. Flombaum CD, Mouradian JA, Casper ES, et al. Thrombotic microangiopathy as a complication of long-term therapy with gemcitabine. Am J Kidney Dis 1999;33:555–62.
12. ten Bokkel Huinink WW, Bergman B, Chemaissani A, et al. Single-agent gemcitabine: an active and better tolerated alternative to standard cisplatin-based chemotherapy in locally advanced or metastatic non-small cell lung cancer. Lung Cancer 1999;26:85–94.
13. Fossella FV, Lippman SM, Shin DM, et al. Maximum-tolerated dose defined for single-agent gemcitabine: a phase I dose-escalation study in chemotherapy-naïve patients with advanced non-small cell lung cancer. J Clin Oncol 1997;15:310–6.
14. Ranson M, Davidson N, Nicolson M, et al. Randomized trial of paclitaxel plus supportive care versus supportive care

for patients with advanced non-small cell lung cancer. J Natl Cancer Inst 2000;92:1074–80.

15. Cvitkovic E, Izzo J. The current and future place of vinorelbine in cancer therapy. Drugs 1992;44 (Suppl 4):36–45 [discussion 66–9].

16. Effects of vinorelbine on quality of life and survival of elderly patients with advanced non-small cell lung cancer. The Elderly Lung Cancer Vinorelbine Italian Study Group. J Natl Cancer Inst 1999;91:66–72.

17. Rothenberg ML, Kuhn JG, Burris HA III, et al. Phase I and pharmacokinetic trial of weekly CPT-11. J Clin Oncol 1993;11:2194–204.

18. Sandler A, van Oosterom AT. Irinotecan in cancers of the lung and cervix. Anticancer Drugs 1999;10 Suppl 1:13–7.

19. Fukuoka M, Niitani H, Suzuki A, et al. A Phase II study of CPT-11, a new derivative of camptothecin, for previously untreated non-small cell lung cancer. J Clin Oncol 1992; 10:16–20.

20. Brown JM. SR 4233 (Tirapazamine): a new anticancer drug exploiting hypoxia in solid tumours. Br J Cancer 1993;67:1163–70.

21. Zeman EM, Hirst VK, Lemmon MJ, Brown JM. Enhancement of radiation-induced tumor cell killing by the hypoxic cell toxin SR 4233. Radiother Oncol 1988;12: 209–18.

22. Senan S, Rampling R, Graham MA, et al. Phase I and pharmacokinetic study of tirapazamine (SR 4233) administered every three weeks. Clin Cancer Res 1997;3:31–8.

23. Rodriguez GI, Valdivieso M, Von Hoff DD, et al. A phase I/II trial of the combination of tirapazamine and cisplatin in patients with non-small cell lung cancer [abstract]. Proc Am Soc Clin Oncol 1996;15:382.

24. Treat J, Haynes B, Johnson E, et al. Tirapazamine with cisplatin: a phase II trial in advanced stage non-small cell cancer (NSCLC). Proc Am Soc Clin Oncol 1997;16:455.

25. Miller VA, Pizzo B, Grant SC, et al. Phase II study of tirapazamine, a unique bioreductive agent, with cisplatin in patients with advanced non-small cell lung cancer (NSCLC) [abstract]. Proc Am Soc Clin Oncol 1996;15:403.

26. von Pawel J, von Roemeling R, Gatzemeier U, et al. Tirapazamine plus cisplatin versus cisplatin in advanced non-small cell lung cancer: a report of the international CATAPULT I study group. Cisplatin and tirapazamine in subjects with advanced previously untreated non-small cell lung tumors. J Clin Oncol 2000;18:1351–9.

27. Jassem J. Chemotherapy of advanced non-small cell lung cancer. Ann Oncol 1999;10 (Suppl 6):77–82.

28. Lilenbaum RC, List M, Desch C. Single-agent versus combination chemotherapy in advanced non-small cell lung cancer: a meta-analysis and the Cancer and Leukemia Group B randomized trial. Semin Oncol 1999;26:52–4.

29. Bengtson EM, Rigas JR. A brief historical review of the development of chemotherapy for the treatment of advanced non-small cell lung cancer: Why we should look beyond platinum. Semin Oncol 1999;26:1–6.

30. Shepherd FA. Chemotherapy for non-small cell lung cancer: Have we reached a new plateau? Semin Oncol 1999; 26:3–11.

31. Kris MG. What does chemotherapy have to offer patients with advanced-stage non-small cell lung cancer? Semin Oncol 1998;25:1–4.

32. Rowinsky EK, Chaudhry V, Forastiere AA, et al. Phase I and pharmacologic study of paclitaxel and cisplatin with granulocyte colony-stimulating factor: neuromuscular toxicity is dose-limiting. J Clin Oncol 1993;11:2010–20.

33. Rowinsky EK, Gilbert MR, McGuire WP, et al. Sequences of Taxol and cisplatin: a phase I and pharmacologic study. J Clin Oncol 1991;9:1692–1703.

34. Bonomi P, Kim K, Fairclough D, et al. Comparison of survival and quality of life in advanced non-small cell lung cancer patients treated with two dose levels of paclitaxel combined with cisplatin versus etoposide with cisplatin: results of an Eastern Cooperative Oncology Group trial. J Clin Oncol 2000;18:623–31.

35. Giaccone G, Splinter TA, Debruyne C, et al. Randomized study of paclitaxel-cisplatin versus cisplatin-teniposide in patients with advanced non-small cell lung cancer. The European Organization for Research and Treatment of Cancer Lung Cancer Cooperative Group. J Clin Oncol 1998;16:2133–41.

36. Langer CJ, Leighton JC, Comis RL, et al. Paclitaxel and carboplatin in combination in the treatment of advanced non-small cell lung cancer: a phase II toxicity, response, and survival analysis. J Clin Oncol 1995;13:1860–70.

37. Natale RB. A phase I/II trial of combination paclitaxel and carboplatin in advanced or metastatic non-small cell lung cancer: preliminary results of an ongoing study. Semin Oncol 1995;22:34–7.

38. Johnson DH, Paul DM, Hande KR, et al. Paclitaxel plus carboplatin in advanced non-small cell lung cancer: a phase II trial. J Clin Oncol 1996;14:2054–60.

39. Tsai CM, Chang KT, Chen JY, et al. Cytotoxic effects of gemcitabine-containing regimens against human non-small cell lung cancer cell lines which express different levels of p185neu. Cancer Res 1996;56:794–801.

40. Lund B, Kristjansen PEG, Hansen HH. Clinical and preclinical activity of 2',2'-difluorodeoxycytidine (gemcitabine). Cancer Treat Rev 1993;19:45–55.

41. Soto Parra HJ, et al. Superiority of three-week vs. four-week schedule of cisplatin and gemcitabine: results of a randomized phase II study [abstract]. Proc Am Soc Clin Oncol 2000;19:546a.

42. Cardenal F, Lopez-Cabrerizo MP, Anton A, et al. Randomized phase III study of gemcitabine-cisplatin versus etoposide-cisplatin in the treatment of locally advanced or metastatic non-small cell lung cancer. J Clin Oncol 1999;17:12–8.

43. Crino L, Scagliotti GV, Ricci S, et al. Gemcitabine and cisplatin versus mitomycin, ifosfamide, and cisplatin in advanced non-small cell lung cancer: a randomized phase III study of the Italian Lung Cancer Project. J Clin Oncol 1999;17:3522–30.

44. Sandler AB, Nemunaitis J, Denham C, et al. Phase III trial of gemcitabine plus cisplatin versus cisplatin alone in patients with locally advanced or metastatic non-small cell lung cancer. J Clin Oncol 2000;18:122–30.

45. Schiller JH, Harrington D, Sandler A, et al. A randomized phase III trial of four chemotherapy regimens in advanced non-small cell lung cancer [abstract]. Proc Am Soc Clin Oncol 2000;19:1a.

46. Le Chevalier T, Brisgand D, Douillard JY, et al. Randomized study of vinorelbine and cisplatin versus vindesine and cisplatin versus vinorelbine alone in advanced non-small cell lung cancer: results of a European multicenter trial including 612 patients. J Clin Oncol 1994;12:360–7.

47. Kelly K, Crowley J, Bunn P, et al. A randomized phase III trial of paclitaxel plus carboplatin (PC) versus vinorelbine

plus cisplatin (VC) in untreated advanced non-small cell lung cancer (NSCLC): a Southwest Oncology Group (SWOG) trial. Proc Am Soc Clin Oncol 1999;18.

48. Vansteenkiste J, Vandebroek J, Nackaerts K, et al. Symptom control in advanced non-small cell lung cancer: a multicenter prospective randomized phase III study of single agent gemcitabine versus cisplatin-vindesine [abstract]. Proc Am Soc Clin Oncol 2000;19:488a.

49. DeVore RF, Johnson DH, Crawford J, et al. Phase II study of irinotecan plus cisplatin in patients with advanced non-small cell lung cancer. J Clin Oncol 1999;17:2710–20.

50. Nagao K. A phase II study of irinotecan combined with cisplatin in non-small cell lung cancer. CPT-11 Lung Cancer Study Group. Gan To Kagaku Ryoho 2000;27:413–21.

51. Masuda N, Fukuoka M, Negoro S, et al. Randomized trial comparing cisplatin (CDDP) and irinotecan (CPT-11) versus CDDP and vindesine versus CPT-11 alone in advanced non-small cell lung cancer, a multicenter phase III study [abstract 1774]. Proc Am Soc Clin Oncol 1999; 18:459a.

52. Miller VA, Rigas JR, Pisters KM, et al. Ifosfamide plus high-dose cisplatin in patients with non-small cell lung cancer previously treated with chemotherapy [published erratum appears in Am J Clin Oncol 1996;19(6):637]. Am J Clin Oncol 1995;18:303–6.

53. Burris H, Eckardt J, Fields S, et al. Phase II trial of taxotere in patients with non-small cell lung cancer. Proc Am Soc Clin Oncol 1993;12.

54. Fossella FV, Lee JS, Berille J, Hong WK. Summary of phase II data of docetaxel (Taxotere), an active agent in the first- and second-line treatment of advanced non-small cell lung cancer. Semin Oncol 1995;22:22–9.

55. Robinet G, Kleisbauer JP, Thomas P, et al. Phase II study of docetaxel (Taxotere) in first- and second-line NSCLC Proc Am Soc Clin Oncol 1997;16.

56. Gandara DR, Vokes E, Green M, et al. Docetaxel (Taxotere) in platinum-treated non-small cell lung cancer (NSCLC): confirmation of prolonged survival in a multicenter trial. Proc Am Soc Clin Oncol 1997;16.

57. Fossella FV, DeVore R, Kerr RN, et al. Randomized phase III trial of docetaxel versus vinorelbine or ifosfamide in patients with advanced non-small cell lung cancer previously treated with platinum-containing chemotherapy regimens. The TAX 320 Non-Small Cell Lung Cancer Study Group. J Clin Oncol 2000;18:2354–62.

58. Miller V, Fossella F, DeVore R, et al. Docetaxel (D) benefits lung cancer symptoms and quality of life (QOL) in a randomized phase III study of non-small cell lung cancer (NSCLC) patients previously treated with platinum-based therapy. Proc Am Soc Clin Oncol 1999;18.

59. Shepherd FA, Dancey J, Ramlau R, et al. Prospective randomized trial of docetaxel versus best supportive care in patients with non-small cell lung cancer previously treated with platinum-based chemotherapy. J Clin Oncol 2000;18:2095–103.

60. Dancey J, Shepherd F, Ramlau R, et al. Quality of life (QOL) assessment in a randomized study of taxotere (TAX) versus best supportive care (BSC) in non-small cell lung cancer (NSCLC) patients (pts) previously treated with platinum-based chemotherapy. Proc Am Soc Clin Oncol 1999;18.

61. McKay CE, Hainsworth JD, Burris HA, et al. Weekly docetaxel in the treatment of elderly patients with advanced non-small cell lung cancer: A Minnie Pearl Cancer Research Network Phase II Trial [abstract]. Proc Am Soc Clin Oncol 2000;19:502a.

62. Crino L, Mosconi AM, Scagliotti G, et al. Gemcitabine as second-line treatment for advanced non-small cell lung cancer: A phase II trial. J Clin Oncol 1999;17:2081–5.

63. Rosvold E, Langer CJ, Schilder R, et al. Salvage therapy with gemcitabine in advanced non-small cell lung cancer (NSCLC) progressing after prior carboplatin-paclitaxel. Proc Am Soc Clin Oncol 1998;17.

64. Sculier JP, Lafitte JJ, Berghmans T, et al. A phase II trial testing gemcitabine as second-line chemotherapy for non-small cell lung cancer. The European Lung Cancer Working Party. 101473.1044@compuserve.com. Lung Cancer 2000;29:67–73.

65. Saitoh Y, Fujisawa T, Shiba M, et al. Prognostic factors in surgical treatment of solitary brain metastasis after resection of non-small cell lung cancer. Lung Cancer 1999;24: 99–106.

66. de Perrot M, Licker M, Robert JH, Spiliopoulos A. Long-term survival after surgical resections of bronchogenic carcinoma and adrenal metastasis. Ann Thorac Surg 1999;68:1084–5.

67. Anderson H, Cottier B, Nicholson M, et al. Phase III study of gemcitabine versus best supportive care in advanced non-small cell lung cancer. J Int Assoc Study Lung Cancer 1997;18:A24.

68. Cerny T, Wanders J, Kaplan S, et al. Taxotere is an active drug in non-small cell lung (NSCLC) cancer: A phase II trial of the early clinical trials group (ECTG). Proc Am Soc Clin Oncol 1993;12:331.

69. Fossella FV, Lee JS, Murphy WK, et al. Phase II study of docetaxel for recurrent or metastatic non-small cell lung cancer. J Clin Oncol 1994;12:1238–44.

70. Francis P, Rigas JR, Kris MG, et al. Phase II trial of docetaxel (Taxol) in patients with stage III and IV non-small cell lung cancer. J Clin Oncol 1994;12:1232–7.

71. Miller VA, Rigas JR, Francis PA, et al. Phase II trial of a 75-mg/m^2 dose of docetaxel with prednisone premedication for patients with advanced non-small cell lung cancer. Cancer 1995;75:968–72.

72. Kunitoh H, Watanabe K, Onoshi T, et al. Phase II trial of docetaxel in previously untreated advanced non-small cell lung cancer: a Japanese cooperative study. J Clin Oncol 1996;14:1649–55.

73. Abratt RP, Bezwoda WR, Falkson G, et al. Efficacy and safety profile of gemcitabine in non-small cell lung cancer: A phase II study. J Clin Oncol 1994;12:1535–40.

74. Anderson H, Lund B, Bach F, et al. Single-agent activity of weekly gemcitabine in advanced non-small cell lung cancer: a phase II study. J Clin Oncol 1994;12:1821–6.

75. Le Chevalier T, Gottfried M, Gatzemeier U, et al. Confirmatory activity of gemcitabine in non-small cell lung cancer (NSCLC). Eur J Cancer 1993;29A(Suppl 6):160.

76. Takada M, Negoro S, Kudo S, et al. Activity of gemcitabine in non-small cell lung cancer: results of the Japan gemcitabine group (A) phase II study. Cancer Chemother Pharmacol 1998;41:217–22.

77. Depierre A, Lemaire E, Dabouis G, et al. A phase II study of navelbine (vinorelbine) in the treatment of non-small cell lung cancer. Am J Clin Oncol 1991;14:115–9.

78. Yokoyama A, Furuse K, Niitani H. Multi-institutional phase II study of navelbine (vinorelbine) in non-small cell lung cancer. Proc Am Soc Clin Oncol 1992;11:287.

79. Crawford J, O'Rourke M, Schiller JH, et al. Randomized trial of vinorelbine compared with fluorouracil plus leucovorin in patients with stage IV non-small cell lung cancer [see comments] [published erratum appears in J Clin Oncol 1996;14(12):3175]. J Clin Oncol 1996;14:2774–84.

80. Gridelli C, Perrone F, Gallo C, et al. Vinorelbine is well tolerated and active in the treatment of elderly patients with advanced non-small cell lung cancer. A two-stage phase II study. Eur J Cancer 1997;33:392–7.

81. Chang AY, Kim K, Glick J, et al. Phase II study of taxol, merbarone, and piroxantrone in stage IV non-small cell lung cancer: The eastern cooperative oncology group results. J Natl Cancer Inst 1993;85:388–94.

82. Murphy WK, Fossella FV, Winn RJ, et al. Phase II study of Taxol in patients with untreated advanced non-small cell lung cancer. J Natl Cancer Inst 1993;85:384–8.

83. Ruckdeschel J, Wagner H Jr, Williams C, et al. Second-line chemotherapy for resistant, metastatic non-small cell lung cancer (NSCLC): the role of Taxol (TAX), Proc Am Soc Clin Oncol 1994;13.

84. Hainsworth JD, Thompson DS, Greco FA. Paclitaxel by 1-hour infusion: an active drug in metastatic non-small cell lung cancer. J Clin Oncol 1995;13:1609–14.

85. Alberola V, Rosell R, Gonzalez-Larriba JL, et al. Single agent Taxol, 3-hour infusion, in untreated advanced non-small cell lung cancer. Ann Oncol 1995;6(Suppl 3):49–52.

86. Millward MJ, Bishop JF, Friedlander M, et al. Phase II trial of a 3-hour infusion of paclitaxel in previously untreated patients with advanced non-small cell lung cancer. J Clin Oncol 1996;14:142–8.

87. Sekine I, Nishiwaki Y, Watanabe K, et al. Phase II study of 3-hour infusion of paclitaxel in previously untreated non-small cell lung cancer. Clin Cancer Res 1996;2:941–5.

88. Negoro S, Fukuoka M, Niitani H. A phase II study of CPT-11, a camptothecin derivative, in patients with primary lung cancer. CPT-11 Cooperative Study Group. Gan To Kagaku Ryoho 1991;18:1013–19.

89. Nakai H, Fukuoka M, Furuse K, et al. An early phase II study of CPT-11 for primary lung cancer. Gan to Kagaku Ryoho 1991;18:607–12.

90. Baker L, Khan R, Lynch T. Phase II study of irinotecan (CPT-11) in advanced non-small cell cancer (NSCLC) [abstract 1658]. Proc Am Soc Clin Oncol 1997;16:461a.

91. Doulliard J, Ibrahim N, Riviere A. Phase II study of CPT-11 (irinotecan) in non-small cell lung cancer [abstract 1118]. Proc Am Soc Clin Oncol 1995;14:365a.

92. Georgoulias V, Kouroussis C, Androulakis N, et al. Front-line treatment of advanced non-small cell lung cancer with docetaxel and gemcitabine: a multicenter phase II trial. J Clin Oncol 1999;17:914–20.

93. Frasci G, Lorusso V, Panza N, et al. Gemcitabine plus vinorelbine versus vinorelbine alone in elderly patients with advanced non-small cell lung cancer. J Clin Oncol 2000;18:2529–36.

94. Kosmidis PA, Bacoyiannis C, Mylonakis N, et al. A randomized phase III trial of paclitaxel plus carboplatin versus paclitaxel plus gemcitabine in advanced non-small cell lung cancer. A preliminary analysis [abstract 1908]. Proc Am Soc Clin Oncol 2000;19:488a.

95. Miller VA, Krug LM, Ng KK, et al. Phase II trial of docetaxel and vinorelbine in patients with advanced non-small lung cancer. J Clin Oncol 2000;18:1346–50.

96. Rebattu P, Quantin X, Morere J, et al. A phase II study of docetaxel and gemcitabine combination in patients with non-small cell lung cancer [abstract 2124]. Proc Am Soc Clin Oncol 2000;19:539a.

97. Fossella FV, Lee JS, Shin DM, et al. Phase II study of docetaxel for advanced or metastatic platinum-refractory non-small cell lung cancer. J Clin Oncol 1995;13:645–51.

98. Nakamura Y, Kunitoh H, Aono H, et al. A phase II trial of low-dose docetaxel (DCT) 60 mg/m^2 in platinum-pretreated advanced non-small cell lung cancer (NSCLC) Proc Am Soc Clin Oncol 1999;18.

99. Alexopoulos K, Kouroussis C, Androulakis N, et al. Docetaxel and granulocyte colony-stimulating factor in patients with advanced non-small cell lung cancer previously treated with platinum-based chemotherapy: a multicenter phase II trial. Cancer Chemother Pharmacol 1999;43:257–62.

100. Murphy WK, Winn RJ, Huber M, et al. Phase II study of Taxol (T) in patients (pt.) with non-small cell lung cancer (NSCLC) who have failed platinum (P) containing chemotherapy (CTX), Proc Am Soc Clin Oncol 1994;13.

101. Socinski MA, Steagall A, Gillenwater H. Second-line chemotherapy with 96-hour infusional paclitaxel in refractory non-small cell lung cancer: report of a phase II trial. Cancer Invest 1999;17:181–8.

102. Hainsworth JD, Thompson DS, Greco FA. Paclitaxel by 1-hour infusion: an active drug in metastatic non-small cell lung cancer. J Clin Oncol 1995;13:1609–14.

103. Garfield DH, Dakhil SR, Whittaker TL, Keller AM. Phase II randomized multicenter trial of two dose schedules of gemcitabine as second-line therapy in patients with advanced non-small cell lung cancer (ANSCLC). Proc Am Soc Clin Oncol 1998;17.

104. Guerra JA, Arcediano A, Lianes P, et al. Improvement of disease-related symptoms with second line of gemcitabine in advanced non-small cell lung cancer (NSCLC), Ann Oncol 1998;9(Suppl 4).

105. Baas P, Codrington H, Muller M, et al. Second line gemcitabine (GEM) therapy in non-small cell lung cancer (NSCLC) stage IIIB and IV. Proc Am Soc Clin Oncol 1999;18.

106. Reddy G, Gandara D, Edelman M, et al. Gemcitabine (GEM) in platinum (PLAT) treated non-small cell lung cancer (NSCLC). Proc Am Soc Clin Oncol 1999;18.

107. Rossi A, Perrone F, Barletta E, et al. Activity of gemcitabine (GEM) in cisplatin-pretreated patients with advanced non-small cell lung cancer (NSCLC): a phase II trial. Proc Am Soc Clin Oncol 1999;18.

108. Belani CP, Natale RB, Lee JS, et al. Randomized phase III trial comparing cisplatin/etoposide versus carboplatin/paclitaxel in advanced and metastatic non-small cell lung cancer[abstract 1751]. Proc Am Soc Clin Oncol 1998;17:455a.

109. Gatzemeier U, von Pawel J, Gottfried M, et al. Phase III comparative study of high-dose cisplatin versus a combination of paclitaxel and cisplatin in patients with advanced non-small cell lung cancer [abstract 1748]. Proc Am Soc Clin Oncol 1998;17:454a.

110. Wozniak AJ, Crowley JJ, Balcerzak SP, et al. Randomized trial comparing cisplatin with cisplatin plus vinorelbine in the treatment of advanced non-small cell lung cancer: a Southwest Oncology Group study. J Clin Oncol 1998;16:2459–65.

11

Palliative and Definitive Local Therapies in the Treatment of Recurrent or Metastatic Lung Cancer

KENNETH ROSENZWEIG, MD

ROBERT J. GINSBERG, MD

Following definitive treatment of locoregional lung cancer, be it surgery or chemoradiation, local, regional, and distant recurrences are common. In most instances, this represents an incurable situation, but local palliation is worthwhile. On rare occasions, definitive curative therapy can be attempted. When patients present with symptomatic metastases, these metastatic areas may require local treatment if symptoms are not alleviated with chemotherapy.

Locoregional Recurrences

Nodal Disease

Following surgical resection, local and regional lymph node recurrences are not uncommon. On very rare occasions, this recurrence is limited to intrapulmonary or hilar nodal disease. Following appropriate staging, re-resection with curative intent occasionally may be warranted. This may require a completion pneumonectomy and/or hilar and mediastinal lymph node dissection. If a complete resection results, patients can be afforded long-term cure in up to one-third of cases.[1,2]

With more extensive nodal recurrence in the mediastinum or supraclavicular regions, incurable but treatable symptoms are related to tracheal, esophageal, or superior vena caval involvement. External beam radi-

ation therapy is commonly used for palliation. There have been a number of trials that have documented its palliative benefit.[3–6] Hypofractionation (high dose per fraction with fewer fractions given) has the advantage of allowing for a shorter, less expensive treatment course with a quicker palliative response. However, standard palliative fractionation of 300 cGy to total doses of 3,000 cGy to 3,900 cGy appears to offer a survival advantage.[7]

The radiation therapy portals for palliative thoracic radiotherapy typically consist of opposed anterior and posterior fields. The radiation volume encompasses the tumor, the mediastinum, the ipsilateral hilum, and possibly the supraclavicular area.

Superior Vena Cava Syndrome

Superior vena cava (SVC) syndrome is caused by compression and obstruction of the superior vena cava by surrounding lymph nodes, or less commonly by the primary tumor, and is characterized by venous distension, facial edema, headache, tachypnea, cyanosis, and plethora[8] (Figure 11–1, A). Rarely can surgical excision and reconstruction be employed. Palliative radiation therapy may help relieve the symptoms[9] (Figure 11–1, B).

The exact indications for intraluminal stenting of the superior vena cava when SVC syndrome occurs have yet to be defined. Certainly, this percutaneous approach can immediately relieve symptoms and is being used increasingly in the actual management of this complication, often supplemented by radiotherapy (Figures 11–2, *A* and *B*).

Airway and Esophageal Compression

When esophageal or tracheal compression occurs, endoluminal stenting utilizing endoscopic techniques can be valuable and is often employed in combination with palliative radiotherapy[10–14] (Figure 11–3, *A* and *B*).

Recurrent Nerve Palsy

Recurrent nerve palsy, usually due to nodal compression, can be debilitating—affecting speech, swallowing function, and ventilatory function. When symptomatic, the affected vocal cord can easily be medialized by simple surgical maneuvers carried out under local anesthesia.[15] Bilateral nerve palsy causes adducted cords and may require a permanent tracheostomy in order to avoid airway obstruction.

Pleura and Chest Wall

Solitary pleural and chest wall recurrences are usually harbingers of a more diffuse process within the pleural space. Most frequently, these present as malignant pleural effusions significant enough to cause symptoms. Since most of these patients have already been treated with either surgical resection or radiotherapy, these pleural effusions, if symptomatic, may be difficult to treat. Pleural drainage and pleurodesis is worthwhile when the lung can be re-expanded, utilizing talc either at the bedside or intra-operatively as an insufflation. Previously, tetracycline and bleomycin were used for pleurodesis (fusion of the two pleural surfaces), but talc has proven to be more effective.[16] More recently, ambulatory chronic pleural drainage has been used with efficacy when the lung cannot be re-expanded. This is an outpatient procedure, utilizing a small catheter attached to a drainage bag that is emptied intermittently. This has proven to be a worthwhile approach.[17] Painful pleural or chest wall lesions can be palliated with local irradiation. Focal lesions can occasionally be excised.

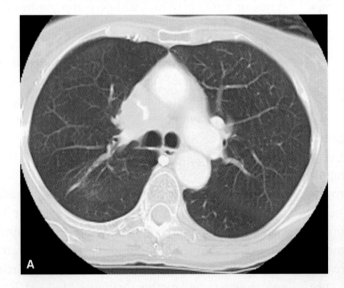

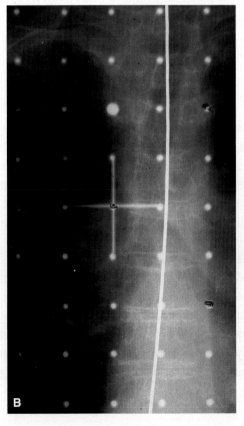

Figure 11–1. *A,* CT scan of patient with SVC syndrome. This axial slice from a chest CT with contrast shows a large right paratracheal mass pressing on the superior vena cava allowing only a thin ribbon of contrast-enhanced serum through the vessel (*arrow*). *B,* Simulation film of palliative thoracic radiation therapy of the patient in *A.* The cross hairs represent the isocenter and the rectangle represents the treatment field. The white cross-hatched area will be blocked form the radiation field. The dots are reference markers that are 2 cm apart. Note that the lesion seen in *A* is included in the treatment field with a margin.

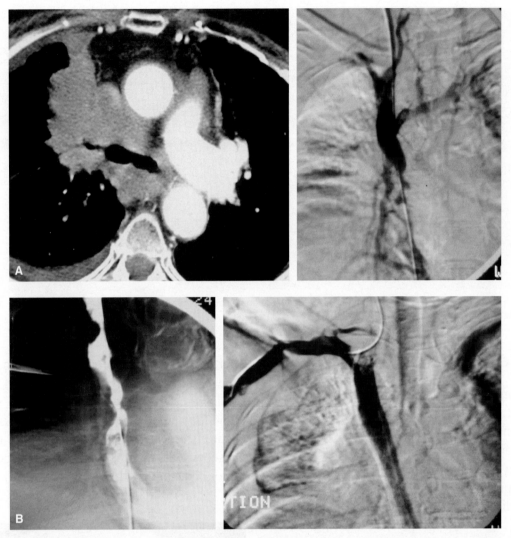

Figure 11–2. A CT scan image (*left*) and venogram (*right*) demonstrating complete SVC obstruction due to lymphadenopathy (Courtesy of Dr. Murray Asch). *B,* Partial SVC obstruction (*left*) relieved by endovascular stenting (*right*) (Courtesy of Dr. Murray Asch).

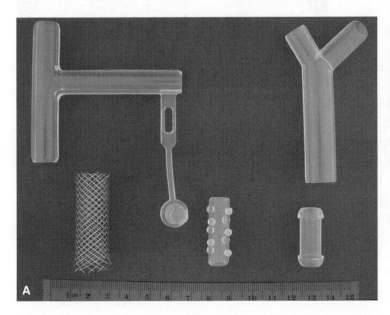

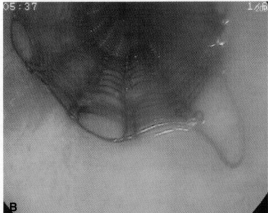

Figure 11–3. *A,* A variety of plastic and expandable wire mesh stents used to relieve airway obstruction. *B,* An endobronchial expandable stent relieves esophageal compression secondary to subcarinal lymphadenopathy.

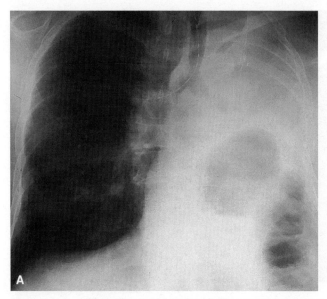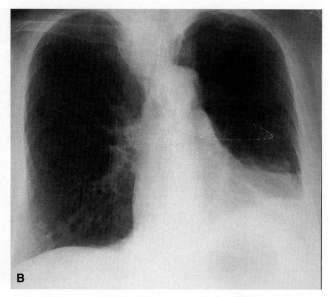

Figure 11–4. *A,* A recurrence following lobectomy causing complete obstruction of the remaining left lower lobe; *B,* Treated successfully by endoscopic laser ablation and brachytherapy.

Endobronchial Recurrences

On occasion, a solitary intrabronchial mucosal or submucosal recurrence at the resection margin or elsewhere may be the only site of recurrent disease. Patients should be considered for curative re-resection whenever possible if there is no evidence of regional spread to lymph nodes or of distant metastatic disease. When this is not an option, endoscopic salvage is appropriate, utilizing bronchoscopy and tumor ablative maneuvers such as mechanical débridement, Yag laser débridement, or hematoporphyrin therapy.[18–20] These approaches can be complimented or substituted by the use of intraluminal brachytherapy or external beam radiotherapy[21–26] (Figures 11–4 and 11–5).

In performing intraluminal brachytherapy, fiberoptic bronchoscopy is performed, usually under local anesthesia, and the lesion is identified (Figure 11–6, *A*). The area to be treated should extend 2 cm distal and proximal to the lesion in order to prevent under-dosing. These positions are marked with externally placed radiopaque markers (Figure 11–6, *B*). A catheter is placed through the bronchoscope and positioned in the area to be treated (Figure 11–6, *C*). This position is confirmed with fluoroscopy (Figure 11–6, *D*). The treatment subsequently takes place when the high-dose rate brachytherapy source travels through the catheter to the site of the lesion after all personnel have exited the room. Treatment time is approximately 2 minutes, with the source dwelling at different locations in the catheter to allow for a homogeneous dose distribution. The procedure is repeated 1 week and 2 weeks later. Bronchoscopy will identify progressive response in the tumor bed (Figure 11–6, *E* and 11–6, *F*).

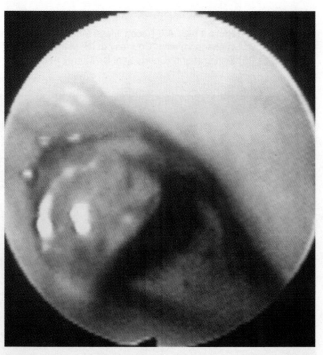

Figure 11–5. An endobronchial recurrence suitable for laser or mechanical débridement.

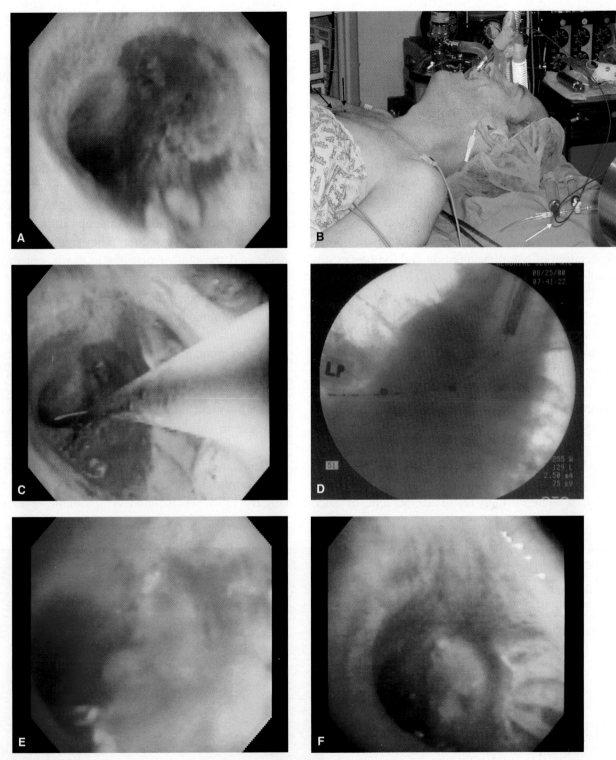

Figure 11–6. *A,* Endobronchial tumor. Photograph taken during bronchoscopy of a lesion in the left main stem bronchus causing hemoptysis. *B,* Endobronchial brachytherapy. The patient is under general anesthesia in the operating room during endobronchial brachytherapy. The brachytherapy catheter (*white arrow*) emanates from the high-dose rate brachytherapy afterloading system (*bottom right-hand corner*) and terminates at the site being treated as seen in *C.* External radio-opaque markers (*black arrow*) are used to confirm the position of the catheter fluoroscopically. When the patient is treated, the radioactive source travels from the afterloading system through the catheter into the patient after medical personnel have left the operating room. *C,* Catheter placement. Bronchoscopic view of the placement of the endobronchial brachytherapy catheter. *D,* Fluoroscopy of the catheter placement. Fluoroscopy confirms the correct placement of the endobronchial catheter. Radio-opaque, non-radioactive "dummy" seeds (*single arrow*) are placed in the catheter to help plan treatment. The external radio-opaque markers (*double arrow*) are visible on fluoroscopy and help determine what volume of endobronchus is treated. *E,* One week later. The lesion 1 week later already shows some necrosis and regression. *F,* Two weeks later. The lesion continues to regress with a white necrotic crust.

Distant Metastases

On occasion, solitary distant metastases will occur metachronously. These may include ipsilateral or contralateral metastasis within the lung or a single lesion within other organs. It has been the approach at Memorial Sloan-Kettering Cancer Center that such solitary lesions, if these can be proven solitary by appropriate staging techniques, including PET scanning, should be considered for definitive curative therapy. With solitary cerebral metastases, either surgical excision or stereotactic radiosurgery can be employed for definitive management with some expectation of complete ablation and long-term survival.[24] Solitary organ metastases elsewhere, including the ipsilateral or contralateral lung, should be approached surgically when possible. High-dose definitive radiotherapy may also be employed with some expectation of complete control and should be employed when surgical therapy is not an option. The results of metastectomy for solitary brain lesions treated either by surgical excision or stereotactic radiosurgery will yield a 15 to 20 percent 5-year survival. Similarly, other solitary organ metastases (lung, adrenal, spleen, bone) have been treated with either surgery or curative radiotherapy. Once again, it appears that 15 to 20 percent of such

patients will be afforded long-term survival if indeed these metastases are solitary.[27–29]

Multiple brain metastases are typically treated with whole brain radiation therapy (WBRT), (Figure 11–7). Typically, a dose of 3,000 cGy in 10 fractions is given, although other fraction schedules (5,040 cGy in 28 fractions, 20 Gy in 5 fractions, etc.) have been explored. A randomized study from Patchell and colleagues demonstrated that surgical resection of brain metastases prior to WBRT prolonged survival.[30] A subsequent study from Patchell's group examined the role of whole brain radiation therapy in patients who underwent surgical resection. They found that WBRT decreased the rate of neurologic death, but did not have an effect on overall survival.[31]

Non-small cell lung cancer can metastasize to a variety of other organs. For non-solitary asymptomatic metastatic disease, the usual approach is expectant management or chemotherapy. Common multiagent chemotherapy regimens used include carboplatin/paclitaxel, which has been shown to have equivalent outcomes to other regimens with a decrease in side effects.[32] Symptomatic metastases can be palliated by local radiation.

Bone metastases are often diagnosed by bone scan (Figure 11–8, *A*), PET scan, CT Scan or MRI (Figure 11–8, *B*). Isolated symptomatic lesions are

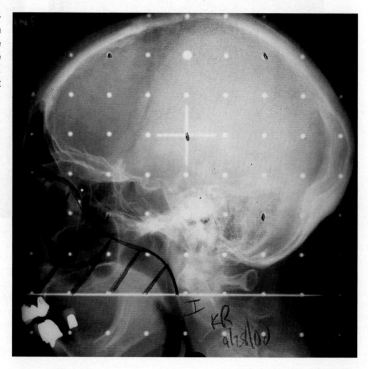

Figure 11–7. Whole brain radiation therapy. This is the simulation film of a patient with brain metastases to be treated with whole brain radiation therapy. The cross hairs represent the isocenter and the rectangle represents the treatment field. The red cross-hatched area will be blocked form the radiation field. The dots are reference markers that are 2 cm apart. Note that the entire brain is in the treatment field, including the retinas.

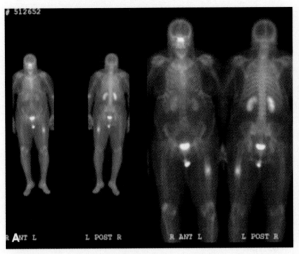
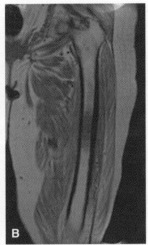
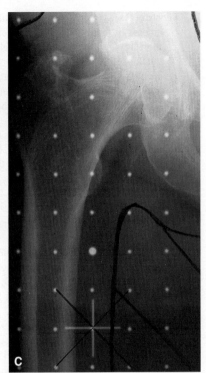

Figure 11–8. *A*, Bone scan. This patient complained of left leg pain and bone scan showed a metastatic lesion in the femur (*arrow*) extending toward the acetabulum. *B*, MRI. The patient in A underwent magnetic resonance imaging which confirmed the presence of a midshaft bone metastasis. *C*, Simulation film for treatment of bone metastases in the patient in *A* and *B*. The cross hairs represent the isocenter and the rectangle represents the treatment field. The red cross-hatched area will be blocked form the radiation field. The dots are reference markers that are two centimeters apart. The lesion and the entire acetabulum is included in the treatment.

managed with palliative courses of radiation (eg, 30 Gy in 10 fractions), (Figure 11–8, *C*). Impending or symptomatic spinal cord compression may require surgical decompression, but most frequently is treated with similar palliative radiotherapy. Destructive lesions in weight-bearing areas may require orthopedic intervention.

CONCLUSIONS

Locoregional disease recurrence is best palliated using surgical or radiotherapeutic maneuvers. Symptoms due to metastatic disease are often treatable by chemotherapy—but when this fails, local radiotherapy can be very effective. Very occasionally, solitary sites of local or distant recurrence can be treated curatively by surgery or radiotherapy.

REFERENCES

1. Rignard JF, Icard P, Magdeleina TP, et al. Completion pneumonectomy: experience in 80 patients. J Thorac Cardiovasc Surg 1999;117:1095.
2. Muysoms FE, de la Riviera AB, Defaun JJ, et al. Completion pneumonectomy: Analysis of operative mortality and survival. Ann Thorac Surg 1998;66:1165–9.
3. Carroll M, Morgan SA, Yarnold JR, et al. Prospective evaluation of a watch policy in patients with inoperable non-small cell lung cancer. Eur J Cancer Clin Oncol 1986;22: 1353.
4. Bleehan N. Inoperable non-small cell lung cancer (NSCLC): a Medical Research Council randomized trial of palliative radiotherapy with two fractions or ten fractions. Br J Cancer 1991;63:265.
5. Teo P, Tai T, Choy D, Tsui K. A randomized study on palliative radiation therapy for inoperable non-small cell carcinoma of the lung. Int J Radiat Oncol Biol Phys 1988;14:867.
6. Simpson J, Francis M, Perez-Tamayo R, et al. Palliative radiotherapy for inoperable carcinoma of the lung: final report of the RTOG multi-institutional trial. Int J Radiat Oncol Biol Phys 1988;11:751.
7. Macbeth FR, Bolger JJ, Hopwood P. Randomized trial of palliative two-fraction versus more intensive 13-fraction radiotherapy for patients with inoperable non-small cell lung cancer and good performance status. Clin Oncol 1996;8:167.
8. Ahmann F. A reassessment of the clinical implications of the superior vena cava syndrome. J Clin Oncol 1984;2:961.
9. Armstrong B, Perez C, Simpson J, et al. Role of irradiation in the management of superior vena cava syndrome. Int J Radiat Oncol Biol Phys 1987;13:531.
10. Nesbitt JC, Carrasco H. Expandable stents in thoracic endoscopy. Chest Surg Clin N Am 1996;(6):305–28.
11. Zannini P, Mellonni G, Chiasa G, et al. Self-expanding stents in the treatment of tracheobronchial obstruction. Chest 1994;86–90.
12. Sawada, Tanigawa N, Kobayashi M, et al. Malignant tracheobronchial obstructive lesions: treatment with self-expandable metallic stents. Radiology 1993;188:205–8.
13. Morgan RA, Ellul JPM, Denton ERE, et al. Malignant esophageal fistulae and perforations: management with plastic-covered metallic endoprothesis.

14. Ginsberg RJ, Koorst RJ. Surgical palliation of inoperable carcinoma of the esophagus. In: Shields TW, editor. General thoracic surgery, 5th ed. Philadelphia (PA): Lippincott, 2000. p. 1947–57.

15. Kraus DH, Ali MK, Ginsberg RJ, et al. Vocal cord medialization for unilateral vocal cord paralysis associated with intrathoracic malignancies. J Thorac Cardiovasc Surg 1996;11:334–41.

16. Kennedy L, Saha S. Talc pleurodesis for the treatment of pneumothorax in pleural effusion. Chest 1994;106:12–5.

17. Putnam JB, Walsh GL, Swisher SG. Outpatient management of malignant pleural effusion by a chronic indwelling pleural catheter. Ann Thorac Surg 2000;69:369–75.

18. Hayata Y, Kato H, Konaka C, et al. Photodynamic therapy (PDT) in early stage lung cancer. Lung Cancer 1993;9:287–294.

19. Cortese BA, Edell ES. Role of phototherapy, laser therapy, brachytherapy and prosthetic stents in the management of lung cancer. Clin Chest Med 1993;1:149–59.

20. Colt HG. Laser bronchoscopy. Chest Surg Clin N Am 1996;277–91.

21. Speiser RB, Spratling L. Remote after loading brachytherapy for the local control of bronchogenic carcinoma. Int J Radiat Oncol Biol Phys 1993;25:4579–87.

22. Spratling L, Speiser BL. Endoscopic brachytherapy. Chest Surg Clin N Am 1996;6:293–303.

23. Miller JI Jr, Phillips TW. Neodymium: YAG laser and brachytherapy in the management of inoperable bronchogenic carcinoma. Thorac Surg 1990;50:190–6.

24. Raben A, Mychalczak B. Brachytherapy for non-small cell lung cancer and selected neoplasms of the chest. Chest 1997;112:276S.

25. Langendijk J, Tjwa M, de Jong J, et al. Massive haemoptysis after radiotherapy in inoperable non-small cell lung carcinoma: Is endobronchial brachytherapy really a risk factor? Radiother Oncol 1998;49:175.

26. Huber R, Fischer R, Hautmann H, et al. Does additional brachytherapy improve the effect of external irradiation? A prospective randomized study in central lung tumors. Int J Radiat Oncol Biol Phys 1997;38:533.

27. Burt M, Wronski M, Arbett E, et al. Resection of brain metastases for non-small cell lung carcinoma: results of therapy. J Thorac Cardiovasc Surg 1992;103:399.

28. Raviv G, Klein E, Yallin A, et al. Surgical treatment of solitary adrenal metastases from lung cancer. J Surg Oncol 1990;43:124.

29. Luketich JD, Martini N, Ginsberg RJ, et al. Successful treatment of solitary extracranial metastases from non-small cell lung cancer. Ann Thor Surg 1995;60:1609–11.

30. Patchell R, Tibbs P, Walsh J, et al. A randomized trial of surgery in the treatment of single metastases to the brain. N Engl J Med 1990;322:494.

31. Patchell RA, Tibbs PA, Regine WF, et al. Postoperative radiotherapy in the treatment of single metastases to the brain: a randomized trial. JAMA 1998;280:1485–9.

32. Schiller JH, Harrington D, Sandler A, et al. A randomized phase III trial of four chemotherapy regimens in advanced non-small cell lung cancer. Proc ASCO 2000;19:1a.

12

Small Cell Lung Cancer

LEE M. KRUG, MD

Small cell lung cancer (SCLC) is a unique form of lung cancer with a fascinating natural history. It was previously termed oat cell carcinoma due to the distinctive, small, round shape of the cancer cells. SCLC displays an aggressive growth pattern, a propensity to metastasize, and a remarkable responsiveness to chemotherapy (Figure 12–1). Although patients can be cured, most die from disease progression due to the rapid development of drug resistance. For this reason, the median survival for patients with metastatic SCLC remains disappointing at 10 months.[1] This is not substantially different from that of patients with advanced non-small cell lung cancer, a disease much less responsive to chemotherapy. Despite great strides in chemotherapy and radiation, the overall survival rate for patients with SCLC has not changed in the last 20 years.[1]

SCLC accounts for approximately 20 percent of lung cancers diagnosed in the United States in 2001.[2,3] Of all the histologic subtypes of lung cancer, SCLC has the greatest association with tobacco use, such that at least 98 percent of patients with SCLC have a history of smoking.[4,5] This makes SCLC one of the most preventable cancers. The parallel between the declining trend in smoking and the decreased incidence of SCLC since the early 1980s supports this notion.[6]

CLINICAL FEATURES

The symptoms from SCLC are similar to those of non-small cell lung cancer. Local symptoms usually predominate due to the frequent medial location of the primary tumor. Patients often present with shortness of breath, cough, hemoptysis, chest pain, or superior vena cava syndrome. SCLC tends to metastasize early in its course, which causes a variety of other symptoms. About half of the patients with

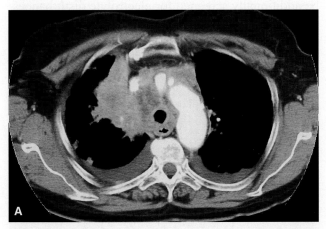 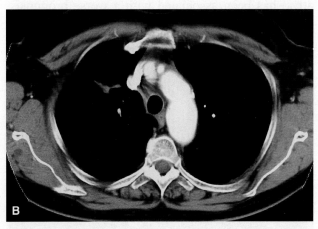

Figure 12–1. This CT scan of a patient with SCLC demonstrates typical features of this disease. *A*, On the presenting CT scan, note the central location of the mass, which caused SVC syndrome, and the presence of a pleural effusion. *B*, After six cycles of etoposide and cisplatin, a follow-up CT scan shows a major response, with just minimal tumor evident and resolution of the pleural effusion. Unfortunately, the patient relapsed a few months later with metastases to the bone and brain.

SCLC will develop central nervous system metastases during the course of their illness, which may cause confusion, motor deficits, or seizures. In rare cases, symptoms related to paraneoplastic syndromes may occur, including muscle weakness, hypokalemia, hyperglycemia, neuropathy, ataxia, or hyponatremia.

DIAGNOSIS

Obtaining an adequate pathologic sample is essential for confirming a diagnosis and distinguishing SCLC from non-small cell carcinoma. Under the microscope, small cell carcinoma appears as small round cells with darkly staining nuclei and scant cytoplasm (Figure 12–2, A). Because the tumor is thought to arise from basal neuroendocrine or Kulchitsky's cells, chromogranin and synaptophysin stains are routinely positive (Figure 12–2, B) and neurosecretory granules can be detected by electron microscopy. In a small percentage of cases, a mixed subtype of SCLC and non-small cell lung carcinoma is detected. No premalignant histology or molecular marker has been identified for SCLC. Because of the strong association with smoking, the absence of a smoking history should raise suspicions about the diagnosis.

Well known molecular abnormalities occur with remarkably high frequency in SCLC.[7] Loss of alleles on chromosome 3p has been observed in greater than 90 percent of cases. The *FHIT* (fragile histidine triad) gene is localized in this region and its deletion can stimulate DNA synthesis and proliferation. Amplification of the *MYC* oncogene (10 to 40%) has been associated with a worse prognosis.

The tumor suppressor genes, *RB* and *P53*, are altered in 80 to 90 percent. CKIT and its ligand stem cell factor likely play an important role in autocrine growth stimulation in SCLC.[8] In one study, 25 of 31 (81%) of SCLC lines and 12 of 13 (93%) human tumor specimens expressed CKIT.[9] These molecular changes may provide opportunities to combat this disease with targeted biologic therapies in the future.

STAGING

The staging of SCLC has been simplified to include two stages—limited or extensive—traditionally defined using the Veterans Administration Lung Study Group criteria.[10] Limited-stage disease is confined to one hemithorax and encompassed in a single radiation port (Figures 12–3, A and B). Patients with extensive-stage SCLC generally have disease that has spread outside of the chest. Common sites of metastasis include the brain (Figure 12–4), liver, bone, and bone marrow. Patients with involved ipsilateral supraclavicular lymph nodes are generally considered limited stage, while patients with malignant pleural effusions are considered extensive stage.

A thorough work-up is necessary to determine the stage of disease. This may include a bone scan, MRI of the brain, and possibly a bone marrow biopsy (Figure 12–5). PET scanning is being studied as an adjunct to this evaluation. Once a test identifies someone as having extensive disease, the remainder of the work-up is superfluous unless it is being done to evaluate a particular symptom. All patients should be additionally screened for electrolyte disturbances.

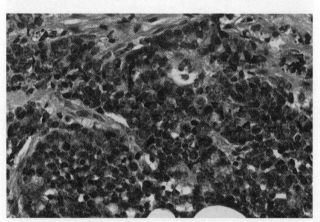
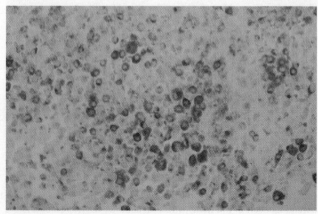

Figure 12–2. This hematoxylin and eosin-stained specimen *(left)* demonstrates the small round blue cells with scanty cytoplasm typical for SCLC. The chromogranin stain *(right)* is diffusely positive.

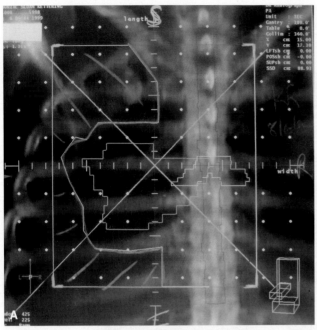

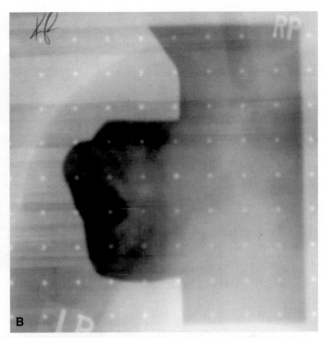

Figure 12–3.   *A* and *B*, Radiation port films for a patient with limited-stage small cell lung cancer. The treatment plan includes the right hilar mass and the mediastinum up to the supraclavicular region.

Clinical factors that impact prognosis include stage, performance status, age, gender, and the presence of paraneoplastic syndromes. Several laboratory values have shown significance in predicting poor prognosis, including low serum sodium, and high-lactate dehydrogenase.[11]

About one-third of patients with SCLC present with limited-stage disease. For these patients, long-term survival is a potential, occurring in a small proportion. If cured, these patients require surveillance for second primary malignancies such as *non-small cell lung cancer*, particularly if they continue to smoke.[12]

CHEMOTHERAPY

Chemotherapy is the mainstay form of treatment. Radiation also plays a role, serving as "consolidation" therapy for individauls with limited stage disease. For patients with extensive-stage disease, chemotherapy alone is the standard of care (Figure 12–6).

Initial Therapy

It was not until combination chemotherapy became available in the 1970s that oncologists improved survival in SCLC from weeks to months. Over the next

20 years, a number of single agents were identified as having significant antitumor activity in SCLC, including cisplatin, carboplatin, cyclophosphamide,

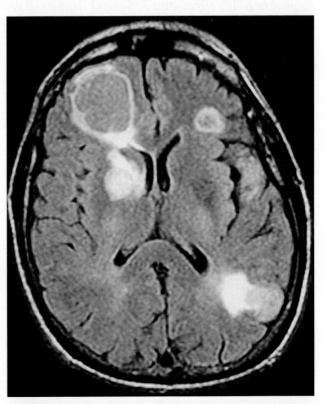

Figure 12–4.   MRI demonstrating brain metastases in a patient with SCLC.

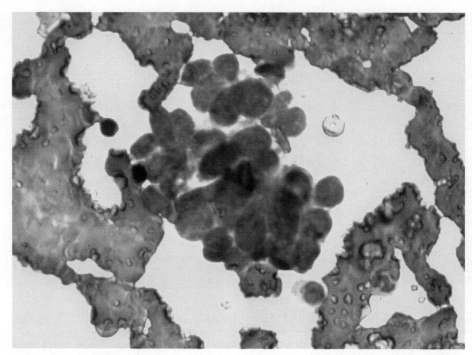

Figure 12–5.   A cluster of SCLC tumor cells from a bone marrow aspirate. This patient had a work-up including an MRI of the brain and a bone scan that were negative for metastases. However, based on the positive bone marrow findings, she was diagnosed with extensive-stage disease and treated with chemotherapy alone.

doxorubicin, etoposide, ifosfamide, methotrexate, lomustine, and vincristine.[5] Several studies have shown that combination therapy is clearly beneficial over single agents, achieving response rates in the range of 80 percent. The most widely used combinations for SCLC are etoposide plus cisplatin (EP) and cyclophosphamide, doxorubicin, and vincristine (CAV) ± etoposide (Table 12–1).

Etoposide plus cisplatin has become a standard regimen for front-line therapy of SCLC, in part because it is better tolerated than doxorubicin-containing regimens when given with radiation therapy. To avoid the toxicities of cisplatin, namely nausea, vomiting, ototoxicity, and peripheral sensory neuropathy, many oncologists have substituted carboplatin. Carboplatin is easier to administer and does not require aggressive hydration or diuresis. Although non-hematologic toxicities are reduced, however, carboplatin does cause cumulative myelosuppression, anemia, and thrombocytopenia. Several phase II trials have evaluated carboplatin in combination with etoposide for the treatment of SCLC. Response rates are similar to those with cisplatin, ranging from 50 to 63 percent in patients with exten-

sive disease. The Hellenic Cooperative Oncology Group reported a randomized phase III trial comparing cisplatin with carboplatin.[13] Overall response

Table 12–1. COMMON CHEMOTHERAPY REGIMENS FOR SMALL CELL LUNG CANCER	
Regimens	**Acceptable Doses**
EP	
Etoposide	100–120 mg/m² days 1–3
Cisplatin	60 mg/m² day 1
or	
Carboplatin	300 mg/m² day 1, or AUC 5
CAV	
Cyclophosphamide	1,000 mg/m² day 1
Doxorubicin	45 mg/m² day 1
Vincristine	2 mg day 1
CAE	
Cyclophosphamide	1,000 mg/m² day 1
Doxorubicin	45 mg/m² day 1
Etoposide	50 mg/m² days 1–5
CAVE	
Cyclophosphamide	1,000 mg/m² day 1
Doxorubicin	50 mg/m² day 1
Vincristine	1.5 mg/m² day 1
Etoposide	50 mg/m² days 1–5
Topotecan	1.5 mg/m² days 1–5

Modified from Ihde DC, et al. Small cell lung cancer. In: DeVita VT, Hellman S, Rosenberg SA, editors. Cancer: principles and practice of oncology. Philadelphia (PA): JB Lippincott Co; 1997. p. 925.

rates, complete response rates, and median survival did not differ significantly in the two arms. Infections, nausea and vomiting, renal and neurologic toxicities, and allergic reactions were significantly more frequent in the cisplatin arm.

Newer Agents

A number of other chemotherapeutic drugs which have known activity in non-small cell lung cancer have also demonstrated activity in SCLC, including paclitaxel, docetaxel, irinotecan, topotecan, gemcitabine, and vinorelbine. For newly diagnosed patients with SCLC, none of these agents has shown adequate effectiveness as monotherapy; thus, various combinations are under study. Single agents are appropriate in patients treated palliatively for relapse.

The taxanes, paclitaxel and docetaxel, act by inhibiting microtubule depolymerization thereby disrupting cell division. Paclitaxel has demonstrated activity both in untreated and previously treated patients with SCLC. An Eastern Cooperative Group trial administered paclitaxel at 250 mg/m² over 24 hours every 3 weeks and demonstrated a response rate of 34 percent.[14] Grade IV leukopenia occurred

in 56 percent of patients. The North Central Cancer Treatment Group used the same schedule but added prophylactic G-CSF.[15] Over half of the patients in that study responded, but the median response duration was a short 3 months. In a phase II study with paclitaxel, 175 mg/m² over 3 hours every 3 weeks in previously treated patients, the response rate was 29 percent. Docetaxel has yielded modest response rates in two phase II trials.[16,17]

Several studies have been conducted to determine whether the addition of paclitaxel to the standard regimens of etoposide and cisplatin or carboplatin improves outcomes. A randomized trial of 133 previously untreated patients with limited or extensive-stage disease compared etoposide and cisplatin with etoposide, cisplatin, and paclitaxel.[18] The trial was stopped early after an interim analysis identified eight toxic deaths in the paclitaxel arm versus none in the control arm. The response and survival rates were the same in both arms. A randomized study of etoposide and carboplatin with or without paclitaxel continues.[19]

Irinotecan, a topoisomerase I inhibitor best known for its activity in colon cancer, has single-agent activity in SCLC,[20] but has gained particular

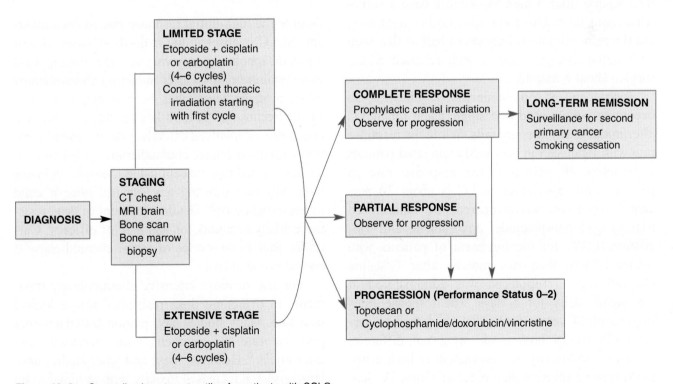

Figure 12–6. Generalized treatment outline for patients with SCLC.

attention in combination with cisplatin. In a Japanese phase III trial, patients with extensive-stage SCLC were randomized to receive either etoposide plus cisplatin, or irinotecan 60 mg/m^2 days 1, 8, and 15 plus cisplatin 60 mg/m^2 day 1.[21] The trial was stopped early after a second interim analysis revealed a significant survival advantage with irinotecan plus cisplatin. U.S. cooperative group trials are now planned to confirm this result.

Although permutations of older regimens have been tested, including adding more drugs or escalating doses, little improvement has been made in response or survival over earlier reports of these therapies.[22] At this time, etoposide plus cisplatin or carboplatin is recommended for initial treatment of SCLC.

Relapsed Disease

As previously discussed, the majority of SCLC patients relapse within a few months of completing their initial chemotherapy. The outcome of patients in this situation strongly depends on the duration of response. Patients who relapse within 3 months are termed "refractory" and respond to further treatment in less than 10 percent of cases. "Sensitive" patients who relapse after 3 months or more have a somewhat more favorable result with further treatment, but the response rate is only about half of that seen with initial therapy. Patients with relapsed SCLC survive about 6 months.

Topotecan, a topoisomerase I inhibitor, is becoming widely used as a single agent for SCLC after initial chemotherapy fails. While the response rate with topotecan in previously untreated patients approaches 40 percent,[23] the response rate in patients with progressive SCLC is about 20 percent.[24] Topotecan was compared in a randomized trial to cyclophosphamide, doxorubicin, and vincristine (CAV) for the treatment of patients who relapsed more than two months after first-line chemotherapy.[25] Topotecan was administered at 1.5 mg/m^2 daily for 5 days. The response rates (topotecan 24 versus CAV 18%) and median survival (25 weeks both arms) were not different. Hematologic toxicity was prominent in both arms, but was more severe with topotecan. Grade IV neutropenia occurred in about 70 percent of patients in both arms. Of the patients treated with topotecan, over half required red blood cell transfusions and 20 percent required platelet transfusions. This compared to red cell transfusions in 27 percent and platelet transfusions in 2 percent of patients treated with CAV. A patient questionnaire revealed that symptomatic improvement was greater with topotecan. This trial led to the approval of topotecan by the FDA for use in patients with SCLC progressing after initial chemotherapy. The myelosuppression with topotecan may require dose reductions or growth factor support.

Other options for treatment are also now available, and include any of the chemotherapy drugs described above, such as the taxanes, gemcitabine, or vinorelbine. Gemcitabine uniquely has demonstrated some efficacy in refractory patients who relapsed within 3 months of initial therapy.[26] Vinorelbine has a response rate of about 15 percent in relapsed patients, and has shown responses in patients previously treated with vincristine.[27,28] However, for fit patients who have failed one prior regimen, topotecan or CAV is recommended.

STRATEGIES TO PREVENT RELAPSE

Despite the high initial response rate to chemotherapy, SCLC relapses in the majority of cases, resulting in disappointing survival rates. Developing ways to maintain remission after induction chemotherapy or chemoradiotherapy has been a major research focus. Because of SCLC's known chemosensitivity, one approach involved extending the treatment duration with maintenance chemotherapy. At least 11 trials have tested this concept using multiple regimens with only two showing any survival benefit amid increased toxicity.[29] The development of drug resistance likely accounts for this lack of efficacy. Currently, four to six cycles of initial chemotherapy is considered standard.

The use of more intensive chemotherapy treatments to overcome drug resistance was a logical next step. Many studies have demonstrated a higher response rate for regimens with increased dose intensity.[30–32] However, these and other studies have largely shown increased toxicity with minimal to no improvement in survival. Advances in growth factors and antibiotics allowed even higher doses of chemotherapy to be administered, in particular when given with autologous stem-cell rescue. As with other diseases such as lymphoma, myeloma, breast cancer, and non-seminomatous germ cell tumors, investigators used these techniques to further increase dose intensity when treating SCLC. At least 36 studies have looked at high-dose chemotherapy with autologous bone marrow or stem-cell rescue in SCLC.[33] Studies have been done in various settings, including relapsed or refractory disease, initial treatment, or after response to first-line therapy. In one trial, 45 patients with a complete or partial response to induction chemotherapy were randomized to receive either conventional or high doses of cyclophosphamide, BCNU, and VP-16.[34] Although median relapse-free survival improved from 10 to 28 weeks with the high-dose therapy, patients in both groups relapsed at the primary site and median overall survival was not statistically different (68 weeks versus 55 weeks, p = 0.13). Four patients died from treatment-related toxicity. This trial and others emphasize that a small fraction of patients can complete high-dose chemotherapy, treatment-related mortality is significant, and survival remains poor.[35] High-dose chemotherapy is not recommended for SCLC.

THORACIC IRRADIATION

Small cell lung cancer has long been known to be exquisitely sensitive to radiation therapy. However, the fact that SCLC is a systemic disease with a high metastatic rate raised doubts as to any advantage that irradiation, a local therapy, would add. Indeed, randomized trials in patients with extensive-stage disease demonstrated no improvement in survival when radiation was added to chemotherapy due to relapse at metastatic sites.[36] In patients with limited-stage disease, thoracic irradiation had a greater rationale, but establishing a clear survival advantage proved difficult. After 13 randomized trials were performed with conflicting results, a meta-analysis of the data confirmed a small but significant improvement in survival for patients treated with radiation therapy.[37] Overall survival at 3 years improved by 5 percent with younger patients receiving the greatest benefit.

The timing of radiation therapy has been an issue of much controversy. Clearly, toxicity is increased when chemotherapy and radiation are used together. This was evident in two trials utilizing cyclophosphamide and doxorubicin-based chemotherapy that showed no difference between concomitant or sequential radiation.[38,39] On the other hand, because of the aggressive nature of SCLC, radiation therapy should theoretically be added early in the treatment to allow the greatest advantage. The National Cancer Institute of Canada compared radiation therapy given concurrently with chemotherapy starting with the second cycle, with radiation given with the final cycle of chemotherapy.[40] Progression-free survival and overall survival were favored in the early radiation treatment arm, although complete remission rates did not differ in the two groups. Severe toxicities were similar in both arms. An overall analysis of several large trials suggests that early radiation results in superior survival.[41]

Twice-daily fractionation has gained attention as a way of potentially improving the results with radiation therapy. Because SCLC is sensitive to radiation even at low doses, administering smaller fractions of radiation more often could theoretically have an antitumor effect while sparing normal tissues. In one trial, twice-daily radiation to a dose of 4,500 cGy given concomitantly with etoposide and cisplatin resulted in a 5-year survival rate of 23 percent compared with 16 percent for daily radiation treatment (p = 0.04).[42] Esophagitis did occur more frequently in the twice-daily radiation arm, but this was reversible.

In summary, thoracic radiation provides a small survival advantage to patients with limited-stage SCLC. Younger patients receiving concomitant radiation early in the course of chemotherapy will likely gain the greatest benefit.

SURGERY

Surgery alone is inadequate therapy for SCLC. In the Medical Reseach Council study conducted in the 1960s, surgery resulted in a 2-year survival rate of less than 2 percent.[43] Subsequent trials from the 1970s showed that even the addition of chemotherapy that would be considered inadequate by today's standards improves the outcome of patients after surgery.[5] Although a select group of patients may benefit from resection, such as patients with disease confined to the lung (N0M0)[44] or patients with a mixed histology with non-small cell lung cancer, surgery is not appropriate for most patients due to the high rate of early metastasis.

The University of Toronto Lung Oncology Group has one of the largest published retrospective series with surgery in the management of SCLC.[45] They reported on 119 patients who had surgery included as part of their multimodality therapy for limited-stage SCLC. Seventy-nine patients had surgery followed by adjuvant chemotherapy, and 40 patients had treatment in the opposite order. This extensive experience yielded several conclusions. Most importantly, just as with non-small cell lung cancer, patients with mediastinal lymph node (N2) involvement did not gain much benefit from surgery. The median survival for patients with stage I disease was not reached and the projected 5-year survival rate was 51 percent. On the other hand, patients with stage II or III disease had median survivals of 19.1 and 19.4 months and 5-year survivals of 28 percent and 19 percent respectively. The sequence of treatment did not affect survival. It is difficult to determine whether patients with stage I disease truly benefited from surgery, or whether their high survival rate was due simply to a more favorable tumor biology.

The Lung Cancer Study Group, the Eastern Cooperative Oncology Group (ECOG), and the European Organization for Research and Treatment of Cancer (EORTC) combined their efforts in an Intergroup randomized study to determine the role of surgery after initial chemotherapy in patients with limited-stage SCLC. Three-hundred and forty-eight patients were registered and treated with five cycles of cyclophosphamide, doxorubicin, and vincristine. The patients who responded were then randomized to thoracotomy or no surgery. All patients were then to receive thoracic and brain irradiation. Only 146 patients were randomized such that 70 had an operation. Many patients either refused randomization, or were inoperable for various reasons. Neither survival nor local recurrence rates differed by treatment arm.

Based on these data, surgery has a minimal role in the management of SCLC and should only be considered in a multimodality treatment plan for patients with stage I SCLC. If a peripheral nodule is found to be small cell carcinoma at the time of thoracotomy, surgeons are advised to complete a lobectomy and lymph node dissection. Chemotherapy or chemoradiation can then be administered post-operatively.

PROPHYLACTIC CRANIAL IRRADIATION

The central nervous system is a common place of metastasis for SCLC, occurring in up to 50 percent of cases in autopsy series.[46] Because the blood-brain barrier provides a sanctuary from the effects of chemotherapy, radiation was studied as a way of

Table 12–2. ENDOCRINE AND NEUROLOGIC PARANEOPLASTIC SYNDROMES ASSOCIATED WITH SMALL CELL LUNG CANCER	
Syndrome	Tumor Factor
Endocrine	
Cushing's syndrome	Adrenocorticotropic hormone (ACTH)
Syndrome of inappropriate antidiuretic hormone secretion	Argenine vasopressin or atrial natriuretic peptide
Hypercalcemia	Parathyroid hormone-related protein
Neurologic	
Central nervous system	
Encephalomyelitis	Anti-Hu antibody
Myoclonus-opsoclonus	
Cancer-associated retinopathy	Cancer-associated retinopathy antibodies
Peripheral nervous system	
Subacute sensory neuronopathy	Anti-Hu antibody
Subacute motor neuropathy	Anti-Hu antibody
Autonomic neuropathy (intestinal pseudo-obstruction, Ogilvie's syndrome)	Antibodies against myenteric plexuses
Neuromuscular junction	
Lambert-Eaton syndrome	Antibodies against presynaptic voltage-gated calcium channels

decreasing the risk of brain metastases. A meta-analysis of early trials of prophylactic cranial irradiation (PCI) revealed that the benefit was greatest in patients with a complete response to chemotherapy; other patients succumbed to systemic disease.[47] More randomized trials followed, evaluating the efficacy of PCI in patients with a complete response and a subsequent meta-analysis summarized the results.[48] PCI not only decreased the incidence of brain metastasis (relative risk 0.46, p < 0.001), but also increased the disease-free survival (relative risk or recurrence or death 0.75, p < 0.001) and the overall survival (15% versus 21% at 3 years). This effect was seen regardless of stage in subgroup analysis though patients with extensive disease comprised a small percentage. With increasing doses of radiation, the rate of local control improved but survival was not affected.

The concern for diminished cognitive function after brain irradiation gives many oncologists pause in recommending this treatment, especially in patients with extensive-stage disease. The argument holds that the PCI only changes the pattern of relapse, and that radiation can be administered when brain metastases are discovered. However, other factors may contribute to cognitive impairment in these patients, such as chemotherapy effects or subtle paraneoplastic syndromes. In fact, in one randomized trial, neuropsychologic function and the rate of brain CT scan abnormalities did not differ between patients who received or did not receive PCI.[49] Thus, PCI, to a dose of 2,500 to 3,000 cGy, is recommended for patients with a complete response to chemotherapy, irregardless of stage.

PARANEOPLASTIC SYNDROMES

Paraneoplastic syndromes result from tumor-secreted peptides or immune responses acting on sites distant from the tumor, which present primarily as endocrine or neurologic syndromes (Table 12–2). In SCLC these are rare, although a large proportion of patients may have subclinical hormone production or subtle neurologic deficits.

About 5 percent of patients with SCLC will develop Cushing's syndrome from ectopic ACTH production. The resultant cortisol excess leads to hypokalemia, hyperglycemia, myopathy, and edema.[50] SCLC tumors may also cause a syndrome of inappropriate antidiuretic hormone secretion (SIADH) which can result in severe hyponatremia. Treatment of hyponatremia depends on the severity of the symptoms, but typically entails water restriction. Demeclocycline, a tetracycline antibiotic which can cause a counteracting nephrogenic diabetes insipidus, has also been used. After management of these disorders as is medically appropriate, initiation of anti-tumor therapy is paramount. Patients with endocrine manifestations of their disease generally have a worse prognosis and have more frequent complications of treatment.[11]

Multiple neurologic disorders have been associated with SCLC. These syndromes can antedate the cancer diagnosis and can be debilitating. Patients with paraneoplastic neurologic syndromes are more likely to have limited disease and survive longer than those without.[11,51] Anti-Hu antibodies directed against a nuclear protein in dorsal root ganglion cells have been detected in some patients with neurologic symptoms.[52] These patients may exhibit sensory or motor neuropathy, dementia, tremor, or cerebellar dysfunction. Although these syndromes may improve somewhat with treatment of the malignancy, many patients are left with residual neurologic deficits.

Lambert-Eaton (or myasthenic) syndrome is a paraneoplastic neurologic syndrome associated with SCLC which is caused by IgG antibodies that block voltage-gated release of acetylcholine from nerve terminals. This differs from myasthenia gravis, a syndrome associated with thymoma, in which antibodies are directed against acetylcholine receptors. These two disorders can be distinguished clinically. Patients with Lambert-Eaton syndrome present more commonly with proximal muscle weakness and less often with ptosis or swallowing difficulties. They have autonomic symptoms (eg, dry mouth, impotence) and absent deep tendon reflexes. Strength and reflexes increase after exercise. Patients with myasthenia, on the other hand, have no autonomic symptoms and grow weaker with exercise. In Lambert-Eaton syndrome, electromyography causes an increase in muscle action potentials with repetitive stimulation whereas in myasthenia this results in decreasing responses. Acetylcholinesterase inhibitors, which are used to treat myasthenia, have little effect in Lambert-

Eaton syndrome though 3,4-diaminopyridine, which augments release of acetylcholine, is beneficial.[53]

CONCLUSION

Small cell lung cancer remains a deadly disease due to metastasis, drug resistance, and relapse. Chemotherapy is the mainstay of treatment. Thoracic irradiation improves survival in patients with limited-stage disease. Prophylactic cranial irradiation improves survival in patients who achieve a complete response. Because a plateau has been reached in the effectiveness of our current treatments, only new strategies targeted against the tumor's unique biology are likely to improve outcomes for SCLC patients. The ultimate goal, however, must be prevention through smoking cessation.

ACKNOWLEDGMENTS

I appreciate the assistance of Dr. Kenneth Rosenzweig, Dr. Maureen Zakowski, and Dr. Peter Maslak for providing various photos. Dr Mark Kris and Dr Jerry Azzoliassisted with editing.

REFERENCES

1. Chute JP, Venzon DJ, Hankins L, et al. Outcome of patients with small cell lung cancer during 20 years of clinical research at the US National Cancer Institute. Mayo Clin Proc 1997;72:901–12.
2. Ries LAG, Hankey BF, Miller BA, et al. Cancer statistics review 1973–1988. Bethesda (MD): National Cancer Institute; 1991.
3. Greenlee RT, Hill-Harmon MB, Murray T, Thun M. Cancer statistics, 2001. CA Cancer J Clin 1999;51:15–36.
4. Khuder SA. Effect of cigarette smoking on major histological types of lung cancer: a meta-analysis. Lung Cancer 2001; 31:139–48.
5. Ihde DC, Pass HI, Glatstein E. Small cell lung cancer. In: DeVita VT, Hellman S, Rosenberg S, editors. Cancer: principles and practice of oncology. 5th ed. Philadelphia (PA): JB Lippincott Co; 1997. p. 911–49.
6. Travis WD, Lubin J, Ries L, Devesa S. United States lung carcinoma incidence trends. Cancer 1996;77:2464–70.
7. Salgia R, Skarin AT. Molecular abnormalities in lung cancer. J Clin Oncol 1998;16:1207–17.
8. Krystal GW, Hines SJ, Organ CP. Autocrine growth of small cell lung cancer mediated by coexpression of c-*kit* and stem cell factor. Cancer Res 1996;56:370–6.
9. Sekido Y, Obata Y, Ueda R, et al. Preferential expression of c-kit protooncogene transcripts in small cell lung cancer. Cancer Res 1999;51:2416–9.
10. Zelen M. Keynote address on biostatistics and data retrieval. Cancer Chemother Rep 1973;(3)4:31–42.
11. Yip D, Harper PG. Predictive and prognostic factors in small cell lung cancer: current status. Lung Cancer 2000;28: 173–85.
12. Tucker M, Murray N, Shaw E, et al. Second cancers related to smoking and treatment for small cell lung cancer. J Natl Cancer Inst 1997;89:1782–8.
13. Skarlos DV, Samantas E, Kosmidis P, et al. Randomized comparison of etoposide-cisplatin vs. etoposide-carboplatin and irradiation in small-cell lung cancer. A Hellenic Cooperative Oncology Group study. Ann Oncol 1994;5:601–7.
14. Ettinger DS, Finkelstein DM, Sarma RP, Johnson DH. Phase II study of paclitaxel in patients with extensive-disease small cell lung cancer: an Eastern Cooperative Oncology Group study. J Clin Oncol 1995;6:1430–5.
15. Kirschling RJ, Grill JP, Marks RS, et al. Paclitaxel and G-CSF in previously untreated patients with extensive stage small-cell lung cancer: a phase II study of the North Central Cancer Treatment Group. Am J Clin Oncol 1999;22:517–22.
16. Smyth JF, Smith IE, Sessa C, et al. Activity of docetaxel (Taxotere) in small cell lung cancer. The Early Clinical Trials Group of the EORTC. Eur J Cancer 1994;30A:1058–60.
17. Hesketh PJ, Crowley JJ, Burris HA, et al. Evaluation of docetaxel in previously untreated extensive-stage small cell lung cancer: a Southwest Oncology Group phase II trial. Cancer J Sci Am 1999;5:237–41.
18. Mavroudis D, Papadakis E, Veslemes M, et al. A multicenter randomized clinical trial comparing paclitaxel-cisplatin-etoposide versus cisplatin-etoposide as first-line treatment in patients with small-cell lung cancer. Ann Oncol 2001;12:463–70.
19. Birch R, Greco FA, Hainsworth J, et al. Preliminary results of a randomized study comparing etoposide and carboplatin with or without paclitaxel in newly diagnosed small cell lung cancer [abstract]. Proc Am Soc Clin Oncol 2000:1918.
20. Masuda N, Fukuoka M, Kusunoki Y, et al. CPT-11: a new derivative of camptothecin for the treatment of refractory or relapsed small-cell lung cancer. J Clin Oncol 1992;10: 1225–9.
21. Negoro S, Noda K, Nishiwaki Y, et al. A randomized phase III study of irinotecan and cisplatin versus etoposide and cisplatin in extensive-disease small cell lung cancer: Japan Clinical Oncology Group Study (JCOG 9511). World Conference on Lung Cancer 29 (p 1):30 (abstr 95), 2000 (abstr).
22. Sierocki JS, Hilaris BS, Hopfan S, et al. Cis-Dichlorodiamineplatinum (II) and VP-16-213: an active induction regimen for small cell carcinoma of the lung. Cancer Treat Rep 1979;63:1593–7.
23. Schiller JH, Kim K, Hutson P, et al. Phase II study of topotecan in patients with extensive-stage small cell carcinoma of the lung: an Eastern Cooperative Oncology Group trial. J Clin Oncol 1996;14:2345–52.
24. Ardizzoni A, Hansen H, Dombernowsky P, et al. Topotecan, a new active drug in the second-line treatment of small-cell lung cancer: a phase II study in patients with refractory and sensitive disease. J Clin Oncol 1997;15:2090–6.
25. von Pawel J, Schiller JH, Shepherd FA, et al. Topotecan versus cyclophosphamide, doxorubicin, and vincristine for

the treatment of recurrent small-cell lung cancer. J Clin Oncol 1999;17:658–67.

26. van der Lee I, Smit EF, van Putten JW, et al. Single-agent gemcitabine in patients with resistant small-cell lung cancer. Ann Oncol 2001;12:557–61.

27. Furuse K, Kubota K, Kawahara M, et al. Phase II study of vinorelbine in heavily previously treated small cell lung cancer. Japan Lung Cancer Vinorelbine Study Group. Oncology 1996;53:169–72.

28. Jassem J, Karnicka-Mlodkowska H, van Pottelsberghe C, et al. Phase II study of vinorelbine (Navelbine) in previously treated small cell lung cancer patients. EORTC Lung Cancer Cooperative Group. Eur J Cancer 1993;29A:1720–2.

29. Sandler AB. Current management of small cell lung cancer. Semin Oncol 1997;24:463–76.

30. Johnson DH, Einhorn LH, Birch R, et al. A randomized comparison of high-dose versus conventional-dose cyclophosphamide, doxorubicin, and vincristine for extensive-stage small cell lung cancer: A phase III trial of the Southeastern Cancer Study Group. J Clin Oncol 1987;5:1731–8.

31. Arriagada R, Le Chevalier T, Pignon J, et al. Initial chemotherapeutic doses and survival in patients with small cell lung cancer. N Engl J Med 1993;329:1848–52.

32. Ihde DC, Mulshine JL, Kramer BS, et al. Prospective randomized comparison of high-dose and standard-dose etoposide and cisplatin chemotherapy in patients with extensive-stage small cell lung cancer. J Clin Oncol 1994;12:2022–34.

33. Elias A. Dose-intensive therapy in small cell lung cancer. Chest 1998;113:S101–S106.

34. Humblet Y, Symann M, Bosly A, et al. Late intensification chemotherapy with autologous bone marrow transplantation in selected small cell carcinoma of the lung: a randomized study. J Clin Oncol 1987;5:1864–73.

35. Krug LM, Grant SC, Miller VA, et al. Strategies to eradicate minimal residual disease in small cell lung cancer: high-dose chemotherapy with autologous bone marrow transplantation, matrix metalloproteinase inhibitors, and BEC2 plus BCG vaccination. Semin Oncol 1999;5(Suppl 15):55–61.

36. Williams C, Alexander M, Glatstein EJ, Daniels JR. The role of radiation therapy in combination with chemotherapy in extensive oat cell cancer of the lung: a randomized study. Cancer Treat Rep 1977;61:1427–31.

37. Pignon JP, Arriagada R, Ihde DC, et al. A meta-analysis of thoracic radiotherapy for small-cell lung cancer. N Engl J Med 1992;327:1618–24.

38. Perry MC, Eaton WL, Propert KJ, et al. Chemotherapy with or without radiation therapy in limited small cell carcinoma of the lung. N Engl J Med 1987;316:912—8.

39. Gregor A, Drings P, Burghouts J, et al. Randomized trial of alternating versus sequential radiotherapy/chemotherapy in limited-disease patients with small cell lung cancer: a European Organization for Research and Treatment of Cancer Lung Cancer Cooperative Group Study. J Clin Oncol 1997;15:2840–9.

40. Murray N, Coy P, Pater JL, et al. Importance of timing for thoracic irradiation in the combined modality treatment of limited-stage small cell lung cancer. J Clin Oncol 1993; 11:336–44.

41. Murray N, Coldman A. The relationship between thoracic irradiation timing and long-term survival in combined modality therapy of limited stage small cell lung cancer [abstract]. Proc Am Soc Clin Oncol 1995;14:A1099.

42. Turrisi AT III, Kim K, Blum R, et al. Twice-daily compared with once-daily thoracic radiotherapy in limited small cell lung cancer treated concurrently with cisplatin and etoposide. N Engl J Med 1999;340:265–71.

43. Fox W, Scadding JG. Medical Research Council comparative trial of surgery and radiotherapy for primary treatment of small-celled or oat-celled carcinoma of the bronchus: ten-year follow-up. Lancet 1973;2:63–5.

44. Shepherd FA, Ginsberg RJ, Patterson GA, et al. A prospective study of adjuvant surgical resection after chemotherapy for limited small cell lung cancer: a University of Toronto Lung Oncology Group Study. J Thorac Cardiovasc Surg 1989;97:177–86.

45. Shepherd FA, Ginsberg RJ, Feld R, et al. Surgical treatment for limited small-cell lung cancer: The University of Toronto Lung Oncology Group experience. J Thorac Cardiovasc Surg 1991;101:385–93.

46. Hirsch FR, Paulson OB, Hansen HH, Vraa-Henssen J. Intracranial metastases in small cell carcinoma of the lung: correlation of clinical and autopsy findings. Cancer 1982; 50:2433–7.

47. Rosen ST, Makuch RW, Lichter AS, et al. Role of prophylactic cranial irradiation in preventing central nervous system metastases in small cell lung cancer: potential benefit restricted to patients with complete response. Am J Med 1983;74:615–24.

48. Auperin A, Arriagada R, Pignon J, et al. Prophylactic cranial irradiation for patients with small cell lung cancer in complete remission. N Engl J Med 1999;341:476–84.

49. Arriagada R, Le Chevalier T, Borie F, et al. Prophylactic cranial irradiation for patients with small cell lung cancer in complete remission. J Natl Cancer Inst 1995;87:183–90.

50. Shepherd FA, Laskey J, Evans WK, et al. Cushing's syndrome associated with ectopic corticotropin production and small cell lung cancer. J Clin Oncol 1992;10:21–7.

51. Maddison P, Newsom-Davis J, Mills KR, Souhami RL. Favourable prognosis in Lambert-Eaton myasthenic syndrome and small cell lung carcinoma [letter]. Lancet 1999;353:117.

52. Graus F, Cordon-Cardo C, Posner JB. Neuronal antinuclear antibody in sensory neuronopathy from lung cancer. Neurology 1985;35:538–43.

53. Sanders DB, Massey JM, Sanders LL, Edwards LJ. A randomized trial of 3,4-diaminopyridine in Lambert-Eaton myasthenic syndrome. Neurology 2000;54:603–7.

13

The Future

ROBERT J. KORST, MD
MARK G. KRIS, MD

Despite optimal treatment with conventional therapies, survival following the diagnosis of lung cancer is poor, with less than 15 percent of patients diagnosed with non-small cell lung cancer (NSCLC) surviving more than 5 years. Given the shortcomings of surgery, radiotherapy, and chemotherapy, research efforts are focusing on not only novel treatment strategies, but also more sensitive and specific techniques of early detection. Although some of these strategies appear promising, prevention may represent the best strategy to attack this deadly disease, since most cases of lung cancer are associated with chronic cigarette smoking.[1]

LUNG CANCER PREVENTION

Cigarette Smoking

Over the past three decades, a high percentage of the adult population has been successful in quitting smoking. The prevalence of cigarette smoking peaked in the late 1960s at approximately 50 percent of adults. Currently, this figure has fallen to 26 percent, reflecting increased public awareness concerning the hazards of smoking.[2] Although these figures appear encouraging, it takes many years of smoking abstinence to reduce the lung cancer risk in patients with long-term smoking histories.[3] In fact, more cases of lung cancer are currently diagnosed in former smokers than active smokers.[4] In addition, the prevalence of smoking may actually be increasing among children and adolescents,[5] a disturbing fact since 80 percent of chronic smokers begin before the age of 18.[6] Clearly, future efforts regarding smoking cessation need to be geared toward the younger segment of the population.

Chemoprevention

Administration of various substances to inhibit the carcinogenic process and prevent the development of cancer is referred to as chemoprevention. Cancer development is thought to be a multi-step process involving a series of genetic mutations resulting in progressively more advanced levels of cellular abnormalities. These mutations may involve oncogenes, tumor supressor genes, growth factors and their receptors, as well as loss of heterozygosity at several loci.[7] Chemopreventive agents seem to be most effective in the early stages of carcinogenesis, before moderate degrees of dysplasia develop.

Clinical trials in the chemoprevention of lung cancer have mainly focused on retinoids and beta-carotene. Several trials investigating the efficacy of various retinoids conducted mainly in smokers with sputum atypia have been conducted, but the results have been negative or mixed.[8] Although the retinoids were administered orally in these studies, some experimental evidence in animals suggests that inhaled retinoids may be a better option.[9] Epidemiologic data has suggested that beta-carotene may have chemopreventive effects in the lung, since a positive correlation has been demonstrated between reduced lung cancer risk and the consumption of beta-carotene-rich foods.[10] Similar to retinoids, however, clinical trials involving beta-carotene as a lung cancer chemopreventive agent in smokers have, for the most part, been disappointing. In fact, two randomized studies demonstrated an increased risk of developing lung cancer among smokers taking beta-carotene.[11,12] This finding was less pronounced in patients who were not active smokers.

Future directions in the realm of chemoprevention for lung cancer will involve agents that have been shown to be effective in preventing lung tumors in animal models. These include glucocorticoids,[13] nonsteroidal anti-inflammatory drugs (NSAIDs),[14] isothiocyanate,[15] and green tea.[16] These compounds have all shown protective effects against the development of carcinogen-induced lung tumors in rodents and need to be investigated in the clinical setting.

EARLY DETECTION/SCREENING

Survival following treatment of lung cancer is clearly better with earlier stages of the disease. For this reason, the ability to detect lung cancer in its early, asymptomatic stages would seem to be important in reducing the mortality from this disease.

Screening for lung cancer in male cigarette smokers has been evaluated by four randomized controlled trials using sputum cytology and chest radiography.[17–20] The interpretation of the data from these studies has been the subject of much controversy, but current recommendations are that mass screening for lung cancer is not beneficial because a reduction in disease-specific mortality has not been demonstrated. In recent years, however, more sophisticated techniques have emerged which are begining to show promise in the early detection of occult lung cancers.

Fluorescence Bronchoscopy

Conventional white-light bronchoscopy (WLB) notoriously lacks the sensitivity to detect most dysplastic lesions and carcinomas in situ in the tracheobronchial tree.[21] To improve the ability to detect these preinvasive lesions, fluorescence bronchoscopy takes advantage of the decrease in autofluorescence intensity exibited by neoplastic tissues compared with normal tissues when exposed to blue light (442 nm). This modality is discussed further elsewhere in this text.

Sputum Analysis

Both the Memorial Sloan-Kettering Lung Project and the Johns Hopkins Lung Project suggested that routine screening with sputum cytology combined with chest radiography fared no better than chest radiography alone in reducing mortality from lung cancer. To improve the sensitivity of sputum analysis in detecting early lung cancers, several new techniques are being investigated.

Immunostaining of exfoliated bronchial epithelial cells is a technique that is receiving attention as a method of detecting preclinical lung cancer. In a retrospective study which evaluated 62 dysplastic sputum specimens archived from the Johns Hopkins Lung Project using immunostaining for a nuclear ribonucleoprotein (hnRNP A2/B1), an 88 percent diagnostic accuracy was found in predicting the development of lung cancer a full 2 years prior to the clinical presentation.[22] In a prospective study, the same technique predicted the development of second primary lung cancers in patients with previously resected stage I tumors with a sensitivity of 77 percent and a specificity of 82 percent.[23] With the unraveling of the molecular biology of lung cancer will come newer, more accurate markers which may enable investigators to detect preclinical epithelial changes with great accuracy.

Genetic mutations involved in the carcinogenic process can also be characterized using polymerase chain reaction (PCR)-based assays. Since approximately two-thirds of human lung cancers contain mutations in the *p53* tumor suppressor gene, this is an attractive target for early detection. Similarly, *K-ras* mutations are found in nearly one-third of patients with non-small cell lung cancer, making this a useful oncogene. These mutations have been detected using PCR in sputum samples obtained prior to clinical diagnosis in patients with adenocarcinoma of the lung.[24] Unfortunately, these mutations are not present in all lung cancers, and several different mutations of these genes exist in this disease, which can make their detection cumbersome in routine practice. In addition, smokers without lung cancer may harbor these genetic abnormalities in their sputum, limiting the specificity of this technique.[25]

The evaluation of genetic abnormalities in exfoliated bronchial epithelial cells requires that the mutated cells be present in expectorated sputum. This limits the usefulness of these techniques since a significant number of early lung cancers are peripheral in location, and malignant or dysplastic cells may not be produced in the sputum. A new approach that may circumvent this problem is to look for morphologic changes in genetically normal cells which may be induced by a neighboring cancer. These malignancy-associated changes (MACs) can be quantitated by computer-assisted image analysis. In a retrospective analysis of archived sputum from the Mayo Lung Project, MACs correctly identified 74 percent of the subjects who later went on to develop cancer.[26] MACs have also been identified in bronchial biopsies from the contralateral lung in patients with lung cancer.[27] Future sputum analysis may combine the use of MACs with the previously mentioned molecular techniques to heighten the sensitivity of preclinical lung cancer detection.

Low-Dose Helical Computed Tomography

Low-radiation-dose helical computed tomography (low-dose CT) is presently being evaluated as a screening tool for lung cancer. This technique provides a means of screening for small, peripheral tumors that may not exfoliate cells into expectorated sputum. Scans of the entire chest are typically completed within a single breath-hold (approximately 20 seconds) with a "slice thickness" of one centimeter. When non-calcified nodules are found, further work-up commences.

The Early Lung Cancer Action Project (ELCAP) has reported the results of baseline (prevalence) screening using this technique in 1,000 subjects over 60 years of age with a history of smoking.[28] Twenty-three percent had non-calcified nodules seen on low-dose CT, while only 7 percent were detected on standard chest radiography. These subjects then underwent a standard, high-resolution CT scan of the chest, and further diagnostic work-up hinged on the results of this study. Of the 233 subjects in whom non-calcified nodules were found, biopsies were taken from 28, with malignant diagnoses in 27. The remaining subjects who had nodules confirmed on high-resolution CT are being followed with serial CT scans.

Since most incidental nodules seen on low-dose CT are small, it is anticipated that if malignancy is found, cure rates will be substantially higher in these patients than those who have their tumors found after symptoms arise. Critics of this screening technique claim that low-dose CT is overly sensitive. Although the cost of the screening CT is low, the cost of the subsequent diagnostic studies may be significant—a potential problem since the majority of nodules found on low-dose CT appear not to be malignant. Before this screening technique can be widely adapted, long-term follow-up of the patients with nodules found on low-dose CT needs to be reported.

NOVEL THERAPEUTIC STRATEGIES

Treatment strategies for patients with lung cancer continue to evolve, with novel approaches designed to address all stages of disease (Tables 13–1 and 13–2). In addition to these novel strategies, however, chemotherapeutic agents continue to evolve as well, with newer drugs being more active against the tumor and less toxic to the host.

Photodynamic Therapy for Early Lung Cancer

With the emphasis placed on early detection of lung cancer, curative therapy may be able to be tailored to these smaller, earlier cancers. Curative photodynamic therapy (PDT) represents an approach specifically geared toward the definitive treatment of early, endobronchial lesions. This modality involves the use of a systemically administered photosensitizing agent which is taken up preferentially by the malignant cells and then activated by a specific

Table 13–1. NOVEL THERAPEUTIC STRATEGIES UNDER INVESTIGATION FOR NSCLC	
Strategy	Target Population
Photodynamic therapy	Early, node-negative, endobronchial tumors
Minimally invasive resections	Early-stage, resectable tumors
Novel molecular therapies	All stages
Immunotherapy	All stages
Gene therapy	All stages

Table 13–2. NOVEL MOLECULAR THERAPIES FOR NSCLC

Target	Strategy
Growth factor receptors (EFGR, *HER2*)	MAb to receptors Block signal transduction
Angiogenesis	Block VEGF Block VEGF receptor Thalidomide Angiostatin/endostatin MMP inhibition
rAS mutations	Immunotherapy Block FT

EFGR = Epidermal Growth Factor Receptor; MAb = Monoclonal Antibodies; VEGF = Vascular endothelial growth factor; MMP = Matrix metalloproteinases; FT = farnesyl transferase

wavelength of light, which is administered using a low-energy laser. This modality is discussed in further detail elsewhere in this text.

Minimally Invasive Surgical Techniques

Video-assisted surgical approaches (VATS) are currently being used to treat a number of thoracic diseases, usually benign. The VATS approach has been reported for the performance of anatomic lobectomy for NSCLC as well. The first reported VATS lobectomy was performed in 1993, and since then, over 1,200 cases have been reported in the literature.[29] Although variations in this technique exist, the most commonly used approach involves a small thoracotomy (5 to 6 cm) and three smaller (1 cm) port sites. The 5 to 6 cm "utility" thoracotomy is necessary for specimen removal, however, the ribs are typically not spread. Advocates of VATS lobectomy argue that this technique minimizes postoperative pain, the operative stress response, as well as duration of hospital stay. Concerns about the oncologic integrity of these minimally invasive techniques exist, and have focused on incisional tumor recurrence, as well as the adequacy of the lymph node dissection that is performed.

Several large series of patients undergoing VATS lobectomy have suggested that postoperative pain as well as the length of hospital stay may be reduced compared to historic controls who underwent traditional lobectomy.[29] However, this has not been consistently demonstrated. In the two randomized trials comparing VATS lobectomy with thoracotomy and lobectomy that exist to date, no consistent benefits

could be seen, although these studies had a small sample size.[30,31] Advocates of VATS lobectomy claim that the same operation is being performed with the minimally invasive approach as is done in the standard "open" procedure. This remains in question, especially since chest tube and air leak duration seem to be less in VATS patients, implying that less dissection is being performed.

In summary, VATS lobectomy is technically a safe procedure and may play a role in the management of early, peripheral lung cancers in the future, provided that a consistent benefit for the patient can be appreciated and the oncologic principles of the operation are not violated. A multicenter randomized trial evaluating the efficacy of mediastinal lymph node dissection in patients with early-stage NSCLC is currently underway. If it is shown that complete mediastinal lymph node dissection does not improve survival and does not need to be performed in patients with small, peripheral tumors, perhaps a VATS lobectomy would be appropriate therapy, since hilar and mediastinal dissection would be minimized, allowing earlier chest tube removal and earlier hospital discharge.

Therapy Targeting Growth Factors

Autocrine growth factors play key roles in the proliferation, longevity, and survival of normal and neoplastic cells. In each case, a peptide ligand binds to the receptor, triggering a cascade of activity within the cell. The mechanisms underlying these intracellular events, broadly termed signal transduction, are complex and incompletely understood. The net result of these processes is the arrival of information within the cell nucleus, where growth and division are controlled. We now have pharmacologic agents that can block these events, either by the use of monoclonal antibodies that attach to the extracellular ligand-binding sites (such as cetuximab with EGFR, and trastuzumab with *HER2*) or bind to the ligands themselves (such as rhuMAb VEGF that attaches to VEGF).[32] An alternative strategy disrupts signaling by blocking other critical sites on the receptor such as tyrosine kinase enzymes, as in the case of compounds like ZD1839 and CP-358,744. The availability of these pharmacologic agents, as well as their specificity, raise the possibility that we soon will have therapies specifically targeting lung cancer.

Epidermal Growth Factor Receptor (EGFR)

The epidermal growth factor receptor (EGFR) is a glycoprotein spanning the cytoplasmic membrane with an extracellular binding region and an endo-domain containing tyrosine kinase activity. When ligands like epidermal growth factor (EGF) or transforming growth factor-α (TGF-α) bind to the receptor, EGFR kinases auto-phosphorylate tyrosine residues, leading to a chain of events resulting in proliferation. EGF receptors are found on normal cells of the skin, cornea, kidney, ovaries, cardiac conduction system, and liver. EGF receptors are often overexpressed on malignant cells including those of non-small cell lung cancer. In a series of primary tumor specimens, EGF receptor was *expressed* in 93 percent and TGF-α in 86 percent. The EGF receptor was *overexpressed* in 45 percent and TGF-α in 61 percent.[33] EGF receptor ecto-domain can be detected in the urine of 50 percent of NSCLC patients.[34] These associations of EGFR with lung cancer have led to the hypothesis that EGFR blockade can arrest the growth of lung cancer. This concept has fostered the development of monoclonal antibodies that attach to the extracellular binding region and blockade of the tyrosine kinases found in the receptor's endo-domain. The monoclonal antibody cetuximab (C225) and the EGFR tyrosine kinase inhibitors CP-358,774 and ZD1839 (Iressa) have been the most extensively studied therapies of this class in humans. Each blocks EGF receptor activation by EGF and TGF-α, and inhibits proliferation of human cell lines and xenografts. Regressions of established human tumor xenografts which overexpress the EGF receptor have occurred.[35] CP-358,774 and cetuximab block cell-cycle progression and induce apoptosis.[36,37] Anti-tumor effects of these EGFR blockers are enhanced when they are combined with cytotoxic chemotherapy.[38–40] Mouse monoclonal antibody 225[41] and its human/chimeric form cetuximab have been tested in man. Dose-dependent tumor uptake has been observed with radiolabeled antibody. CP-358,774[42] and ZD1839[43,44] are being evaluated in patients. Each EGFR blocker has demonstrated few adverse effects. Reversible skin rashes and diarrhea appear dose-dependent. Durable objective regressions have been reported in patients with chemotherapy-refractory non-small cell lung cancer treated with ZD1839 alone.

Anti-P185 *HER2*/Trastuzumab(Herceptin)

Human epidermal growth factor receptor-2 (*HER2*), also known as c-*erb*B-2, is a proto-oncogene located on chromosome 17q21.[45] Homologous to the rat gene *neu*, *HER2* encodes a transmembrane glycoprotein receptor with tyrosine kinase activity called P185 *HER2* (*HER2* protein). Several lines of evidence support a direct role for P185 *HER2* expression in tumor pathogenesis.[46–48] Specific antibodies to the extracellular domain of the membrane-based protein encoded by the *neu* gene or the human *HER2* gene inhibit the growth of tumors that express the gene.[49] These data are consistent with a direct role for *HER2* in both malignant transformation and enhanced tumorigenicity, and establish *HER2* protein as a target for cancer therapy.

HER2 overexpression in lung cancer occurs in 20 to 25 percent of cases.[50,51] As with breast cancer, clinical data[52,53] suggest that *HER2* overexpression in lung cancer may indicate a worse prognosis. In a study of surgical samples assessed for *HER2* protein by immunohistochemical analysis,[53] 30 percent of the samples were positive, including 38 percent of adenocarcinomas, and 36 percent of squamous carcinomas. In a multivariate analysis, expression of P185 *HER2* was associated with shorter survival. The level of P185 expression independently predicted recurrence rate, disease-free survival, and time-to-recurrence in patients who underwent resection.[52] Other authors have refuted the prognostic value of *HER2*.[54–56] Tumors with *HER2* protein overexpression are more likely to demonstrate drug resistance, making treatment with chemotherapy less efficacious. In 20 NSCLC cell lines, the sensitivity to chemotherapy correlated with the degree of *HER2* expression.[57] Chemoresistance has been demonstrated in *HER2*/*neu*-transfected human lung cancer cell lines.[58]

Monoclonal antibodies were produced against the extracellular domain of the *HER2* receptor to inhibit the proliferation of human tumor cells overexpressing P185 *HER2*. They inhibited the growth of human NSCLC cell lines that naturally expressed or were transfected with P185 *HER2*.[59] When the antibody is given with either cisplatin or paclitaxel, synergistic anticancer effects occur.

Trastuzumab (Herceptin®) binds the extracellular domain of the *HER2* receptor. Phase II trials demonstrated durable remissions in patients with breast cancer. When trastuzumab was given with chemotherapy, more patients had major responses, and both time-to-progression and one-year-survival were improved. With lung tumors demonstrating a degree of *HER2* protein overexpression similar to that seen in breast cancer patients, many investigators have postulated that trastuzumab can improve outcomes in individuals with non-small cell lung cancer. This hypothesis is now being tested.

Anti-Angiogenesis

For tumors to grow larger than a few millimeters they must induce the growth of new blood vessels within the tumor mass, a process called angiogenesis. These new capillaries are derived from normal vessels and are composed of non-neoplastic endothelial cells. Several tumors secrete endothelial-specific growth factors which drive neovascularization, one example of which is vascular endothelial growth factor (VEGF). Endothelial cells migrate into the tumor by exiting their native vessel and then dissolving a passage through the extracellular matrix using proteolytic enzymes such as matrix metalloproteinases (MMPs). Micro vessel count (MVC) is a marker of this process, and a higher MVC may portend a worse prognosis following complete surgical resection of NSCLC.[60–62] Disruption of tumor angiogenesis represents a potential therapeutic target. Examples of strategies designed to inhibit angiogenesis include: monoclonal antibodies binding directly to VEGF; VEGF receptor antagonists; MMP inhibitors (MMPIs); thalidomide; and endogenous molecules such as angiostatin and endostatin. Many of these agents are in clinical trials from phase I to III.

The greatest experience has accumulated with three of the MMP inhibitors: marimastat, BAY 12-9566, and AG 3340. These compounds are bioavailable orally and are well tolerated. These agents have undergone phase I testing. The major toxicities of AG 3340 and marimastat are arthralgias and myalgias, while those of BAY 12-9566 are thrombocytopenia and elevations in transaminases. A phase III trial of marimastat in SCLC has completed accrual, as has a phase III trial of AG 3340 in advanced NSCLC. Results are expected soon. A study of marimastat in patients with stage-III NSCLC who have minimal residual disease following standard combined-modality therapy is ongoing.

Thalidomide is an agent known to have anti-angiogenic properties, which may account for its teratogenicity. Its major side effect is sedation, to which tolerance develops. A phase II trial of thalidomide in patients with multiple myeloma that had relapsed following transplant has been published.[63] Increased bone marrow vascularity is known to impart a poor prognosis in this disease, suggesting that an agent that inhibits angiogenesis could be of value. A clinically significant reduction in serum paraproteins was seen in 32 percent of patients. The usefulness of thalidomide in lung cancer patients is under study.

Angiostatin and endostatin are peptide fragments of the larger endogenous molecules plasminogen and collagen XVIII, respectively. They likely function as natural inhibitors of angiogenesis. Preclinical studies have shown that administration of these compounds can lead to inhibition of tumor growth. More impressively, repeated administration of endostatin has led to complete tumor regression in mouse models.[64] Resistance to the effect of this compound did not develop despite repeated administration.[65] Phase I trials of endostatin are underway.

Ras Mutations

Ras proteins are guanine nucleotide-binding proteins that are encoded by three *ras* proto-oncogenes: *Hras*, *Kras* and *Nras*. These proteins play a key role in signal transduction pathways, trafficking proliferative signals to the nucleus from a variety of cell-surface receptor tyrosine kinases. Increased *ras* function, arising from a *ras*-point mutation that leads to a constitutively active protein, results in unregulated growth and cell transformation. Up to one-third of all non-small cell lung cancers (predominantly adenocarcinomas) harbor a point mutation in *Kras*, most commonly at codon 12. The presence of mutated *Kras* has been associated with a poorer outcome following surgical resection in some[66,67] but not all[68,69] series. Anticancer therapies that specifically target *ras* are being investigated.

For activation, *ras* must undergo several post-translational modifications, the first of which is farnesylation, catalyzed by the enzyme farnesyltransferase (FT). Inhibition of FT results in impaired *ras* maturation and disruption of signal transduction. A review of the biology of FT inhibitors and *ras* has been recently published.[70] FT-inhibiting molecules have been identified and synthesized. In vitro studies have shown that these can lead to loss of the malignant phenotype when added to cultured transformed cells.[71] FT inhibitors are felt to be "cytostatic," as their removal from the culture medium results in reversion of cells to the malignant phenotype.[71] These compounds have shown anti-tumor activity against a number of human xenograft models,[70] without overt toxicity. FT inhibitors are the subjects of early clinical trials. Their relative lack of toxicity preclinically promotes their study in combination with standard cytotoxic chemotherapy. In addition, synergistic anti-tumor effects have been observed in vitro when FT inhibitors are combined with chemotherapeutic agents like paclitaxel.[72]

Another targeted approach recognizes the fact that *ras*-point mutations encode proteins unique to the tumor. Since they are not present in normal tissues, tumor-specific peptides represent a potential target for immunotherapy. With vaccination, the patient's immune system might be induced to generate a response against the mutated *RAS* protein. Knowledge of the precise mutation in an individual patient's tumor is required so that a specific peptide vaccine could be administered. There is data to support that mutated *Kras* protein product can be immunogenic.[73] A pilot trial of vaccine therapy following complete surgical resection of mutated *ras*-containing NSCLC is currently accruing patients at Memorial Sloan-Kettering Cancer Center.

Immunotherapy

The common goal of all immunotherapeutic strategies is to harness agents of the immune system (cells, molecular agents) to kill host tumor cells. These strategies can be categorized as shown in Figure 13–1. Active immunotherapy implies that the

host's immune system is stimulated to mount a response against the tumor. These responses may represent either nonspecific augmentation or specific tumor antigen-directed responses.

Nonspecific active immunotherapy for lung cancer has been investigated extensively, using such stimulants as neutralized infectious agents, levamisole, and intravenous cytokines, both alone and in combination with other conventional therapies.[74] The majority of these phase II and phase III studies failed to demonstrate a beneficial effect of nonspecific immune stimulation, with some agents actually worsening survival in the randomized setting.[75] The future of nonspecific active immunotherapy most likely lies in combined therapy strategies where it can be used to augment a specific immunotherapy response. In addition, nonspecific therapies (ie, cytokine therapy) may be more beneficial, and less toxic to the host, if they could be localized to either the tumor or involved immune tissues, sparing "bystander" organs.

Tumor cells are characterized by the expression of proteins resulting from mutated genes, as well as the overexpression of certain non-mutated genes. Consequently, tumor cells differ from normal cells with respect to both the quality and quantity of many gene products. These mutated or dysregulated gene products may be recognized as foreign by the host immune system, forming the basis of active, specific immunotherapy.

With more sophisticated molecular technology, both tumor-specific antigens (TSA, found only on

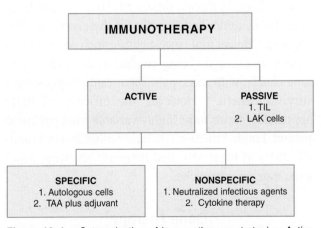

Figure 13–1. Categorization of immunotherapy strategies. Active strategies induce tumor-specific immunity in the tumor-bearing host, while passive strategies involve the transfer of activated immune cells into the tumor-bearing host.

tumor cells) as well as tumor-associated antigens (TAA, found on both tumor and select normal cells) are being characterized for a wide variety of tumor types. Lung cancer tumor antigens, however, tend to be heterogeneous, poorly immunogenic, and poorly defined, making certain specific immunotherapy strategies more difficult to accomplish. Despite this, some such "vaccination" strategies have been investigated in clinical trials, but with mixed results. Examples include immunization with autologous tumor cells or lung cancer tumor-associated antigen combined with a nonspecific immune adjuvant.[76] Current and future investigative efforts will be geared toward the further characterization of lung cancer tumor antigens, augmenting tumor antigen presentation, as well as immunization with other specific peptides known to be mutated in lung tumors (*Kras*, *p53*). "Combination" strategies utilizing both specific (tumor antigens, tumor cells) and more powerful nonspecific (cytokine) approaches are also being evaluated.

Passive immunotherapy involves the activation of the immune reagent(s) prior to administration into the tumor-bearing host. The adoptive transfer of activated lymphocytes represents one such strategy that has been evaluated in many different tumor types, including lung cancer. Lymphokine-activated killer (LAK) cells are obtained from tumor-bearing hosts, amplified in vitro using high concentrations of IL-2, followed by injection back into the host in conjunction with IL-2. Similarly, tumor-infiltrating lymphocytes (TILs) can be harvested from surgical specimens, amplified and even genetically modified in vitro, and injected back into the host. In theory, these cells have already been activated by tumor antigens prior to their removal from the host. Clinical trials investigating such passive techniques are currently being conducted in patients with lung cancer, with some published results suggesting a survival benefit.[77] However, the efficacy of these approaches seems to be highly variable from patient to patient. Future directions include further in-vitro modifications of these activated lymphocytes using novel gene transfer approaches.

Gene Therapy

The transfer of exogenous genes to tumors and/or the tumor-bearing host to induce tumor regression is presently the subject of intensive research. Several different strategies are being evaluated in the lung cancer arena. The suicide gene/pro-drug strategy involves the transduction of tumors with a gene encoding an enzyme that converts a relatively nontoxic pro-drug to a toxic metabolite, theoretically limiting toxicity to the host. Neighboring, non-transduced tumor cells are also killed (bystander effect). Examples that have been used to treat lung tumors in preclinical models include the *Escherichia coli* cytosine deaminase gene/5-fluorocytosine combination and the herpes simplex virus thymidine kinase gene followed by ganciclovir therapy. Although this is mainly a local strategy, some studies have documented development of systemic, specific tumor immunity in animal models.

The replacement of normal tumor suppressor genes and inhibition of oncogenes represents another approach for lung cancer gene therapy. Encouraging preclinical results utilizing wild-type *p53*-replacement gene therapy has led to the initiation of a phase I clinical trial in patients with advanced non-small cell lung cancer.[78] Again, this strategy is mainly a local one, and the bystander effect may not be as pronounced as with suicide gene therapy. *p53* gene transfer may also enhance radiosensitivity in transduced tumor cells, as do certain suicide gene therapy approaches, as well as the use of radiation-sensitive promoter regions in the vector construct. This augmentation of radiosensitivity represents another potentially useful gene therapy strategy which may be applicable in lung cancer.

Gene therapy has also been used to inhibit angiogenesis and cause tumor regression in preclinical models of lung cancer. Vascular endothelial growth factor (VEGF) production and activity can be inhibited using a number of different strategies, including antisense gene transfer. The antisense approach involves engineering target cells to produce singlestranded DNA or RNA that is complementary to the mRNA of various tumor-promoting genes, including angiogenesis agents and receptors, oncogenes, and drug resistance genes. In its current state, this strategy is mainly a local one, with the targeting of metastatic disease remaining unsolved.

Gene-based immunotherapy is perhaps the most actively investigated application of gene therapy in the realm of cancer research. The overwhelming theoretical advantage of using gene therapy for the manipulation of the systemic immune response to tumors is the potential for the eradication of metastatic disease. These strategies have focused mainly on the enhancement of tumor antigen presentation as well as the transfer of genes encoding for cytokines to various cell targets, and combinations of these approaches. Unfortunately, lung cancer tumor antigens are poorly characterized and heterogeneous, making strategies using specific tumor antigens difficult. As a result, investigators are now focusing on ways to release lung tumor antigens in vivo in order to upregulate the antitumor immune response.

Although these strategies have been effective in causing tumor regression in animal models, a major hurdle to be overcome is that of gene delivery. To date, no gene therapy strategy specifically and efficiently targets tumor cells, including metastatic disease, while sparing normal tissue.

REFERENCES

1. Shopland DR, Fyre J II, Pechacek TF. Smoking attributable cancer mortality in 1991: Is lung cancer now the leading cause of death among smokers in the United States? J Natl Cancer Inst 1991;83:1142–7.

2. Cigarette smoking among adults-United States, 1992, and changes in the definition of current cigarette smoking. MMWR Morb Mortal Wkly Rep 1994;43:

3. United States Department of Health and Human Services. The health benefits of smoking cessation: a report of the Surgeon General. 1990;142(5):993–4.

4. Tong L, Spitz MR, Fueger JJ, Amos CA. Lung cancer in former smokers. Cancer 1996;78:1004–10.

5. The Centers for Disease Control and Prevention. Cigarette smoking among high school students—11 states, 1991–1997. J Sch Health 1999;69(8):303–6.

6. Cigarette smoking among high school students—11 states, 1991–1997. MMWR Morb Mortal Wkly Rep 1999; 48:686–92.

7. Minna JD. The molecular biology of lung cancer pathogenesis. Chest 1993;103:449–56.

8. You M, Bergman G. Preclinical and clinical models of lung cancer chemoprevention. Hematol Oncol Clin North Am 1998;12:1037–53.

9. Miller VA, Brooks A, Benedetti F, et al. Inhaled retinoids for the prevention of respiratory tract cancers [abstract #727]. Lung Cancer 1997;18 Suppl 1:186.

10. Willett WM, McMahon B. Diet and cancer: an overview. N Engl J Med 1984;310:633–8.

11. The Alpha-Tocopherol, Beta-Carotene Cancer Prevention Study Group. The effect of vitamin E and beta-carotene on the incidence of lung cancer and other cancers in male smokers. N Engl J Med 1994;330:1029–35.

12. Omenn GS, Goodman GE, Thornquist MD, et al. Effects of a combination of beta-carotene and vitamin A on lung cancer and cardiovascular disease. N Engl J Med 1996;334: 1150–5.

13. Wattenberg LW, Estensen RD. Chemopreventive effects of *myo*-inositol and dexamethasone on benzo[a]pyrene and 4-(methylnitrosoamino)-1-(3-pyridyl)-1-butanone-induced pulmonary carcinogenesis in female A/J mice. Cancer Res 1996;56:5132–5.

14. Jalbert G, Castonguay A. Effects of NSAIDs on NNK-induced pulmonary and gastric tumorigenesis in A/J mice. Cancer Lett 1992;66:21–8.

15. Morse MA, Amin SG, Hect SS, Chung FL. Effect of aromatic isothiocyanates on tumorigenicity, O^6-methylguanine formation, and metabolism of the tobacco-specific nitrosamine 4-(methylnitrosoamino)-1-(3-pyridyl)-1-butanone in A/J mouse lung. Cancer Res 1989;49:2894–7.

16. Xu Y, Ho CT, Amin SG, et al. Inhibition of tobacco-specific nitrosamine-induced lung tumorigenesis in A/J mice by green tea and its major polyphenol as antioxidants. Cancer Res 1992;52:3875–9.

17. Fontana RS, Sanderson DR, Woolner LB, et al. Lung cancer screening: the Mayo program. J Occup Med 1986;28: 746–50.

18. Kubik A, Parkin DM, Khlat M, et al. Lack of benefit from semi-annual screening for cancer of the lung: follow-up report of a randomized controlled trial on a population of high-risk males in Czechoslovakia. Int J Cancer 1990;45: 26–33.

19. Melamed MR, Flehinger BJ, Zaman MB, et al. Screening for early lung cancer: results of the Memorial Sloan-Kettering study in New York. Chest 1984;86:44–53.

20. Tockman MS. Survival and mortality from lung cancer in a screened population. The Johns Hopkins Study. Chest 1986;89:S325–6.

21. Woolner LB, Fontana RS, Cortese DA, et al. Roentgenographically occult lung cancer: pathologic findings and frequency of multicentricity during a 10-year period. Mayo Clin Proc, 1984;59:453–66.

22. Tockman MS, Gupta PK, Myers JD, et al. Sensitive and specific monoclonal antibody recognition of human lung cancer antigen on preserved sputum cells: a new approach to early lung cancer detection. J Clin Oncol 1988;6:1685–93.

23. Tockman MS, Mulshine JL, Piantadosi S, et al. Prospective detection of preclinical lung cancer: results from two studies of heterogeneous nuclear ribonucleoprotein A2/B1 overexpression. Clin Cancer Res 1997;3(12 Pt 1):2237–46.

24. Mao L, Hruban RH, Boyle JO, et al. Detection of oncogene mutations in sputum precedes diagnosis of lung cancer. Cancer Res 1994;54:1634–7.

25. Mao L, Lee JS, Kurie JM, et al. Clonal genetic alterations in the lungs of current and former smokers. J Natl Cancer Inst 1997;89:857–62.

26. Payne PW, Sebo TJ, Doudkine A, et al. Sputum screening by quantitative microscopy: a re-examination of a portion of the National Cancer Institute Cooperative Early Lung Cancer Study. Mayo Clin Proc 1997;72:697–704.

27. MacAualay C, Lam S, Payne PW, et al. Malignancy-associ-

ated changes in bronchial epithelial cells in biopsy specimens. Anal Quant Cytol Histol 1995;17:55–61.

28. Henschke CI, McCauley DI, Yankelevitz DF, et al. Early Lung Cancer Action Project: overall design and findings from baseline screening. Lancet 1999;354:99–105.

29. McKenna RJ. The current status of video-assisted thoracic surgery lobectomy. Chest Surg Clin N Am 1998;8:775–85.

30. Giudicelli R, Thomas P, Lonjon T, et al. Video-assisted mini-thoracotomy versus muscle-sparing thoracotomy for performing lobectomy. Ann Thorac Surg 1994;58:712–7.

31. Kirby TJ, Mack MJ, Landreneau RJ, Rice TW. Lobectomy—video-assisted thoracic surgery versus muscle-sparing thoracotomy. A randomized trial. J Thorac Cardiovasc Surg 1995;109:99–1001.

32. DeVore R, Fehrenbacher L, Herbst R, et al. A randomized phase II trial comparing rhuMAb VEGF (recombinant humanized monoclonal antibody to vascular endothelial cell growth factor) plus carboplatin/paclitaxel (CP) alone in patients with stage IIIB/IV NSCLC. Proc Am Soc Clin Oncol 19, 2000. [In press]

33. Rusch V, Baselga J, Cordon-Cardo C, et al. Differential expression of the epidermal growth factors receptor and its ligands in primary non-small cell lung cancers and adjacent benign lung. Cancer Res 1993;53:2379–85.

34. Witters LM, Curley EM, Kumar R, et al. Epidermal growth factor receptor ectodomain in the urine of patients with squamous cell carcinoma. Clin Cancer Res 1995;1:551–7.

35. Woodburn JR, Barker AJ, Gibson KH, et al. ZD1839, an epidermal growth factor tyrosine kinase inhibitor selected for clinical development [abstract #4251]. Proc Am Assoc Cancer Res 1997;38:633.

36. Moyer JD, Barbacci EG, Iwata KK, et al. Induction of apoptosis and cell cycle arrest by CP-358, 774, an inhibitor of epidermal growth factor receptor tyrosine kinase (EGFR-TK). Cancer Res 1997;57:4838–48.

37. Huang SM, Bock JM, Harari PM. Epidermal growth factor receptor blockade with C225 modulates proliferation, apoptosis, and radiosensitivity in squamous cell carcinomas of the head and neck. Cancer Res 1999;59:1935–40.

38. Baselga J, Norton L, Masui H, et al. Antitumor effects of doxorubicin in combination with anti-epidermal growth factor receptor monoclonal antibodies. J Natl Cancer Inst 1993;85(16):1327–33.

39. Fan Z, Baselga J, Masui H, Mendelsohn J. Antitumor effect of anti-epidermal growth factor receptor monoclonal antibodies plus cis-diamminedichloroplatinum on well established A431 cell xenografts. Cancer Res 1993;53:4637–42.

40. Sirotnak FM, Miller VA, Scher HI, et al. Efficacy of cytotoxic agents against human tumor xenografts is markedly enhanced by co-administration of ZD1839 (Iressa), an inhibitor of EGF receptor tyrosine kinase [abstract #98]. Clin Cancer Res 1999; Suppl 5:3749.

41. Divgi CR, Kris M, Real FX, et al. Phase I and imaging trial of indium 111-labeled anti-epidermal growth factor receptor monoclonal antibody 225 in patients with squamous cell lung carcinoma. J Natl Cancer Inst 1991;83:97–104.

42. Karp D, Silberman SL, Csudae R, et al. Phase I dose escalation study of epidermal growth factor receptor (EGFR) tyrosine kinase (TK) inhibitor CP-358,774 in patients with advanced solid tumors. [abstract # 1499]. Proc Am Soc Clin Oncol 1999;18:388a.

43. Kris M, Ranson M, Ferry D, et al. Phase I study of oral ZD1839 (Iressa), a novel inhibitor of epidermal growth factor receptor tyrosine kinase (EGFR-TK): evidence of good tolerability and activity [abstract #99]. Clin Cancer Res 1999; Suppl 5:3749–50.

44. Baselga J, LoRusso P, Herbst R, et al. A pharmacokinetic/pharmacodynamic trial of ZD1839 (Iressa), a novel oral epidermal growth factor receptor tyrosine kinase (EGFR-TK) inhibitor, in patients with 5 selected tumor types (a phase I/II trial of continuous once-daily treatment [abstract #29]. Clin Cancer Res 1999; Suppl 5:3736.

45. Coussens L, Yang-Feng TL, Liao YC, et al. Tyrosine kinase receptor with extensive homology to EGF receptor shares chromosomal location with neu oncogene. Science 1985; 230:1132–9.

46. DiFiore PP, Pierce JH, Kraus MH, et al. ErbB-2 is a potent oncogene when overexpressed in NIH/3T3 cells. Science 1987;237:178–82.

47. Hudziak RM, Schlessinger J, Ullrich A. Increased expression of the putative growth factor receptor p18HER2 causes transformation and tumorigenesis of NIH 3T3 cells. Proc Natl Acad Sci U S A 1987;84:7159–63.

48. Muller W, Sinn E, Patengale P, et al. Single-step induction of mammary adenocarcinoma in transgenic mice bearing the activated c-NEU oncogene. Cell 1988;54:105–15

49. Drebin JA, Winget M, Greene MI. Monoclonal antibodies specific for the neu oncogene product directly mediate anti-tumor effects in vivo. Oncogene 1988;2:387–94.

50. Pastorino U, Sozzi G, Miozzo M, et al. Genetic changes in lung cancer. J Cell Biochem 1993; Suppl 17F:237–48.

51. Salgia R, Skarin AT. Molecular abnormalities in lung cancer. J Clin Oncol 1998;16:1207–17.

52. Diez M, Pollan M, Maestro M, et al. Prediction of recurrence by quantification of p185neu protein in non-small cell lung cancer tissue. Br J Cancer 1997;75:684–9.

53. Kern JA, Schwartz DA, Nordberg JE, et al. P185neu expression in human lung adenocarcinomas predicts shortened survival. Cancer Res 1990;50:5184–7.

54. Greatens TM, Niehans GA, Rubins JB, et al. Do molecular markers predict survival in non-small cell lung cancer? Am J Respir Crit Care Med 1998;157:1093–7.

55. MacKinnon M, Kerr KM, King G, et al. P53, c-erbB-2, and nm23 expression have no prognostic significance in primary pulmonary adenocarcinoma. Eur J Cardiothorac Surg 1997;11:838–42.

56. Pfeiffer P, Clausen PP, Andersen K, Rose C. Lack of prognostic significance of epidermal growth factor receptor and the oncoprotein p185HER-2 in patients with systemically untreated non-small cell lung cancer: an immunohistochemical study on cryosections. Br J Cancer 1996; 74:86–91.

57. Tsai C, Chang K, Perng R, et al. Correlation of intrinsic chemoresistance of non-small-cell lung cancer cell lines with HER-2/neu gene expression but not with ras gene mutations. J Natl Cancer Inst 1993;85:897–901.

58. Tsai C, Yu D, Chang K, et al. Enhanced chemoresistance by elevation of p185neu levels in HER-2/neu-transfected human lung cancer cells. J Natl Cancer Inst 1995;87:682–4.

59. Kern J, Torney L, Weiner D, et al. Inhibition of human lung cancer cell line growth by an anti-p185HER2 antibody. Am J Respir Cell Mol Biol 1993;9:448–54.

60. Shibusa T, Shijubo N, Abe S. Tumor angiogenesis and vascular endothelial growth factor expression in stage I lung adenocarcinoma. Clin Cancer Res 1998;4:1483–7.

61. Fontanini G, Lucchi M, Vignati S, et al. Angiogenesis as a prognostic indicator of survival in non-small cell lung carcinoma: a prospective study. J Natl Cancer Inst 1997; 89:881–6.

62. Angeletti CA, Lucchi M, Fontanini G, et al. Prognostic significance of tumoral angiogenesis in completely resected late stage lung carcinoma (stage IIIA-N2). Cancer 1996; 78:409–15.

63. Singhal S, Mehta J, Desikan R, et al. Antitumor activity of thalidomide in refractory multiple myeloma. N Engl J Med 1999;341:1565–71.

64. O'Reilly MS, Boehm T, Shing Y, et al. Endostatin: an endogenous inhibitor of angiogenesis and tumor growth. Cell 1997;88:277–85.

65. Boehm T, Folkman J, Browder T, O'Reilly MS. Antiangiogenic therapy of experimental cancer does not induce acquired drug resistence. Nature 1997;390:404–7.

66. Slebos R, Kibbelaar R, Dalesio O. K-RAS oncogene activation as a prognostic marker in adenocarcinoma of the lung. N Engl J Med 1990;323:561–5.

67. Sugio K, Ishida T, Yokoyama H, et al. Ras gene mutations as a prognostic marker in adenocarcinoma of the human lung without lymph node metastasis. Cancer Res 1992; 52:2903–6.

68. Graziano SL, Gamble GP, Newman NB, et al. Prognostic significance of K-ras codon 12 mutations in patients with resected stage I and II non-small cell lung cancer. J Clin Oncol 1999;17:668–75.

69. Keohavong P, DeMichele MAA, Melacrinos AC, et al. Detection of K-ras mutations in lung carcinomas: relationship to prognosis. Clin Cancer Res 1996;2:411–8.

70. Rowinsky EK, Windle JJ, Von Hoff DD. Ras protein farnesyltransferase: a strategic target for anticancer therapeutic development. J Clin Oncol 1999;17:3631–52.

71. Prendergast GC, Davide JP, de Solms SJ, et al. Farnesyltransferase inhibition causes morphological reversion of ras-transformed cells by a complex mechanism that involves regulation of the actin cytoskeleton. Mol Cell Biol 1994; 14:4193–202.

72. Moasser MM, Sepp-Lorenzino L, Kohl NE, et al. Farnesyl transferase inhibitors cause enhanced mitotic sensitivity to Taxol and epothilones. Proc Nat Acad Sci U S A 1998; 95(4):1369–74.

73. Gjertsen MK, Bakka A, Breivik J, et al. Vaccination with mutant ras peptides and induction of T-cell responsiveness in pancreatic carcinoma patients carrying the corresponding ras mutation. Lancet 1995;346:1399–400.

74. Al-Moundhri M, O'Brien M, Souberbielle BE. Immunotherapy in lung cancer. Br J Cancer 1998;78:282–8.

75. Holmes EC, Hill LD, Gail M. A randomized comparison of the effects of adjuvant therapy on resected stages II and III non-small cell carcinoma of the lung. The Lung Cancer Study Group. Ann Surg 1985;202:335–41.

76. Takita H, Holinshead AC, Adler RH, et al. Adjuvant, specific, active immunotherapy for resectable squamous cell lung carcinoma: A 5-year survival analysis. J Surg Oncol 1991; 46:9–14.

77. Kimura H, Yamaguchi Y. Adjuvant chemo-immunotherapy after curative resection of stage II and IIIA primary lung cancer. Lung Cancer 1996;14:301–14.

78. Roth JA, Swisher SG, Merritt JA, et al. Gene therapy for non-small cell lung cancer: a preliminary report of a phase I trial of adenoviral p53 gene replacement. Semin Oncol 1998;25(3 Suppl 8):33–7.

Index

Page numbers followed by f indicate figure; those followed by t indicate table.